Biomarkers in Heart Failure

Guest Editor

EUGENE BRAUNWALD, MD

HEART FAILURE CLINICS

www.heartfailure.theclinics.com

Consulting Editors
RAGAVENDRA R. BALIGA, MD, MBA
JAMES B. YOUNG, MD

Founding Editor
JAGAT NARULA, MD, PhD

October 2009 • Volume 5 • Number 4

SAUNDERS an imprint of ELSEVIER, Inc.

W.B. SAUNDERS COMPANY
A Division of Elsevier Inc.

1600 John F. Kennedy Boulevard • Suite 1800 • Philadelphia, Pennsylvania 19103-2899

http://www.theclinics.com

HEART FAILURE CLINICS Volume 5, Number 4
October 2009 ISSN 1551-7136, ISBN-13: 978-1-4377-1446-3, ISBN-10: 1-4377-1446-3

Editor: Barbara Cohen-Kligerman
Developmental Editor: Theresa Collier

Heart Failure Clinics (ISSN 1551-7136) is published quarterly by Elsevier Inc., 360 Park Avenue South, New York, NY 10010-1710. Months of publication are January, April, July, and October. Business and editorial offices: 1600 John F. Kennedy Boulevard, Suite 1800, Phliadelphia, PA 19103-2899. Customer service office: 11830 Westline Industrial Drive, St. Louis, MO 63146. Periodicals postage paid at New York, NY, and additional mailing offices. Subscription prices are USD 193.00 per year for US individuals, USD 320.00 per year for US institutions, USD 67.00 per year for US students and residents, USD 232.00 per year for Canadian individuals, USD 367.00 per year for Canadian institutions, USD 247.00 per year for international individuals, USD 367.00 per year for international institutions, and USD 85.00 per year for Canadian and foreign students/residents. To receive student and resident rate, orders must be accompanied by name of affiliated institution, date of term, and the *signature* of program/residency coordinator on institution letterhead. Orders will be billed at individual rate until proof of status is received. Foreign air speed delivery is included in all *Clinics* subscription prices. All prices are subject to change without notice. **POSTMASTER:** Send address changes to *Heart Failure Clinics*, Elsevier Journals Customer Service, 11830 Westline Industrial Drive, St. Louis, MO 63146. **Customer Service: 1-800-654-2452 (US and Canada). From outside of the US and Canada, call 314-453-7041. Fax: 314-453-5170. For print support, E-mail: JournalsCustomerService-usa@elsevier.com. For online support, E-mail: JournalsOnlineSupport-usa@elsevier.com.**

Reprints. For copies of 100 or more of articles in this publication, please contact the Commercial Reprints Department, Elsevier Inc., 360 Park Avenue South, New York, NY 10010-1710. Tel.: 212-633-3812; Fax: 212-462-1935; E-mail: reprints@elsevier.com.

Heart Failure Clinics is covered in *MEDLINE/PubMed (Index Medicus).*

Cover artwork courtesy of Umberto M. Jezek.

Printed and bound by CPI Group (UK) Ltd, Croydon, CR0 4YY

Transferred to Digital Print 2011

Contributors

CONSULTING EDITORS

RAGAVENDRA R. BALIGA, MD, MBA
Assistant Chief, Division of Cardiovascular
Medicine, and Professor of Internal Medicine,
The Ohio State University, Columbus, Ohio

JAMES B. YOUNG, MD
Chairman and Professor, Department
of Medicine, Lerner College of Medicine; and
George and Linda Kaufman Chair, Cleveland
Clinic Foundation, Case Western Reserve
University, Cleveland, Ohio

GUEST EDITOR

EUGENE BRAUNWALD, MD
Distinguished Hersey Professor of Medicine,
Harvard Medical School; Chairman, TIMI Study
Group, Brigham and Women's Hospital,
Boston, Massachusetts

AUTHORS

STEFAN D. ANKER, MD, PhD
Department of Cardiology, Applied Cachexia
Research, Charité Medical School, Campus
Virchow-Klinikum, Berlin, Germany; and
Centre for Clinical and Basic Research,
IRCCS San Raffaele, Rome, Italy

GUIDO BOERRIGTER, MD
Cardiorenal Research Laboratory, Division of
Cardiovascular Diseases, Mayo Clinic College
of Medicine, Rochester, Minnesota

JOHN C. BURNETT, JR, MD
Marriott Family Professor of Cardiovascular
Research, Cardiorenal Research Laboratory,
Division of Cardiovascular Diseases, Mayo
Clinic College of Medicine, Rochester,
Minnesota

LISA C. COSTELLO-BOERRIGTER, MD, PhD
Cardiorenal Research Laboratory, Division
of Cardiovascular Diseases, Mayo Clinic
College of Medicine, Rochester,
Minnesota

JAMES A. DE LEMOS, MD
Division of Cardiology, Department of Internal
Medicine, The University of Texas
Southwestern Medical Center, Dallas, Texas

WOLFRAM DOEHNER, MD, PhD
Department of Cardiology, Applied Cachexia
Research, Charité Medical School, Campus
Virchow-Klinikum, Berlin, Germany

MARK H. DRAZNER, MD, MSc
Division of Cardiology, Department of Internal
Medicine, The University of Texas
Southwestern Medical Center, Dallas, Texas

SACHIN GUPTA, MD
Division of Cardiology, Department of Internal
Medicine, The University of Texas
Southwestern Medical Center, Dallas, Texas

TOR-ARNE HAGVE, MD, PhD
Professor of Medicine, Faculty Division,
Akershus University Hospital, University of
Oslo; and Consultant, Center of Laboratory
Medicine, Akershus University Hospital,
Lorenskog, Norway

JOSHUA M. HARE, MD
Professor, Department of Medicine, Cardiovascular Division, University of Miami Miller School of Medicine; and Director, Interdisciplinary Stem Cell Institute, University of Miami, Miami, Florida

JAMES L. JANUZZI, JR, MD
Associate Professor of Medicine, Division of Cardiology, Department of Medicine, Massachusetts General Hospital, Harvard Medical School, Boston, Massachusetts

RAHUL KAKKAR, MD
Division of Cardiology, Department of Medicine, Massachusetts General Hospital, Boston, Massachusetts

TIBOR KEMPF, MD
Research Fellow, Department of Cardiology and Angiology, Hans-Borst Center for Heart and Stem Cell Research, Hannover Medical School, Hannover, Germany

MITJA LAINSCAK, MD, PhD
Division of Cardiology, University Clinic of Respiratory and Allergic Diseases, Golnik, Slovenia

ROBERTO LATINI, MD
Department of Cardiovascular Research, Istituto di Ricerche Farmacologiche "Mario Negri," Milan, Italy

RICHARD T. LEE, MD
Division of Cardiology, Department of Medicine, Brigham and Women's Hospital, Harvard Medical School, Boston, Massachusetts

SERGE MASSON, PhD
Department of Cardiovascular Research, Istituto di Ricerche Farmacologiche "Mario Negri," Milan, Italy

ASIM A. MOHAMMED, MD
Dennis and Marilyn Barry Fellow in Cardiovascular Research, Division of Cardiology, Department of Medicine, Massachusetts General Hospital, Harvard Medical School, Boston, Massachusetts

TORBJØRN OMLAND, MD, PhD, MPH
Professor of Medicine and Chief, Faculty Division, Akershus University Hospital, University of Oslo; and Consultant Cardiologist, Division of Medicine, Akershus University Hospital, Lorenskog, Norway

BERTRAM PITT, MD
Professor of Medicine Emeritus, Department of Medicine, University of Michigan School of Medicine, Cardiovascular Center, Ann Arbor, Michigan

A. MARK RICHARDS, MD, PhD
Professor of Medicine, University Department of Medicine, University of Otago; Professor of Cardiovascular Studies, National Heart Foundation of New Zealand; and Director, Cardioendocrine Research Group, University of Otago, Christchurch, New Zealand

JOERG C. SCHEFOLD, MD
Department of Nephrology and Intensive Care Medicine, Charité Medical School, Campus Virchow-Klinikum, Berlin, Germany

BARRY H. TRACHTENBERG, MD
Fellow, Heart Failure and Transplantation, Department of Medicine, Cardiovascular Division, University of Miami Miller School of Medicine, Miami, Florida

STEPHAN VON HAEHLING, MD
Department of Cardiology, Applied Cachexia Research, Charité Medical School, Campus Virchow-Klinikum, Berlin, Germany

KAI C. WOLLERT, MD
Professor of Medicine, Department of Cardiology and Angiology, Hans-Borst Center for Heart and Stem Cell Research, Hannover Medical School, Hannover, Germany

FAIEZ ZANNAD, MD, PhD
Director, Inserm, Centre d' Investigation Clinique de Nancy, Hôpital Jeanne d'Arc, Dommartin-les-Toul, France; Head, Centre Hospitalier Universitaire de Nancy, Hôpital Brabois, Hypertension and Heart Failure Unit, Department of Cardiology, Nancy, France; and Professor, Department of Therapeutics, Nancy-Université, Faculté de Médecine, Vandoeuvre-lès-Nancy, France

Contents

A profusion of circulating candidate biomarkers in heart failure is currently being investigated. Although all will advance our insight into the pathophysiology of heart failure, their potential clinical utility will depend on satisfaction of three key criteria. Assays must be accessible, reliable, and affordable. Secondly, the marker must provide information about cardiac function and prognosis not otherwise available. Finally, measurement of the marker must demonstrably lead to improved management and better clinical outcomes. Despite many promising candidates requiring fuller investigation, currently, only the natriuretic peptides satisfy these requirements.

Natriuretic peptides play a central role in cardiovascular, endocrine, and renal homeostasis and can be considered physiologic antagonists to the renin-angiotensin-aldosterone system. ANP and BNP in the circulation are derived primarily from the myocardium, whereas CNP is mainly derived from endothelial cells and the central nervous system. Increased ventricular and atrial diastolic wall stretch augment synthesis and release of BNP and NT-proBNP from cardiomyocytes, and is the principal stimulus controlling BNP production. Circulating BNP and NT-proBNP levels are increased in heart failure in proportion to disease severity, but elevated levels may also be observed in other cardiac and noncardiac disease states, including cardiac arrhythmias, ventricular hypertrophy, myocardial ischemia, pulmonary embolism, acute and chronic cor pulmonale, renal failure, anemia, hyperthyroidism, and sepsis. Fully automated analyses of both BNP and NT-proBNP can be rapidly performed on large hospital-based platforms as well as on small point-of-care devices.

The emergence of BNP or NT-proBNP testing has improved the management of acutely decompensated heart failure patients significantly by aiding in early recognition, prognostication, and treatment. Furthermore, their logical application may not only reduce healthcare costs but also potentially reduce adverse clinical outcomes. This article reviews the understanding of utilizing natriuretic peptide testing to correctly diagnose and manage acute heart failure.

Circulating levels of the BNP system can help in the diagnosis of cardiovascular disease and provide prognostic information not only for patients who have HF but also for the general population and other patient groups. Changes over time also carry prognostic information, and studies are assessing BNP-guided treatment strategies.

With the identification of circulating molecular forms of BNP, new insights regarding the biology of the BNP system are emerging that may improve the diagnostic and prognostic value of BNP. Likewise, accounting for rs198389 (a common single nucleotide polymorphism that increases BNP levels) may help to further refine the use of components of the BNP system as biomarkers.

ST2 and Adrenomedullin in Heart Failure

Rahul Kakkar and Richard T. Lee

ST2 is the receptor for interleukin-33, a cytokine with antihypertrophic and antifibrotic effects on the myocardium. Serum levels of the soluble form of ST2 serve as a biomarker for ventricular biomechanical strain and provide prognostic information in patients who have symptomatic heart failure. Adrenomedullin is a vasoactive peptide whose actions run counter to the physiologic derangements of clinical heart failure. It appears that measurements of serum adrenomedullin levels can be used to identify those patients who have advanced heart failure and who are at increased risk for heart failure–related death.

Biomarkers of Myocyte Injury in Heart Failure

Roberto Latini and Serge Masson

Markers of cardiac myocyte injury have contributed over the years to the diagnosis and to the assessment of size of myocardial infarction. Recent evidence suggests that measurement of the release of cardiac contractile proteins into the bloodstream at lower levels may be useful in the clinical assessment of patients who have acute or chronic heart failure. The advent of a new generation of high-sensitivity immunoassays for cardiac troponins offers challenges for scientists and clinicians and will likely change the understanding and interpretation of cardiac injury.

Growth-Differentiation Factor-15 in Heart Failure

Tibor Kempf and Kai C. Wollert

The stress-responsive transforming growth factor-β–related cytokine, growth-differentiation factor-15 (GDF-15), is emerging as a new biomarker in patients with cardiovascular disease. The circulating levels of GDF-15 are elevated and independently related to an adverse prognosis in acute coronary syndrome and left- or right-sided heart failure. GDF-15 adds significant prognostic information to established clinical and biochemical risk markers in these conditions. Elevated levels of GDF-15 may identify patients who have non–ST-elevation acute coronary syndrome who derive the greatest benefit from an invasive treatment strategy. As with other heart failure biomarkers, including BNP, it is currently not known what specific therapies could be used to reduce the risk associated with elevated levels of GDF-15 in heart failure. Further elucidation of the pathobiology and upstream inducers of this new biomarker may lead to new therapeutic concepts that address the risk associated with elevated GDF-15 levels. A commercial assay for GDF-15 should be available in the near future.

Inflammatory Biomarkers in Heart Failure Revisited: Much More than Innocent Bystanders

Stephan von Haehling, Joerg C. Schefold, Mitja Lainscak, Wolfram Doehner, and Stefan D. Anker

Chronic heart failure is viewed as a state of chronic inflammation. Many inflammatory markers have been shown to be up-regulated in patients who have this condition, but the markers' roles in clinical decision making have not yet been fully elucidated. A panel of biomarkers is likely to have a strong impact on patient management. Inflammatory biomarkers are interesting candidates that could answer specific clinical questions on their own or complement a multi-marker approach. This article provides a broad overview of several inflammatory biomarkers, including the pro-inflammatory cytokines tumor necrosis factor-α, interleukin (IL)-6, IL-1, IL-18, and the soluble receptors TNFR-1, TNFR-2, IL-6R, and gp130. In addition to these acute phase reactants, several adhesion molecules, and lipopolysaccharide-signaling pathways are discussed.

Biomarkers of Oxidative Stress in Heart Failure

Barry H. Trachtenberg and Joshua M. Hare

Oxidative stress is the relative excess of reactive oxygen species (ROS) versus endogenous defense mechanisms. Abundant evidence has demonstrated the role of ROS, along with reactive nitrogen species (RNS), in the pathophysiology of cardiovascular disease, including heart failure. Many biomarkers of oxidative stress have been studied as surrogates of oxidative damage. Recently, markers of impaired nitric oxide signaling have also been identified. Many biomarkers have been associated with prognosis and mortality, and some may even be modified by therapy. However, the clinical utility is limited by less than optimal standardization techniques and the lack of sufficient large-sized, multimarker prospective trials.

Newer Biomarkers in Heart Failure

Sachin Gupta, Mark H. Drazner, and James A. de Lemos

The pathophysiology of heart failure is complex, and the list of biomarkers representing distinct pathophysiologic pathways is growing rapidly. This article focuses on some promising newer biomarkers that have contributed to a better understanding of pathophysiologic mechanisms involved in heart failure but for which less data are currently available: osteoprotegerin, galectin-3, cystatin C, chromogranin A, and the adipokines adiponectin, leptin, and resistin. Despite the intriguing early information from these newer markers, none is ready for routine clinical use. Much additional study is needed to determine how these biomarkers will fit into diagnostic and treatment algorithms for patients who have heart failure.

Biomarkers of Extracellular Matrix Turnover

Faiez Zannad and Bertram Pitt

The extracellular cardiac matrix (ECCM) plays an important role in the support of myocytes and fibroblasts. ECCM turnover is influenced by ischemia, stretch, inflammation, and neurohormonal mediators. Myocardial fibrosis is the consequence of several pathologic processes mediated by mechanical, neurohormonal, and cytokine factors. It is a major determinant of diastolic dysfunction and pumping capacity and may result in tissue heterogeneity, dys-synchrony, and arrhythmias. The measurement of various serum peptides arising from the metabolism of collagen types 1 and 3, of degradation fragments, and of specific metalloproteinases may provide noninvasive assessment of fibrosis. ECCM biomarkers are clinically useful tools, particularly given the potential for cardioprotective and cardioreparative pharmacologic strategies.

Index

Heart Failure Clinics

VISIT THE CLINICS ONLINE!

Access your subscription at:
www.theclinics.com

Editorial

Do Biomarkers Deserve High Marks?

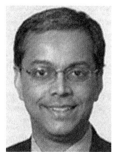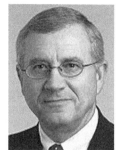

Ragavendra R. Baliga, MD, MBA   James B. Young, MD
Consulting Editors

It seems that the moment of truth for any blood test is if the results can answer the critical questions we all struggle with: What's wrong with the patient? How severe is the difficulty? Tell me what I, as a clinician, should do next? Indeed, biomarkers typically have four main clinical uses:[1] (1) diagnosis, (2) risk stratification, (3) guidance in the selection or titration of therapy in patients with known clinical features of disease,[2] and (4) screening for preclinical disease.[3] So is there a "CBC" or "PSA" for heart failure (HF)? The development of commercially available point-of-service assays for biomarkers, particularly troponins and B-type natriuretic peptide and its inactive N-terminal fragments, has led to a dramatic increase in the number of studies evaluating the potential clinical use of measurement of these biomarkers for all four of these clinical uses and particularly for HF. Biomarkers, along with other diagnostic modalities, may also be used to elucidate pathophysiologic processes, but they are not without limitations, since clinical features are a result of deviations in the dynamic equilibrium between risk factors, precipitating factors, and the body's ability to defend, repair, compensate, and respond to these factors.

The ability of any diagnostic modality, including biomarkers, to enhance the quality and efficacy of clinical care depends on several factors, including pretest probability, sensitivity and specificity, cost, benefits, risks, patient preference, and alternatives (such as continued observation, or proceeding to another test or empirical treatment). Particularly important is the fact that these tests are largely the results of simple blood draws. Problematic,

however, is an error in the test that results in clinical interventions that can actually be harmful, such as the prescription of aggressive diuretic doses in a patient who has "stable" congestive HF with high B-natriuretic peptide levels. Indeed, the pretest probability of the disease requiring clarification needs to be integrated with the test result to determine a revised post-test probability. Bayesian analysis combines these data mathematically to determine a precise probability. An important assumption in the Bayesian model is that a test adds new additional information above and beyond what is already known. Diagnostic studies are most useful when they have the ability to change a probability across a decision-making threshold so that it alters the clinical management of the patient.[4] However, for many conditions, the precise threshold that should guide clinical decision making has not yet been determined. Important principles to consider when evaluating and applying the results of diagnostic studies include: (1) Are the results valid? (2) What are the results? (3) Will the results help me in caring for my patients?[5] Brain natriuretic peptide (BNP) is one biomarker that has been shown to meet these important principles and enhance the quality and efficacy of care in HF.

BNP results in cost savings in the diagnosis of HF. When randomized clinical trials explored a diagnostic strategy, guided by BNP to aid in the diagnosis of HF in patients presenting to the emergency room with shortness of breath, the group that was randomized to have BNP evaluated spent a shorter time in the hospital at lower cost with no increased mortality and morbidity.

Heart Failure Clin 5 (2009) ix–xii
doi:10.1016/j.hfc.2009.05.001
1551-7136/09/$ – see front matter © 2009 Elsevier Inc. All rights reserved.

In one single-blind study of 452 patients,[6] point-of-service BNP in the emergency room decreased the rate of hospitalization by 10%, reduced the median length of stay by 3 days, and reduced the mean total cost of therapy by 1800 dollars with no adverse effects on mortality or the rate of re-hospitalization for HF.

Increasing evidence suggests that BNP is also useful in asymptomatic screening, risk stratification, and cost reduction. In the Framingham Offspring Study, when BNP was evaluated in asymptomatic middle-aged individuals, the investigators found that even small elevations of BNP were independently predictive of mortality, HF, atrial fibrillation, and stroke over a mean follow-up period of 5 years.[3] When screening for asymptomatic left ventricular systolic dysfunction, BNP testing seems to be cost-effective (less than 50,000 dollars per quality-adjusted life years gained) when used in a population with a HF prevalence of at least 1%.

The use of biomarkers to guide therapy is affected by comorbidities. For example, BNP levels in hospitalized patients are often affected by renal function and obesity.[7] Therefore, the management of HF using BNP would require that it be measured with renal function and with consideration of body mass index. In the outpatient setting, the STARS-BNP study showed that titrating therapy to BNP levels <100 pg/mL reduced the composite primary end point of

mortality and hospitalization due to HF compared with guideline-directed therapy;[8] however, not all studies have demonstrated that changes in BNP levels are associated with improved outcomes.[9] Currently, from an economic perspective, data are insufficient to determine whether regular assessment of BNP is cost-effective for outpatient titration.

As the field of biomarkers continues to evolve, it is increasingly clear that a panel of biomarkers may add incremental value in the management of HF. For example, when BNP and troponin (a marker of myocardial necrosis) are both elevated in HF, mortality risk increases 12-fold compared with those with both undetectable cardiac troponin I and lower BNP.[10] Therefore, incorporating a multi-marker approach in the routine evaluation of heart patients should allow clinicians to more accurately identify high risk patients who may derive benefit from intensive management strategies.

Biomarkers may be used as a package or a strategy. For example, integrating echocardiography with BNP has been shown to improve the diagnosis of HF in the emergency room (**Fig. 1**).[11] In patients presenting with shortness of breath, when BNP is below 100 pg/mL, HF is unlikely (<2%), and it is useful in ruling out HF with a negative predictive value of >95%. When the BNP is >500 pg/mL, HF is very likely (95%); very high levels are associated with a positive

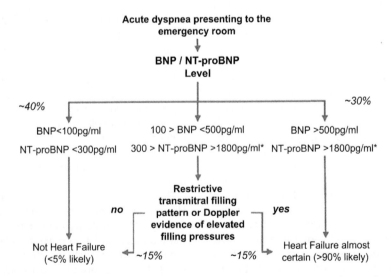

Fig. 1. Combining BNP and echocardiography for diagnosis. Algorithm for integrated use of B-type natriuretic peptide levels and echocardiography for diagnosis of acute heart failure. *Use of age stratified values for amino-terminal pro-B-type natriuretic peptide (NT-proBNP) provides more accurate test performance: <50 years, use NT-proBNP >450 pg/mL; 50 to 75 years, use NT-proBNP >900 pg/mL; >75 years, use NT-proBNP >1,800 pg/mL.[15] (*From* Troughton RW, Richards AM. B-type natriuretic peptides and echocardiographic measures of cardiac structure and function. JACC Cardiovasc Imaging 2009;2(2):216–25; with permission.)

predictive value of >85%. A restrictive transmitral Doppler pattern more accurately differentiates acute HF from noncardiac causes of shortness of breath when BNP is between 100 pg/mL and 500 pg/mL (the intermediate or "grey" zone). The accuracy for early HF diagnosis is improved by up to 30% in patients presenting with acute shortness of breath.[12] Integrating BNP with echocardiography has also been used to more accurately estimate left ventricular filling pressures.[13] Although BNP is associated with increased left ventricular end-diastolic pressure, the relationship is modest and depends on the clinical scenario. In contrast, the accuracy of tissue Doppler in the estimation of left ventricular filling pressures is better validated. Combining both BNP and tissue Doppler should, therefore, provide more value. Several studies have demonstrated that the addition of tissue Doppler to BNP levels significantly increases the ability to identify high-risk patients, including mortality and readmission (**Fig 2**). This is one example showing how biomarkers can be combined with other modalities to provide more powerful risk stratification in HF.

Biomarkers are not without limitations, and the assays have inter- and intra-individual variability. These limitations, therefore, make it important that these results are interpreted in the context of clinical history, physical examination, and bedside tests, such as 12-lead EKG and chest roentgenogram. Occasionally however, biomarkers may have incremental value regardless of the pretest probability. For example, in a patient who has shortness of breath and a very high BNP level,

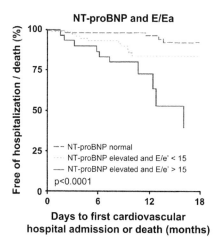

NT-proBNP and E/Ea

Free of hospitalization / death (%)

-- NT-proBNP normal
···· NT-proBNP elevated and E/e' < 15
— NT-proBNP elevated and E/e' > 15
p<0.0001

Days to first cardiovascular hospital admission or death (months)

Fig. 2. Combining BNP and echocardiography for risk stratification. (*From* Whalley GA, Wright SP, Pearl A, et al. Prognostic role of echocardiography and brain natriuretic peptide in symptomatic breathless patients in the community. Eur Heart J 2008;29(4):509–16; with permission.)

Box 1
Biomarkers in Heart Failure

Inflammation*†‡
C-reactive protein
Tumor necrosis factor α
Fas (APO-1)
Interleukins 1, 6, and 18

Oxidative stress*†§
Oxidized low-density lipoproteins
Myeloperoxidase
Urinary biopyrrins
Urinary and plasma isoprostanes
Plasma malondialdehyde

Extracellular-matrix remodeling*†§
Matrix metalloproteinases
Tissue inhibitors of metalloproteinases
Collagen propeptides
   Propeptide procollagen type I
   Plasma procollagen type III

Neurohormones*†§
Norepinephrine
Renin
Angiotensin II
Aldosterone
Arginine vasopressin
Endothelin

Myocyte injury*†§
Cardiac-specific troponins I and T
Myosin light-chain kinase I
Heart-type fatty-acid protein
Creatine kinase MB fraction

Myocyte stress†‡§¶
Brain natriuretic peptide
N-terminal pro–brain natriuretic peptide
Midregional fragment of proadrenomedullin
ST2

New biomarkers†
Chromogranin
Galectin 3
Osteoprotegerin
Adiponectin
Growth differentiation factor 15

* Biomarkers in this category aid in elucidating the pathogenesis of heart failure.
† Biomarkers in this category provide prognostic information and enhance risk stratification.
‡ Biomarkers in this category can be used to identify subjects at risk for heart failure.
§ Biomarkers in this category are potential targets of therapy.
¶ Biomarkers in this category are useful in the diagnosis of heart failure and in monitoring therapy.
From Braunwald E. Biomarkers in heart failure. N Engl J Med 2008;358(20):2148–59; with permission.

echocardiography is indicated even in the absence of abnormalities on physical examination and bedside investigations.

The Braunwald classification of biomarkers[1] for HF divides them into seven categories, including markers of inflammation, oxidative stress, extracellular matrix remodeling, myocyte injury, myocyte stress, neurohormones, and renal dysfunction (**Box 1** and the Preface to this issue). Dr. Braunwald included newer biomarkers in a separate class in the *New England Journal* article. In this issue of *Heart Failure Clinics*, Dr. Braunwald has assembled a panel of experts in this field to discuss biomarkers included in this classification. These experts demonstrate that biomarkers singly, as a panel of markers, or in conjunction with other modalities such as echocardiography are an important addition to the clinical armamentarium and should be a valuable adjunct to a thorough history and clinical evaluation at these points of care. Biomarkers serve to enhance the quality and efficacy of clinical care by helping with triage and risk stratification. In particular, they allow cost reduction of medical care by leading to early initiation of highly effective therapeutic strategies that reduce the risk of complications of the disease process, by reducing or even eliminating the need for other more expensive diagnostic studies, or by establishing an alternative diagnosis that does not require hospitalization.[14] In our opinion, biomarkers do deserve high marks!

Ragavendra R. Baliga, MD, MBA
The Ohio State University
Columbus, OH, USA

James B. Young, MD
Division of Medicine and Lerner College of
Medicine
Cleveland Clinic
Cleveland, OH, USA

E-mail addresses:
Ragavendra.Baliga@osumc.edu (R.R. Baliga)
YOUNGJ@ccf.org (J.B. Young)

REFERENCES

1. Braunwald E. Biomarkers in heart failure. N Engl J Med 2008;358(20):2148–59.
2. Troughton RW, Frampton CM, Yandle TG, et al. Treatment of heart failure guided by plasma aminoterminal brain natriuretic peptide (N-BNP) concentrations. Lancet 2000;355(9210):1126–30.
3. Wang TJ, Larson MG, Levy D, et al. Plasma natriuretic peptide levels and the risk of cardiovascular events and death. N Engl J Med 2004;350(7):655–63.
4. Goldman L. Clinical decision making in primary cardiology. In: Goldman E, editor. Philadelphia: Saunders; 1998. p. 13–26.
5. Richardson WS, Detsky AS. Users' guides to the medical literature. VII. How to use a clinical decision analysis. A. Are the results of the study valid? Evidence-Based Medicine Working Group. JAMA 1995;273(16):1292–5.
6. Mueller C, Scholer A, Laule-Kilian K, et al. Use of B-type natriuretic peptide in the evaluation and management of acute dyspnea. N Engl J Med 2004;350(7):647–54.
7. Maisel A, Mueller C, Adams K Jr, et al. State of the art: using natriuretic peptide levels in clinical practice. Eur J Heart Fail 2008;10(9):824–39.
8. Jourdain P, Jondeau G, Funck F, et al. Plasma brain natriuretic peptide-guided therapy to improve outcome in heart failure: the STARS-BNP Multicenter Study. J Am Coll Cardiol 2007;49(16):1733–9.
9. Pfisterer M, Buser P, Rickli H, et al. BNP-guided versus symptom-guided heart failure therapy: the Trial of Intensified versus Standard Medical Therapy in Elderly Patients With Congestive Heart Failure (TIME-CHF) randomized trial. JAMA 2009;301(4):383–92.
10. Horwich TB, Patel J, MacLellan WR, et al. Cardiac troponin I is associated with impaired hemodynamics, progressive left ventricular dysfunction, and increased mortality rates in advanced heart failure. Circulation 2003;108(7):833–8.
11. Troughton RW, Richards AM. B-type natriuretic peptides and echocardiographic measures of cardiac structure and function. JACC Cardiovasc Imaging 2009;2(2):216–25.
12. Dokainish H, Zoghbi WA, Lakkis NM, et al. Comparative accuracy of B-type natriuretic peptide and tissue Doppler echocardiography in the diagnosis of congestive heart failure. Am J Cardiol 2004;93(9):1130–5.
13. Whalley GA, Wright SP, Pearl A, et al. Prognostic role of echocardiography and brain natriuretic peptide in symptomatic breathless patients in the community. Eur Heart J 2008;29(4):509–16.
14. Schunemann HJ, Oxman AD, Brozek J, et al. Grading quality of evidence and strength of recommendations for diagnostic tests and strategies. BMJ 2008;336(7653):1106–10.
15. Januzzi JL, van Kimmenade R, Lainchbury J, et al. NT-proBNP testing for diagnosis and short-term prognosis in acute destabilized heart failure: an international pooled analysis of 1256 patients: the International Collaborative of NT-proBNP Study. Eur Heart J 2006;27(3):330–7.

Preface

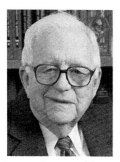

Eugene Braunwald, MD
Guest Editor

Until recently, the classification of heart failure (HF) has focused on the anatomic cause of failure of the cardiac pump (eg, valvular heart disease, hypertension, chronic coronary artery disease, and so forth), the pathophysiology (eg, reduced or normal ejection fraction), and the clinical features (eg, the acuity and severity of the HF). A biomarker profile can be a valuable addition to this approach. The major classes of biomarkers for HF discussed in this issue of *Heart Failure Clinics* are usually considered individually, as they were done so expertly in this issue. However, investigators are finding increasingly that a multimarker strategy may be useful in refining risk stratification in patients who have acute coronary syndrome,[1] and there is a growing interest in utilizing this approach in HF as well.[2]

It has been demonstrated that using troponin together with BNP can achieve a more accurate stratification of risk than can be obtained with either biomarker alone. [3–5] The accuracy of risk prediction was also enhanced when a natriuretic peptide was coupled with other biomarkers of myocardial stress—adrenomedullin[6] and ST-2[7]— as well as with the inflammatory biomarkers C-reactive protein (CRP) and myeloperoxidase.[8] Zathelius and colleagues have shown that the combination of four biomarkers (TnI, NTproBNP, CRP, and cystatin C) improves risk stratification for total cardiovascular mortality in elderly men.[9]

From the foregoing, the next logical step is to obtain a profile using the seven classes of biomarker described in this issue (**Fig. 1**). This profile should provide not only a more accurate risk stratification, but it may provide clues to the pathophysiology of HF in any given patient and point the way to individualized therapy. New approaches to bioinformatics, including the use of neural networks, will be needed to assist in data analysis and its clinical application.

We are now moving rapidly into the proteomic era, which provides a greatly expanded approach to the study of proteins, their variations, and their concentrations. The evaluation of proteins using mass spectrometric analysis coupled with high pressure liquid chromatography is likely to yield totally new classes of biomarkers of HF.[10] Large platforms of hundreds of proteins are likely to provide deeper insights into the detection of ventricular dysfunction, elucidating pathogenesis, and in monitoring the therapy of HF. As a result of these expanding technologies, advances in

BIOMARKER PROFILE IN HEART FAILURE

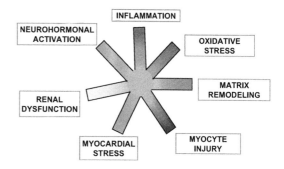

Fig. 1. Seven axes representing the classes of biomarkers discussed in this issue. It is proposed that a representative marker of each class be measured in patients who have established HF, or who are at risk for HF. The resultant biomarker profile should enhance prevention, treatment, and prognostication. Other classes of biomarkers are likely to be added in the future.

Heart Failure Clin 5 (2009) xiii–xiv
doi:10.1016/j.hfc.2009.05.002

biomarkers in the next ten years may be expected to be greater and to have even more impact on the detection, risk assessment, and management of patients who have HF than those advances that have occurred since work in this field began a half of a century ago.

Eugene Braunwald, MD
TIMI Study Group
350 Longwood Avenue
1st Office Floor
Boston, MA 02115, USA

E-mail address:
ebraunwald@partners.org (E. Braunwald)

REFERENCES

1. Sabatine MS, Morrow DA, deLemos J, et al. Multimarker approach to risk stratification in non-ST elevation acute coronary syndromes: Simultaneous assessment of troponin I, C-reactive protein, and B-type natriuretic peptide. Circulation 2002;105:1760–3.
2. Lee DS, Vasan RS. Novel markers for heart failure diagnosis and prognosis. Curr Opin Cardiol 2005; 20:201–10.
3. Horwich TB, Patel J, MacLellan WR, Fonarow GC. Cardiac troponin I is associated with impaired hemodynamics, progressive left ventricular dysfunction, and increased mortality rates in advanced heart failure. Circulation 2003;108:833–8.
4. Miller WL, Hartman KA, Burritt MF, et al. Serial biomarker measurements in ambulatory patients with chronic heart failure. Circulation 2007;116:249–57.
5. Latini R, Masson S, Anand IS, et al. Prognostic value of very low plasma concentrations of troponin T in patients with stable chronic heart failure. Circulation 2007;116:1242–9.
6. Khan SQ, O'Brien RJ, Struck J, et al. Prognostic value of midregional pro-adrenomedullin in patients with acute myocardial infarction. J Am Coll Cardiol 2007;49:1525–32.
7. Januzzi JL, Peacock WF, Maisel AS, et al. Measurement of the interleukin family member ST2 in patients with acute dyspnea. J Am Coll Cardiol 2007;50:607–13.
8. Ng LL, Pathik B, Loke IW, et al. Myeloperoxidase and C-reactive protein augment the specificity of B-type natriuretic peptide in community screening for systolic heart failure. Am Heart J 2006;152:94–101.
9. Zethelius B, Berglund L, Sundstrom J, et al. Use of multiple biomarkers to improve the prediction of death from cardiovascular causes. N Engl J Med 2008;358:2107–16.
10. Arab S, Gramolini AO, Ping P, et al. Cardiovascular proteomics: Tools to develop novel biomarkers and potential applications. J Am Coll Cardiol 2006;48:1733–41.

What We May Expect from Biomarkers in Heart Failure

A. Mark Richards, MD, PhD[a,b,*]

KEYWORDS

- Heart failure • Biomarkers • Diagnosis
- Prognosis • Monitoring • Treatment

Biomarkers are biologic variables, the measurement of which provides information about a condition of interest. In heart failure, biomarkers may include demographic features such as age and gender, cardiac imaging (including ultrasound, radiography, and magnetic resonance scanning), or even determination of a particular genetic polymorphism. However, the term *biomarker* is now customarily applied to circulating serum and plasma analytes beyond the hematology (hemoglobin) and biochemistry (creatinine and electrolytes) included in routine clinical management. This encompasses an expanding array of biochemicals, the levels of which reflect assorted aspects of the pathophysiology of heart failure.

In the larger context of cardiovascular disease, biomarkers that have attained cardinal significance over the last decade include troponins in acute coronary syndromes and the B-type natriuretic peptides in heart failure. The latter illustrate what biomarkers have to offer in heart failure and also demonstrate some shortcomings relative to the notional ideal marker. The B-type peptides and more recently discovered candidate markers are discussed in detail in articles elsewhere in this issue.

CRITERIA FOR CLINICALLY APPLICABLE BIOMARKERS

Recent authoritative commentary[1,2] has suggested criteria or benchmarks for assessment of the clinical utility of biomarkers. The key requirement is that measurement of the biomarker in question should demonstrably facilitate improved clinical management and outcomes in patients with heart failure. For example, the new marker should provide an improvement in diagnostic certainty in comparison, or in combination, with existing diagnostic tests. Alternatively, or in addition, levels of the marker should be closely associated with a defined risk of onset or deterioration in heart failure that, in turn, can be addressed with specific therapy or biomarker-guided triage, or monitoring through serial measurement should enhance clinical outcomes (with reductions in episodes of acute decompensation, reduced heart failure mortality, or enhanced quality of life).

Secondly, the biomarker should provide information not otherwise available. There should be a strong and consistent relationship between marker levels and the diagnosis, prognosis, or both. The marker should improve diagnostic certainty or clinical risk stratification beyond existing tests.

Finally, practical, technical, and commercial issues bear upon the successful application of biomarkers in broad clinical practice. The marker must be subject to assay by accurate, reproducible, and well-supported analytical methods. Stability of the analyte in serum or plasma must be ascertained and sufficient to avoid confounding of results by excessive post-sampling degradation. The assay must be both accessible and affordable. High throughput of results with a rapid

a National Heart Foundation of New Zealand, New Zealand
b University of Otago, Christchurch, New Zealand
* Corresponding author. University Department of Medicine, University of Otago, Christchurch, PO Box 4345, Christchurch 8140, New Zealand.
E-mail address: mark.richards@cdhb.govt.nz

Heart Failure Clin 5 (2009) 463–470
doi:10.1016/j.hfc.2009.04.011
1551-7136/09/$ – see front matter © 2009 Published by Elsevier Inc.

turnaround must be provided at a reasonable cost. As articulated elsewhere in this issue, the B-type natriuretic peptides satisfy criteria as valuable biomarkers that are of use in the clinical management of acute and chronic heart failure. Nevertheless, they fall well short of the perfect biomarker as outlined toward the end of this article.

Among the flood of candidate biomarkers currently receiving attention in the field of heart failure, few will satisfy the criteria summarized previously. In addition to the requisite test performance, clinical practicality and fiscal limitations dictate that the array of markers that become established in everyday clinical practice for the management of heart failure are restrained by appropriately parsimonious algorithms. This requirement in no way detracts from the other major benefit which we may expect from biomarkers in heart failure, that is, pathophysiologic insight. Biomarkers reflect one or more of the many and varied aspects of the complex pathophysiology of heart failure. They potentially offer new information regarding the etiology of the condition and, by reflecting disease processes occurring at whole body, organ, cellular, or intracellular levels, may pinpoint potential novel therapeutic targets. Biomarkers may provide this improved understanding of heart failure and open avenues of therapy without necessarily being particularly powerful diagnostic or prognostic measures.

CATEGORIES OF BIOMARKERS IN HEART FAILURE

Table 1 provides a listing of biomarkers in heart failure broadly grouped according to current, often limited, understanding of their role in the pathophysiology of cardiac failure.

Neurohormones

The best known subgroup is that of the neurohormones, including the cardiac natriuretic peptides, the components of the renin-angiotensin-aldosterone system (RAAS), the catecholamines, arginine vasopressin (AVP), and endothelium-derived vasoactive peptides including endothelin, adrenomedullin, the C-type natriuretic peptides, and the urocortins. These substances are all biologically active endocrine or paracrine or autocrine entities which reflect the systemic or cardiac response to acute or chronic cardiac injury. Some appear to be predominantly compensatory in nature. For example, the cardiac natriuretic peptides facilitate enhanced renal filtration and excretion of sodium while suppressing the vasoconstrictor/sodium-retaining RAAS and exerting a tonic antitrophic effect which abates interstitial scarring and cardiac hypertrophy.

Genetically modified "knockout" models of atrial natriuretic peptide (ANP), B type natriuretic peptide (BNP), or their specific receptors exhibit hypertension, cardiac hypertrophy, and fibrosis together with increased mortality when compared with wild-type animals. The prime secretory stimulus for the cardiac natriuretic peptides is cardiomyocyte stretch; therefore, the increased intracardiac and transmural pressures which characterize all forms of heart failure trigger secretion of the natriuretic peptides. This mechanism underlies the relatively consistent association between plasma concentrations of the B-type natriuretic peptides with the severity of cardiac structural and functional abnormality and with prognosis.[3] Nevertheless, this relationship is modulated and potentially confounded by age, gender, renal function, body mass, hypoxemia, arrhythmia, glucocorticoid and thyroid status, inflammatory states, and severe multisystem disease as seen in severe cases of trauma or sepsis.

Cardiac impairment with associated reductions in regional blood flow together with increased renal, cardiac, and systemic sympathetic drive stimulate the RAAS, which can be viewed as a maladaptive effort to sustain arterial pressure and renal perfusion. This system is diametrically counterpoised to the cardiac natriuretic peptides, and its activation leads to widespread vasoconstriction and sodium retention together with cardiac hypertrophy and fibrosis. Along with activation of the sympathetic nervous system and high levels of circulating catecholamines, the RAAS appears to be a major culprit promoting adverse ventricular remodeling after cardiac injury and facilitating the vicious cycle of spiraling cardiac dysfunction, decompensation, and high mortality observed in chronic heart failure. Plasma levels of norepinephrine, plasma renin activity, and aldosterone are all related to prognosis in chronic heart failure.[4]

AVP is activated in heart failure and may become predominantly regulated by hemodynamic cues and by raised angiotensin II rather than plasma osmolarity. The consequences include inappropriate antidiuresis (which may lead to frank hyponatremia) and increased peripheral vasoconstriction. Endothelin, another potent vasoconstrictor peptide, is produced by the endothelium. Levels are raised and independently related to adverse prognosis in heart failure. Acute blockade of endothelin in heart failure results in beneficial hemodynamic effects (including falls in pulmonary artery and ventricular filling pressures together with increments in cardiac output) proportional to the baseline elevation of endothelin.[5]

Conversely, adrenomedullin, which is also elevated in heart failure and independently related

Table 1
Biomarkers in heart failure

Type of Marker Based on Physiologic Role in Heart Failure	Examples
Neurohormonal markers	
Cardiac natriuretic peptides	B-type natriuretic peptides (BNP1-32, NTproBNP1-76, pro-BNP) ANP, NTproANP, midregion pro-ANP C-type natriuretic peptides (CNP, NTproCNP)
Renin-angiotensin-aldosterone system	Plasma renin activity (PRA) Angiotensin II Aldosterone
Adrenergic nervous system	Norepinephrine Epinephrine
Arginine vasopressin	Arginine vasopressin (AVP) Copeptin
Endothelial-derived peptides	Endothelin 1, big endothelin Adrenomedullin, midregion proadrenomedullin Urocortins I, II, III
Inflammatory markers	
	C-reactive protein Tumor necrosis factor alpha Fas (APO-1) Interleukins 1, 6, and 18
Oxidative stress markers	
	Oxidized low-density lipoproteins Myeloperoxidase Urine biopyrrins Urine and plasma isoprostanes Plasma malondialdehyde Carbonyl proteins
Interstitial matrix remodeling markers	
	Matrix metalloproteinases (MMPs) Tissue inhibitors of metalloproteinases (TIMPs) Propeptide procollagen I Procollagen III
Myocyte injury markers	
	Cardiac troponins I and T Myosin light-chain kinase I Heart fatty acid binding protein Creatine kinase, creatine kinase MB fraction Ischemia modified albumin
Other/new markers	
	ST2 Growth differentiation factor 15 Osteoprotegerin Adiponectin Galectin 3 Coenzyme Q10

to prognosis, is a vasodilator peptide predominantly of endothelial origin. In experimental heart failure, it has a beneficial hemodynamic profile. Despite activating renin, it does not elevate aldosterone levels, and it lowers natriuretic peptide concentrations in parallel with reductions in left atrial pressures.[6]

Plasma levels of the more recently discovered urocortins (members of the corticotrophin-releasing factor peptide family) are increased in heart failure. When administered in experimental heart failure, they exhibit a powerful array of beneficial effects, including minimal lowering of systemic arterial pressure but major reductions in right heart and left ventricular filling pressures, increments in cardiac output while lowering cardiac work in concert with suppression of the RAAS, endothelin, and AVP, and marked improvement in renal filtration. Blockade of urocortin exacerbates the hemodynamic, renal, and neurohormonal features of experimental heart failure, suggesting that endogenous urocortin is a significant contributor to the compensatory response to heart failure.[7]

Markers of Inflammation and Oxidative Stress

A further broad group of markers reflect inflammation and oxidative stress. C-reactive protein (CRP), tumor necrosis factor (TNF) alpha, and other cytokines are increased in heart failure, with higher levels portending a worse prognosis.[1,8–11] Myeloperoxidase activity, urine and plasma isoprostanes, and other markers of oxidative damage similarly rise with increasing severity of heart failure. Investigation of CRP dates back more than 50 years, whereas the associations between the cytokines and the risk of developing heart failure (and with prognosis in established heart failure) have been recognized since the 1990s. These elements of the immune system may exert part of their deleterious effect by triggering expression of adverse neurohormonal factors such as endothelin 1 in addition to more direct promotion of cardiomyocyte necrosis and apoptosis.

Other Markers

The rate and severity of adverse ventricular remodeling (partly reflecting the cardiotoxic effects of neurohormonal and cytokine activation) are mirrored in markers of interstitial matrix degradation and formation. These markers include circulating levels of matrix metalloproteinases, the tissue inhibitors of metalloproteinases, and the procollagens.[12] TNF alpha may drive cardiac dilatation partly through increased expression and activity of metalloproteinases, again illustrating the complex interplay between different elements of the molecular causes of, and responses to, cardiac impairment. Ongoing low-grade apoptosis and necrosis of cardiomyocytes are reflected in myocyte injury markers including troponins I and T, better known for their role in the diagnosis and management of acute coronary syndromes. Troponin levels are prognostic in heart failure.[13]

New markers, many of which are discussed in articles elsewhere in this issue, continue to emerge from diverse aspects of the pathophysiology of heart failure. ST2 is a soluble form of the receptor for interleukin-33. Levels are induced through cardiomyocyte stretch. Interleukin-33 appears to mediate an antifibrotic pathway in the heart.[14,15] In contrast to most markers, coenzyme Q10 is reduced in heart failure, possibly reflecting a fundamental impairment of mitochondrial respiration.[16] Other newcomers include growth differentiation factor 15, osteoprotegerin, adiponectin, galectin 3, and urotensin II.[1,17–20]

ASSESSMENT OF MARKERS

Of the broad and increasing array of markers discussed previously, only the B-type peptides have become established as recommended aids to the diagnosis of acute heart failure.[21] Their independent prognostic power across the spectrum from "silent" risk factor to overt decompensated heart failure is well recognized. Serial measurements appear likely to guide improved management of both acute and chronic heart failure. Baseline plasma B-type peptide levels are now routinely included among recruitment criteria in therapeutic trials, and the response of plasma B-type peptides is a respected secondary end-point in such trials.

Recent evidence suggests that assay of midregion proatrial natriuretic peptide levels has similar diagnostic power for acute heart failure as does assay of the B-type natriuretic peptides. It is also possible that midregion proadrenomedullin levels and ST2 levels are superior to the B-type peptides as indicators of prognosis in acute heart failure. Whether these distinctions in test performance will allow one or more biomarkers to replace the B-type natriuretic peptides or will lead to their use in combination with BNP remains to be seen.

In contrast, all of the other markers identified to date in heart failure have yet to find an established role as diagnostic, prognostic, or management tools. Although the pivotal adverse role of the RAAS and the sympathetic nervous system in the evolution of cardiac failure is undeniable, there is no proven clinical benefit in routine measurement of plasma levels of renin, angiotensin II, aldosterone, or plasma catecholamines for diagnosis, for dictating introduction of therapy, or for monitoring heart failure.

There are some indications that biomarker profiling may assist in more accurate case selection for more effective use of specific therapies. Neurohormonal substudies undertaken in association with early randomized controlled therapeutic trials of angiotensin-converting enzyme inhibition (ACEI) suggested that the greatest benefit accrued to those with higher renin activity and angiotensin II levels.[22] Within the RALES trial of the aldosterone antagonist spironolactone, in patients with severe heart failure, a substudy suggested that benefit was confined to those with elevation of procollagen 3 levels above a certain threshold.[23] Similarly, some evidence from randomized controlled trials suggests that elevation of B-type natriuretic peptides above a certain level predicts beneficial response to the introduction of beta-blocker therapy.[24] Although the introduction of existing treatments is dictated on empiric grounds (derived from the outcomes of randomized controlled trials), it is possible that some future treatments will be subject to more selective prescribing dictated, in part, through biomarker profiling.

Biomarkers to Identify New Therapeutic Targets

The neurohormonal hypothesis of the pathophysiology of heart failure has underpinned major advances in anti–heart failure therapy since the mid-1980s. Its elaboration has rested heavily upon investigation of circulating levels of biomarkers. Interruption of the RAAS using ACEI, angiotensin receptor blockers, and aldosterone antagonists has been rationally based on gathered understanding of the adverse effects of this system in evolving heart failure. This approach has been self-evidently successful.[25] Blockade of adrenergic beta receptors is also a successful therapy with a logical underpinning given the known adverse effects of excess adrenergic drive and circulating catecholamines on cardiac energy balance, peripheral vascular resistance, cellular integrity, and renin secretion in heart failure.[26] Administration of human recombinant BNP (nesiritide) has received approval as treatment in acute decompensated heart failure. Although questions remain to be resolved regarding the effects of this agent on renal function and mortality, it is clear that nesiritide rapidly lowers cardiac filling pressures and relieves dyspnea in acute heart failure.[27] This effect is what would be expected given the known bioactivity of this endogenous peptide and its clear role as part of a beneficial compensatory response to cardiac distress.

Rational pursuit of neurohormonal or other targets has not always borne therapeutic fruit, and the last decade has seen a series of disappointments with experimental treatments based on impeccable logic (and often with compelling background preclinical evidence) that have failed to reduce morbidity or mortality in heart failure. Agents reducing central sympathetic traffic outflow, blockade of TNF alpha, and endothelin antagonists have not proven to be useful.[28–30] Antagonists of AVP have not reduced mortality.[31] Whether manipulation of plasma or tissue levels of urocortin or adrenomedullin or blockade of specific mediators of inflammation/oxidation will prove useful in the treatment of heart failure remains to be discovered. History tells us that, even given excellent understanding of the biology of these entities, only rigorously designed randomized controlled trials can answer such questions.

Multimarker Strategies

Concurrent use of multiple prognostic indicators, each independently associated with outcomes in heart failure, improves risk stratification. For example, combining measurements of one or another B-type natriuretic peptide with radionuclide ventriculography,[3] with genotype, or with estimates of renal function markedly augments risk stratification after myocardial infarction and in acute and chronic heart failure. Combining two or more circulating biomarkers which reflect different aspects of heart failure pathophysiology (eg, BNP and troponin levels) and which are independently associated with important clinical outcomes can improve prognostic power. In a recent assessment of NTproBNP and ST2 levels in patients with acute heart failure presenting to the emergency department, it was apparent that concurrent elevation of both biomarkers conferred a far higher risk of mortality than elevation of either marker alone (**Fig. 1**).[15] Markers predominantly reflecting acute phase responses to cardiac injury may be combined with others reflecting hemodynamic load (cardiomyocyte stretch), potentially giving indications as to the acuity and the severity of the current presentation.

The Perfect Biomarker in Heart Failure

Given our experience to date, what would we wish for in the ideal biomarker in heart failure? It should have a consistent, graded, and specific association with increasing degrees of cardiac impairment and with prognosis. The relationship between increments and decrements in biomarker levels on the one hand and concurrent deterioration and improvement in cardiac function on the other within an individual patient should be consistent. There should be little interindividual variation in this relationship so that level x or increment y of the biomarker has much the same diagnostic and prognostic significance in patient A as in patient B for any given cardiac pathology. There

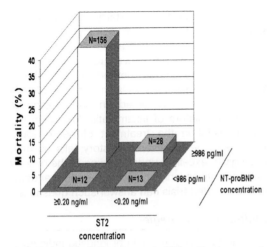

Fig. 1. Mortality (%) at 1 year in 208 patients presenting with acute heart failure according to ST2 and NTproBNP levels. (*From* Januzzi JL Jr, Peacock WF, Maisel AS, et al. Measurement of the interleukin family member ST2 in patients with acute dyspnea: results from the PRIDE (Pro-Brain Natriuretic Peptide Investigation of Dyspnea in the Emergency Department) study. J Am Coll Cardiol 2007;50:607–13; with permission.)

should be a high "signal-to-noise" ratio such that even modestly abnormal cardiac function is associated with raised biomarker levels readily distinguished from the normal range. It should show a clear rise in parallel with the evolving episodes of heart failure which precedes severe symptomatic crises and is of value in triggering an appropriate therapeutic intervention to prevent decompensation and the need for hospital admission. There should be minimal confounding from universal background variables including age, gender, renal function, arterial oxygen saturation, posture, and body mass. Pathology in noncardiac systems (respiratory, endocrine, central nervous system, gastrointestinal tract, and hepatic function) and drug therapy should not disturb the marker beyond the expected signal from any concurrent or secondary change in cardiac function. Assays should be reliable, precise, reproducible, and affordable with high throughput and rapid turnaround available to the clinician. Assay variability (both analytic and biologic) from sources other than a change in cardiac status should be low to allow a low (20% or less) minimal requirement for change carrying a high statistical likelihood of reflecting a clinically relevant shift in cardiac status. The marker should closely reflect a specific pathophysiologic pathway or process for which there is a specific therapeutic response of proven benefit, or serial measurements should enable optimal monitoring and drug titration.

Measurement of the biomarker should demonstrably lead to improved management of heart failure (when compared with the best available treatment without biomarker results), leading to reductions in acute decompensation, admissions to the hospital, the duration of admissions, and heart failure mortality together with sustained or improved quality of life.

SUMMARY

Only a minority of candidate biomarkers will prove to satisfy the three key criteria for widespread clinical application in the day-to-day management of heart failure. These criteria include (1) widely accessible, well-standardized assays capable of high throughput and rapid turnaround; (2) a strong and consistent association of levels of the biomarker with the diagnosis of heart failure and its prognosis; and (3) most importantly, a clinical consequence of measurements which clearly improves diagnosis, management, and outcomes.

We may never enjoy the application of the perfect marker, but we do have the tools to search for and to recognize this particular "holy grail." Combining markers may provide information compensating for the shortcomings of individual tests. New markers may or may not point to new therapeutic targets; however, each emerging biomarker will offer some additional insight into the pathophysiology of heart failure, and even on these grounds alone, their continued investigation is worthwhile.

Currently, the criteria for clinical utility have been met by the B-type natriuretic peptides alone. It is now 20 years since BNP was discovered, with the almost immediate recognition of the association between circulating plasma levels of BNP and the degree of cardiac dysfunction. Thousands of publications addressing the basic science and clinical aspects of the B-type peptides have followed prior to their current acceptance and clinical application. This literature hints at the burden of evidence which will be required of future candidate biomarkers. Fortunately, the pathway from discovery to proof of clinical utility is now well established thanks in large part to the global effort in natriuretic peptide research. The accumulated basic and clinical research experience (including the existing banks of samples from well-characterized patient cohorts) should facilitate more efficient assessment of new candidate biomarkers. The continuing exploration of the genome, coupled with the evolving disciplines of proteomics and metabolomics, ensure that there will be no shortage of newly discovered candidate biomarker molecules for the foreseeable future.[32,33]

REFERENCES

1. Braunwald E. Biomarkers in heart failure. N Engl J Med 2008;358:2148–59.
2. Morrow DA, de Lemos JA. Benchmarks for the assessment of novel cardiovascular biomarkers. Circulation 2007;115:949–52.
3. Richards AM, Nicholls MG, Espiner EA, et al. B-type natriuretic peptides and ejection fraction for prognosis after myocardial infarction. Circulation 2003; 107:2786–92.
4. Latini R, Masson S, Anand I, et al. The comparative prognostic value of plasma neurohormones at baseline in patients with heart failure enrolled in Val-HeFT. Eur Heart J 2004;25:292–9.
5. Kiowski W, Kim J, Oechslin E, et al. Evidence for endothelin-1-mediated vasoconstriction in severe chronic heart failure. Lancet 1995;346:732–6.
6. Rademaker MT, Charles CJ, Lewis LK, et al. Beneficial hemodynamic and renal effects of adrenomedullin in an ovine model of heart failure. Circulation 1997;96:1983–90.
7. Rademaker MT, Charles CJ, Espiner EA, et al. Endogenous urocortins reduce vascular tone and renin-aldosterone/endothelin activity in experimental heart failure. Eur Heart J 2005;26:2046–54.
8. Vasan RS, Sullivan LM, Roubenoff R, et al. Inflammatory markers and risk of heart failure in elderly subjects without prior myocardial infarction: the Framingham Heart Study. Circulation 2003;107: 1486–91.
9. Levine B, Kalman J, Mayer L, et al. Elevated circulating levels of tumor necrosis factor in severe chronic heart failure. N Engl J Med 1990;223: 236–41.
10. Rauchhaus M, Doehner W, Francis DP, et al. Plasma cytokine parameters and mortality in patients with chronic heart failure. Circulation 2000;102:3060–7.
11. Anker SD, von Haehling S. Inflammatory mediators in chronic heart failure: an overview. Heart 2004; 90:464–70.
12. Spinale FG, Coker ML, Krombach SR, et al. Matrix metalloproteinase inhibition during the development of congestive heart failure: effects on left ventricular dimensions and function. Circ Res 1999;85:364–76.
13. Horwich TB, Patel J, MacLellan WR, et al. Cardiac troponin I is associated with impaired hemodynamics, progressive left ventricular dysfunction, and increased mortality rates in advanced heart failure. Circulation 2003;108:833–8.
14. Weinberg EO, Shimpo M, Hurwitz S, et al. Identification of serum soluble ST2 receptor as a novel heart failure biomarker. Circulation 2003;107: 721–6.
15. Januzzi JL Jr, Peacock WF, Maisel AS, et al. Measurement of the interleukin family member ST2 in patients with acute dyspnea: results from the PRIDE (Pro-Brain Natriuretic Peptide Investigation of Dyspnea in the Emergency Department) study. J Am Coll Cardiol 2007;50:607–13.
16. Molyneux SL, Florkowski CM, George PM, et al. Coenzyme Q10: an independent predictor of mortality in chronic heart failure. J Am Coll Cardiol 2008;52:1435–41.
17. Kempf T, von Haehling S, Peter T, et al. Prognostic utility of growth differentiation factor-15 in patients with chronic heart failure. J Am Coll Cardiol 2007; 50:1054–60.
18. van Kimmenade RR, Januzzi JJL, Ellinor PT, et al. Utility of amino-terminal pro-brain natriuretic peptide, galectin-3, and apelin for the evaluation of patients with acute heart failure. J Am Coll Cardiol 2006;48:1217–24.
19. Omland T, Drazner MH, Ueland T, et al. Plasma osteoprotegerin levels in the general population: relation to indices of left ventricular structure and function. Hypertension 2007;49:1392–8.
20. Richards AM, Charles C. Urotensin II in the cardiovascular system. Peptides 2004;25:1795–802.
21. Troughton RW, Richards AM. Outpatient monitoring and treatment of chronic heart failure guided by NT-proBNP measurement. Am J Cardiol 2008; 101(Suppl):72A–5A.
22. Francis GS, Cohn JN, Johnson G, et al. Plasma norepinephrine, plasma renin activity, and congestive heart failure: relations to survival and the effects of therapy in V-HeFT II. Circulation 1993;87:VI40–8.
23. Zannad F, Alla F, Dousset B, et al. Limitation of excessive extracellular matrix turnover may contribute to survival benefit of spironolactone therapy in patients with congestive heart failure: insights from the Randomized Aldactone Evaluation Study (RALES). Circulation 2000;102:2700–6.
24. Richards AM, Doughty R, Nicholls MG, et al. Neurohumoral prediction of benefit from carvedilol in ischemic left ventricular dysfunction. Circulation 1999;99:786–92.
25. The CONSENSUS Trial Study Group Effects of enalapril on mortality in severe congestive heart failure: results of the Cooperative North Scandinavian Enalapril Survival Study (CONSENSUS). N Engl J Med 1987;316:1429–35.
26. Goldstein S, Fagerberg B, Hjalmarson Å, et al. Metoprolol controlled release/extended release in patients with severe heart failure: analysis of the experience in the MERIT-HF study. J Am Coll Cardiol 2001;38:932–8.
27. Publication Committee for the VI. Intravenous nesiritide vs nitroglycerin for treatment of decompensated congestive heart failure: a randomized controlled trial. JAMA 2002;287:1531–40.
28. Swedberg K, Bristow MR, Cohn JN, et al. Effects of sustained-release moxonidine, an imidazoline

agonist, on plasma norepinephrine in patients with chronic heart failure. Circulation 2002;105: 1797–803.

29. Mann DL, McMurray JJV, Packer M, et al. Targeted anticytokine therapy in patients with chronic heart failure: results of the Randomized Etanercept Worldwide Evaluation (RENEWAL). Circulation 2004;109: 1594–602.

30. Kelland NF, Webb DJ. Clinical trials of endothelin antagonists in heart failure: publication is good for the public health. Heart 2007;93:2–4.

31. Konstam MA, Gheorghiade M, Burnett JC Jr, et al. Effects of oral tolvaptan in patients hospitalized for worsening heart failure: the EVEREST outcome trial. JAMA 2007;297:1319–31.

32. Arab S, Gramolini AO, Ping P, et al. Cardiovascular proteomics: tools to develop novel biomarkers and potential applications. J Am Coll Cardiol 2006;48:1733–41.

33. Lewis GD, Ru W, Liu E, et al. Metabolite profiling of blood from individuals undergoing planned myocardial infarction reveals early markers of myocardial injury. J Clin Invest 2008;118:3503–12.

Natriuretic Peptides: Physiologic and Analytic Considerations

Torbjørn Omland, MD, PhD, MPH*, Tor-Arne Hagve, MD, PhD

KEYWORDS

- Natriuretic peptides • Heart • Physiology • Synthesis
- Receptors • Analysis

The concept of the heart as an organ with endocrine function is not new. After discovering that norepinephrine is synthesized in the heart in 1963,[1] Braunwald and colleagues[2] published a paper the following year in the *American Journal of Medicine* entitled: "The heart as an endocrine organ." Although not scientifically documented before this seminal finding, the theory that the heart might possess endocrine functions emerged even earlier. In the 1950s, early electron microscopy investigations demonstrated the presence of electron dense "specific atrial granules" in the atria of the heart, which resemble secretory granules previously identified in endocrine cells.[3] Concomitantly, experiments showed that balloon stretching of the canine left atrium resulted in increased urinary flow.[4] However, the physiologic and pathophysiologic significance of the atrial granules remained obscure until de Bold, more than two decades later, demonstrated that atrial granularity was associated with changes in water and electrolyte balance,[5] and that homogenized atrial tissue injected into rats caused hypotension, diuresis and natriuresis.[6] In contrast, extract of ventricular tissue was ineffective in producing such effects. Based on these observations, de Bold proposed that the natriuretic response was elicited by an "atrial natriuretic factor." In a remarkable series of subsequent scientific achievements, atrial or A-type natriuretic peptide (ANP) was rapidly purified, sequenced and synthesized.[7]

In 1988, researchers from Hisayuki Matsuo's group in Japan identified a peptide sharing structural features and biologic activity with ANP in porcine brain and named it brain natriuretic peptide (BNP).[8] Subsequent experiments soon made it clear that the heart is the main source of BNP in the circulation;[9] B-type natriuretic peptide is currently the most commonly used name of this peptide. Soon after the discovery of BNP, Matsuo's research group identified a third member of the natriuretic peptide family from porcine brain, C-type natriuretic peptide (CNP).[10]

In the late 1980s, it also became clear that the N-terminal fragment of the ANP prohormone, proANP, was circulating in human plasma,[11] and in the mid 1990s, the N-terminal fragment of the BNP prohormone was also detected in the human circulation.[12] This article provides an overview of the physiology of the natriuretic peptides, with an emphasis on BNP and NT-proBNP, and highlights some analytic considerations of significance to the clinician.

PHYSOLOLOGIC CONSIDERATIONS
Natriuretic Peptides

The natriuretic peptide family encompasses several genetically distinct peptide hormones that share structural features (**Fig. 1**), possess important physiologic properties, including natriuresis, diuresis, vasorelaxation, sympatho-inhibition,[13] growth inhibition,[14] and anti-fibrogenic mechanisms,[15] and are central players in cardiovascular, endocrine and renal homeostasis (**Fig. 2**).[16] ANP and BNP in the circulation are

Akershus University Hospital, Lørenskog, Norway
* Corresponding author. Department of Cardiology, Division of Medicine, Akershus University Hospital, NO-1478 Lørenskog, Lørenskog, Norway.
E-mail address: torbjorn.omland@medisin.uio.no (T. Omland).

Heart Failure Clin 5 (2009) 471–487
doi:10.1016/j.hfc.2009.04.005
1551-7136/09/$ – see front matter © 2009 Published by Elsevier Inc.

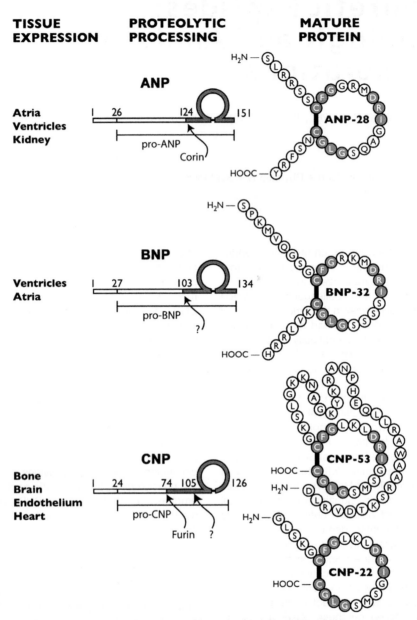

TISSUE EXPRESSION   **PROTEOLYTIC PROCESSING**   **MATURE PROTEIN**

Fig. 1. Natriuretic peptide expression, processing, and structure: ANP, BNP and CNP are expressed as pre-pro-hormones. The signal sequences are removed to form pro-ANP, pro-BNP and pro-CNP. The peptides are further proteolytically processed to form mature peptide hormones. proANP is cleaved by corin. The enzymes responsible for proBNP cleavage are thought to be furin and corin, but this contention has not been definitively verified. proCNP is cleaved by furin in vitro into a 53 amino acid peptide, which is further processed to a 22 amino acid form by an unknown protease. All peptides contain a conserved 17 amino acid disulfide linked ring structure that is required for biologic activity. Invariant residues within the ring structure are shaded. (*From* Potter LR, Abbey-Hosch S, Dickey DM. Natriuretic peptides, their receptors, and cyclic guanosine monophosphate-dependent signaling functions. Endocr Rev 2006 February;27(1):47–2; with permission.)

derived primarily from the myocardium.[9] In contrast, CNP is primarily produced by vascular endothelium cells and in the central nervous system.[17] D-type natriuretic peptide, found in the venom of the green mamba (Dendroaspis angusti-ceps);[18] urodilatin, derived from alternative processing of proANP in the kidney;[19] and the intestinal epithelium-derived peptides guanylin and uroguanylin[20] also share primary structure features with ANP, BNP and CNP. Different natriuretic peptides may—to a variable degree—exert their actions in an autocrine, paracrine, or

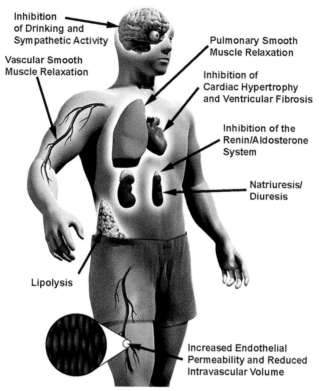

Inhibition
of Drinking and
Sympathetic Activity

Vascular Smooth
Muscle Relaxation

Pulmonary Smooth
Muscle Relaxation

Inhibition of
Cardiac Hypertrophy
and Ventricular Fibrosis

Inhibition of the
Renin/Aldosterone
System

Natriuresis/
Diuresis

Lipolysis

Increased Endothelial
Permeability and Reduced
Intravascular Volume

Fig. 2. Physiologic consequences of NPR-A activation. (*From* Potter LR, Abbey-Hosch S, Dickey DM. Natriuretic peptides, their receptors, and cyclic guanosine monophosphate-dependent signaling functions. Endocr Rev 2006 February;27(1):47–2; with permission.)

endocrine fashion. Biochemical characteristics of ANP, BNP and CNP are summarized in **Table 1**.

Synthesis and Release of B-type Natriuretic Peptide

Human BNP is encoded by a single copy gene located on chromosome 1 and is organized in tandem with the ANP gene. The human BNP gene consists of three exons and two introns;[21] exon 1 encodes the 5' untranslated region and part of pre-proBNP, exon 2 encodes amino acids 45-129, and exon 3 encodes five terminal amino acids plus the 3' untranslated region.[22] Upstream regulatory regions include serum response elements, M-CAT, GATA sites, and an AP1 binding site.[23]

The initial gene product resulting from translation of the BNP gene is a 134 amino acid pre-prohormone, pre-proBNP (see **Fig. 1**). Following the removal of the 26 amino acid signal sequence, a 108 amino acid prohormone, proBNP, is formed. Circulating BNP is a cyclic polypeptide consisting of 32 amino acids; the proteolytic enzymes, furin and corin, are thought to be responsible for specific cleavage of proBNP into the N-terminal

and C-terminal fragments during or shortly after secretion.[24,25] BNP is found predominantly in the 32 amino acid form in the human myocardium, but the intact 108 amino acid precursor peptide, proBNP,[9] as well as other peptide fragments, are also detectable.[26]

Recent studies using Western blot analysis techniques suggest that the existing paradigm of BNP secretion and resulting nomenclature for circulating fragments of the BNP precursor represent an oversimplification. According to these studies, both low-molecular weight (ie, BNP 1-32) and high molecular weight forms, including intact proBNP 1-108, circulate in plasma from heart failure patients.[27] Moreover, recent data suggest that further truncation of BNP 1-32 occurs in the circulation, yielding fragments, including BNP 3-32 or BNP 7-32, that may circulate in higher concentrations than the biologically active BNP 1-32.[28] In advanced heart failure, concentrations of BNP 1-32 may be very low or absent.[29] Likewise, for NT-proBNP, truncation of both the N-terminus and the C-terminus may occur.[30] Finally, both oligomerization[31] and glycosylation[32] of NT-proBNP have been reported. Consequently, what is measured as BNP or NT-proBNP, in fact, may

Table 1
Natriuretic peptides

	ANP	BNP	CNP
Precursor with signal peptide	preproANP (1-151)	preproBNP (1-134)	preproCNP (1-126)
Prohormone	proANP (1-126)	proBNP (1-108)	proCNP (1-103)
Circulating fragments	NT-proANP (proANP 1-98)	NT-proBNP (proBNP 1-76)	NT-proCNP
	ProANP 1-30, proANP 31-67	ProBNP 1-108	CNP 1-22
	ANP (proANP 99-126)	BNP (proBNP 77-108)	CNP 1-53
	—	BNP 3-32, BNP 7-32	—
Clearance	NPR-C, NEP	NPR-C, NEP	NPR-C, NEP
Circulating half-life	3 min	21 min	3 min

Abbreviations: NEP, neutral endopeptidase; NPR-C, natriuretic peptide receptor-C.

be intact proBNP 1-108 or alternative peptide fragments. Characteristics of BNP and NT-proBNP are summarized in **Table 2**.

In humans, BNP is synthesized both in the atrial and in the ventricular myocardium;[33] and secretion is believed to be regulated at the level of gene expression. In contrast to the regulation of granular excretion of ANP, proBNP is only partially stored in granules. BNP is often claimed to be exclusively derived from cardiac ventricles, but, per weight unit, the concentration of BNP is higher in atrial than in ventricular tissue. Given the greater mass of the ventricles than of the atria, the total amount of BNP mRNA may be three times higher in the ventricle than in the atrium, ie, approximately two thirds of circulating BNP may be derived from the ventricles.[34] Catheterization studies in patients with left ventricular hypertrophy have demonstrated that circulating BNP levels reflect atrial pressures and volumes, and that atrial-derived BNP contributes significantly to circulating levels.[35] Conversely, in patients with heart failure and left ventricular systolic dysfunction of moderate to severe degree, ventricular-derived BNP probably predominates in the circulation. Given that the source of BNP in the circulation may depend on various factors, including the severity and etiology of heart disease, BNP should be regarded as a combined atrial and ventricular peptide.

Increased ventricular and atrial diastolic wall stretch augments synthesis and release of BNP from cardiomyocytes, and is commonly considered the principal stimulus controlling BNP production.[34] It remains unclear how cardiomyocytes sense increased strain, but extracellular matrix integrin cell surface attachments may be involved.[36] Cardiomyocyte and cardiac fibroblast production of BNP can further be stimulated by various endocrine, paracrine, and

autocrine substances commonly activated in heart failure.[37] These substances include pro-inflammatory cytokines, including tumor necrosis factor-alpha and vasocontrictor neurohormones, including catecholamines,[38] angiotensin II,[39] and endothelin I.[40] Ischemia may also represent a stimulus for natriuretic peptide production in the heart. Recently, in isolated perfused beating rat atria, adenosine in a dose-dependent fashion induced cAMP dependent ANP release.[41] Adenosine is known to exert cardioprotective actions, including coronary vasodilation and suppression of myocardial contractility, and these effects may potentially be mediated via activation of the natriuretic peptide system. Another endogenous substance that is released from cell membranes during myocardial ischemia is lysophosphatidyl choline. Experimental data suggest that lysophosphatidyl choline modulates the secretion of ANP in response to atrial stretch. However, the suppression of ANP release by lysophosphatidyl choline was attenuated in hypertrophied atria.[42] Conditions associated with increased circulating BNP and NT-proBNP are listed in **Table 3**.

Although the ANP and BNP genes are localized in tandem on the same chromosome, some features of the regulation and induction of BNP and ANP synthesis differ. Experimentally, cardiac overload-induced translation of the ANP gene occurs slowly (ie, days), permitting granular release of ANP, whereas both atrial and ventricular BNP mRNA levels increase rapidly (<1 hr) following acute pressure overload[43] and after experimental myocardial infarction.[44] Accordingly, the kinetics of ANP and BNP release differ in that storage of ANP in secretory granules provides a source for rapid release of this peptide, whereas a higher rate of BNP release generally requires augmented production of BNP mRNA. Augmented BNP

Table 2
Characteristics of BNP and NT-proBNP

Characteristic	BNP	NT-proBNP
Prohormone fragment	C-terminal (proBNP 77-108)	N-terminal (proBNP 1-76) proBNP 1-108
Molecular weight	3.5 kd	8.5 kd
Physiologic activity	Active	Inactive
Clearance mechanisms	Clearance receptors Neutral endopeptidase	Unclear, probably passively removed by multiple organs, including the kidneys
Circulating half-life	21 min	60–120 min
In vitro stability	24 hrs at room temperature	> 3 days at room temperature

Data from Omland T. Advances in congestive heart failure management in the intensive care unit: B-type natriuretic peptides in evaluation of acute heart failure. Crit Care Med 2008;36(Suppl 1):S17–27.

release may require stronger and more prolonged stimulation than that necessary for granular release of ANP. Posture change and intravenous saline loading may thus provoke rapid release of ANP into the bloodstream, leading to higher circulating levels. In contrast, circulating BNP levels remain unaltered after posture change or saline loading.[45] Alternative mechanisms for more rapid release of BNP may, however, exist, as exemplified by a rapid rise in BNP during myocardial ischemia.

Natriuretic Peptide Receptors

Natriuretic peptides exert their physiologic actions via binding to natriuretic peptide receptors (NPRs) located on the cell surface. Three different NPRs have been identified: NPR-A, NPR-B and NPR-C. ANP and BNP associate with NPR-A with high affinity,[46] whereas CNP appear ineffective in exerting biologic effects via NPR-A. Conversely, CNP binds with high affinity to NPR-B.[47] To stimulate guanylyl cyclase activity in cells expressing NPR-B, high pharmacologic concentrations of ANP and BNP must be applied.

NPR-A and NPR-B are expressed widely in the cardiovascular system,[48] lungs, kidneys, skin, platelets, and pre-synaptic sympathetic nerve fibers.[49] NPR-A is the predominant NPR in large blood vessels, whereas NPR-B is found most abundantly in the brain.

The NPRs share structural features and contain an extracellular ligand binding domain, a single transmembrane domain, and NPR-A and NPR-B also contain an intracellular domain, the latter consisting of a kinase homology domain, a hinge region, and a guanylyl cyclase domain.[50] In the absence of a ligand, NPR-A and NPR-B both exist in the form of homodimers or homotetramers.

Conformational change of the receptor is induced by ligand binding. Consecutive signaling via the transmembrane domain is associated with binding of ATP within the phosphorylated kinase homology domain with subsequent phosphorylation as a result. These events are required for receptor activation and cGMP production.[23] A cGMP-dependent protein kinase (PKG) is the principal intracellular mediator of cGMP signals.[51] Elevated cGMP levels intracellularly may activate phosphodiesterase-II, and thereby modulate cyclic nucleotide concentrations.

Recent work has advanced the understanding of how NPR-A and NPR-B activity is modulated. For instance, natriuretic peptides may be able to suppress NPR-A activity via cGMP effects on a specific promoter region on the gene encoding NPR-A.[52] Changes in osmolality may also modulate expression and promoter activity of NPR-A.[23] The cyclosporin receptor cyclophylin A may associate with NPR-A and suppress NPR-A activity.[53] Recently, using radiolabeled analogs, NPR-A binding sites have been visualized in both adult human heart and coronary arteries.[54] Dual immunohistochemistry demonstrated NPR-A on cardiomyocytes, endocardial endothelial cells, and smooth muscle of intramyocardial vessels. The NPR-A density in the myocardium and coronary artery is down-regulated in patients who have severe ischemic heart disease, suggesting a lack of antifibrotic signaling in these patients.

The natriuretic peptide clearance receptor, NPR-C, is structurally distinct from NPR-A and NPR-B; its main function is to clear natriuretic peptides from the circulation.[55] In contrast to NPR-A and NPR-B, NPR-C lacks a large cytoplasmic domain and has no guanylyl cyclase activity. Two different subtypes of NPR-C have

Table 3
Conditions associated with increased circulating BNP and NT-proBNP

Stretch of the atrial and ventricular myocardium (eg, acute and chronic congestive heart failure, acute and chronic cor pulmonale)

Ventricular hypertrophy (eg, hypertensive heart disease)

Volume expansion and consequent elevated pressure/distension (eg, renal or hepatic failure)

Decreased renal clearance (eg, acute and chronic renal failure, advanced age)

Neurohormonal and cytokine stimulation (eg, sepsis, shock)

Myocardial ischemia (eg, unstable angina, acute myocardial infarction)

Hypoxia (eg acute pulmonary embolism, cyanotic congenital heart disease)

Tachycardia (eg, atrial fibrillation, ventricular tachycardia)

Female gender

Data from Omland T. Advances in congestive heart failure management in the intensive care unit: B-type natriuretic peptides in evaluation of acute heart failure. Crit Care Med 2008;36(Suppl 1):S17–27.

been identified. A 77kD subtype appears to be involved in peptide internalization whereas as 67 kD peptide may be involved in natriuretic peptide inhibition of cAMP production.[56] NPR-C is widely distributed, and is found located in vascular endothelium, smooth muscle, cardiac muscle, adrenal glands, kidneys, brain, and adipose tissue.[57] The binding of all natriuretic peptides to NPR-C occurs with high affinity, although the affinity for ANP and CNP is apparently higher than for BNP,[58] which may potentially account for a longer plasma half-life for BNP than for ANP.

Association between natriuretic peptides and the NPRs seems to require an intact ring structure of the natriuretic peptides. Accordingly, disruption of the disulfide bridge responsible for the ring structure results in loss of biologic activity. This phenomenon explains why the N-terminal fragments of the natriuretic peptide prohormones, devoid of any disulfide bridges, are incapable of associating with NPRs.

Natriuretic Peptides Degradation

Circulating levels of N-terminal proBNP exceed those of BNP; because these peptides probably are secreted in a 1:1 ratio, it follows that BNP is cleared more rapidly than NT-proBNP. The plasma half-life of BNP is 21 minutes.[9] Studies in sheep suggest that the half-life of N-terminal proBNP is considerably higher, perhaps as long as 70 minutes.[59]

The main pathways involved in the degradation and clearance of natriuretic peptides from the circulation are NPR-C–mediated endocytosis and subsequent lysosomal degradation and enzymatic degradation by neutral endopeptidase (NEP), a zinc metallopeptidase widely distributed on the surface of endothelial cells, vascular smooth muscle cells, cardiac myocytes, and fibroblasts.[60]

The actions of NEP involve proteolytic cleavage and disulfide bond disruption. In addition, renal impairment is also associated with increased circulating levels of natriuretic peptides and the N-terminal fragments of their prohormones. The inverse association between renal function and natriuretic peptide levels may be caused by one or more of the following factors: decreased renal clearance, increased myocardial stretch secondary to volume overload, and renal impairment associated cardiac dysfunction. Recent data from a large-scale epidemiologic study suggest that neither BNP nor NT-proBNP are associated with renal function in the normal range estimated glomerular filtration rate.[61] Below an estimated glomerular filtration rate threshold of 90 mL/min/1.73 m^2, however, both NT-proBNP and BNP increase in an exponential fashion with decreasing renal function, although the increase is substantially greater for NT-proBNP than for BNP. These associations remain significant after adjustment for potential confounders.[61]

The relative impact of renal function on the clearance of BNP versus NT-proBNP remains controversial. Although it is a common view that NT-proBNP is cleared exclusively by the kidneys, recent mechanistic data suggest that the renal extraction ratios of both BNP and NT-proBNP are approximately similar and in the range between 15% and 20%.[62] Moreover, although natriuretic peptides and N-terminal prohormone fragments can be identified and measured in urine, levels are very low,[63] which suggests that renal filtration is not a major pathway for natriuretic peptide degradation.

An inverse association between BNP levels and body mass index both in healthy subjects and in patients who have acute dyspnea and heart failure has led to speculations that adipose tissue may contribute to degradation of BNP via an NPR-C–

mediated mechanism.[64] However, recent data demonstrate that the association between NT-proBNP and body mass index is as strong as the one between BNP and body mass index.[65] Moreover, both peptides are more strongly associated with lean mass than with fat mass. As NPR-C is not involved in degradation of NT-proBNP, alternative mechanisms that may involve sex steroids, are probably responsible for the association between body mass index and circulating natriuretic peptide concentrations.[65]

Biologic Effects

Cardiovascular system

Effects on vascular tone and permeability ANP and BNP cause arterial and venous vasodilation, lower peripheral vascular resistance, and reduce arterial blood pressure via relaxation of vascular smooth muscle cells in both animal models and in humans (**Fig. 3**).[66] CNP may possess stronger venodilator actions than ANP or BNP.[16] A single intravenous injection of naked human ANP DNA construct is associated with sustained blood pressure lowering in the young, but not adult, hypertensive rat.[67] A long-term beneficial effect of ANP gene therapy, including a sustained decrease in systolic blood pressure, an increase in urinary cGMP production, and decreased heart weight, has been demonstrated,[68] and raises the question of whether ANP gene delivery may represent a future strategy for treatment of arterial hypertension. In addition to potent vasorelaxant actions, ANP and BNP have important effects on capillary permeability. A shift of fluid from the intravascular to the extravascular

compartment, which is secondary to natriuretic peptide-induced increased permeability of the vascular endothelium, may contribute to cardiac preload reduction.[69]

Other studies have also demonstrated lower levels of natriuretic peptides in patients who have the metabolic syndrome,[70] independent of waist circumference,[71] indicating that a relative deficiency of natriuretic peptides may represent a potential link between the metabolic syndrome and hypertension.

Effects on myocardial contractility and relaxation In addition to vascular effects, natriuretic peptides may modulate cardiovascular function via direct effects on the myocardium. ANP, BNP and CNP have been reported to modulate cardiac contractility in experimental studies, but the results are not consistent between studies. In healthy humans, BNP exerts lusitropic effects.[72]

Effects of cell growth and proliferation Natriuretic peptides modulate vascular smooth muscle cell and cardiomyocyte growth, proliferation, and apoptosis.[73] Moreover, natriuretic peptides affect noncardiomyocyte cells in the heart by suppressing cardiac fibroblast proliferation and extracellular matrix secretion.[37] Interestingly, genetic engineering studies of animals with selective deletion of the genes encoding pre-proANP or preproBNP demonstrate that ANP gene knock-out mice develop salt-sensitive hypertension with ventricular hypertrophy,[74] BNP knock-out mice develop cardiac fibrosis but not hypertension or hypertrophy,[75] whereas deletion of the gene-encoding NPR-A results in

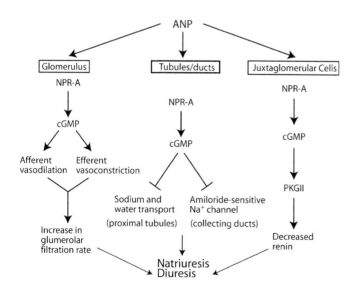

Fig. 3. Natriuretic peptide-dependent smooth muscle relaxation: Stimulation of NPR-A and NPR-B by their respective ligands results in increased intracellular cGMP concentrations. cGMP activates protein kinase GI (PKGI), which phosphorylates target proteins, inhibits the IP_3 receptor, the plasma membrane calcium/ATPase, the sarcoplasmic reticulum calcium/ATPase (SERCA), and the potassium/calcium channel (BK_{Ca}) to decrease intracellular calcium concentrations. PKGI phosphorylation and activation of myosin light chain phosphate (MLCP) increases the calcium levels required for contraction. (*From* Potter LR, Abbey-Hosch S, Dickey DM. Natriuretic peptides, their receptors, and cyclic guanosine monophosphate-dependent signaling functions. Endocr Rev 2006 February; 27(1):47–2; with permission.)

development of salt-resistant hypertension, ventricular hypertrophy and fibrosis.[76] Accordingly, ANP and BNP may play complementary roles in cardiac physiology and pathophysiology. In a coronary ligation model of experimental myocardial infarction in mice, NPR-A gene deletion resulted in increased incidence of heart failure and mortality, as well as a concomitant increase in myocardial expression of ANP, BNP, transforming growth factor beta, and type I collagen.[77] Moreover, a double knockout model with combined deletion of the NPR-A and the angiotensin type I receptor was associated with myocardial hypertrophy and decreased survival even though fibrosis was not present. These findings suggest that the antifibrotic actions of natriuretic peptides are at least partially mediated via inhibition of angiotensin II and they raise the possibility that activation of the natriuretic peptide system after acute ischemic injury is cardioprotective.

By modulating cardiomyocyte growth, fibroblast activation, and the deposition of extracellular matrix, transforming growth factor-beta is a key player in hypertrophic and fibrotic remodeling of the heart in response to cardiac overload. Hypertrophic stimuli result in increased ventricular expression of transforming growth factor-beta and disruption of transforming growth factor-beta signaling reduces pressure overload-induced myofibroblast formation and interstitial fibrosis in the mouse heart.[78] Recent data suggest that ANP binding to NPR-A and subsequent increase in intracellular cGMP and activation of protein kinase G, lead to inhibition of transforming growth factor-beta–induced Smad nuclear translocation, thereby inhibiting cardiac myofibroblast transformation and collagen synthesis.[15]

Genetic studies in humans also support the concept that natriuretic peptides and their receptors are of importance for myocardial hypertrophy. A functional deletion mutation of the 5'-flanking region of the NPR-A gene has been associated with essential hypertension and increased left ventricular mass.[79] Moreover, a promoter ANP gene variant associated with reduced circulating levels of NT-proANP is independently related to increased cardiac mass.[80] In the same study, an allelic variant of the NPR-A gene, potentially associated with decreased receptor activity, was also associated with increased left ventricular mass.

CNP may also inhibit cardiomyocyte growth and potentially modulate ventricular remodeling during the development of heart failure.[81] Partial deficiency of NPR-B in transgenic rats is associated with progressive myocardial hypertrophy and elevated heart rate.[82] Repetitive administration of CNP following experimental myocardial infarction in the rat is associated with reduced dilation and fibrosis of the left ventricle,[83] suggesting that natriuretic peptides may have beneficial effects in the setting of acute ischemic injury. CNP may also exert growth-inhibitory effects on vascular smooth muscle cells[84] and reduce the degree of intimal thickening induced by balloon inflation in the rat carotid artery.[85] Because CNP immunoreactivity is present in atherosclerotic lesions,[86] this peptide has been postulated to play a role in the development of atherosclerosis.

Kidney

As indicated by their names, natriuretic peptides exert natriuretic and diuretic effects in the kidneys (**Fig. 4**). These actions are mediated via combined effects on renal hemodynamics and tubular reabsorption. There also seem to be significant

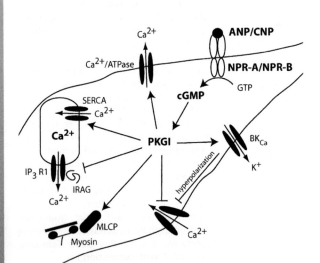

Fig. 4. Natriuretic peptide regulation in the kidney. Renal function is modulated by natriuretic peptides in at least three ways: (1) natriuretic peptides increase the glomerular filtration rate by differentially regulating the tone of the afferent and efferent glomerular arterioles; (2) natriuretic peptides decrease sodium reabsorption in the proximal tubules and collecting ducts; and (3) natriuretic peptides decrease renin secretion from the juxtaglomerular cells. (*From* Potter LR, Abbey-Hosch S, Dickey DM. Natriuretic peptides, their receptors, and cyclic guanosine monophosphate-dependent signaling functions. Endocr Rev 2006 February;27(1):47–2; with permission.)

differences between ANP and BNP: whereas ANP increases glomerular filtration via pressure elevation within the glomerular capillaries,[87] BNP may not augment glomerular filtration.[88] An augmented filtration fraction may be the result of natriuretic peptide-induced mesangial cell relaxation that causes an increase of the effective glomerular filtration area.[89] Moreover, renal effects of natriuretic peptides include direct actions on tubular cells, ie, antagonism of angiotensin II-induced sodium and water reabsorption in the proximal convoluted tubules,[90] inhibition of vasopressin-induced water reabsorption in the cortical collecting ducts,[91] and of sodium reabsorption in the medullary collecting ducts.[92] Contrary to ANP and BNP, CNP does not appear to possess natriuretic effects,[93] whereas urodilatin, a peptide formed by alternative processing of proANP in the distal tubules, may have potent paracrine/autocrine renal effects.

Neuroendocrine and immune system
In addition to direct effects on target organs, including the heart, kidneys and blood vessels, natriuretic peptides synergistically modulate other neuroendocrine systems and the activity of the immune system. One example is inhibition of the renin-angiotensin-aldosterone system by natriuretic peptides on several levels, ie, direct inhibition of renal renin release, and direct and indirect inhibition of aldosterone production (**Fig. 5**). Additional neuroendocrine effects include inhibition of central sympathetic outflow and catecholamine release from peripheral sympathetic neurons,[94] as well as inhibition of endothelin-1 synthesis.[95] Other central nervous system effects of the natriuretic peptides include inhibition of thirst and salt appetite via a NPR-A mediated mechanism[16] and NPR-B mediated inhibition of vasopressin secretion from the posterior lobe of the pituitary.

Natriuretic peptides also possess potent anti-inflammatory actions. Macrophage production of tumor necrosis factor-alpha, as well as adipose tissue production of a wide range of cytokines, chemokines, and adipokines involved in leukocyte recruitment, are suppressed by natriuretic peptides.[96]

ANALYTIC CONSIDERATIONS

The aim of this section is to provide the clinician with an overview of the most important pre-analytical, analytical, and postanalytical factors of significance for the correct interpretation of BNP and NT-proBNP test results.

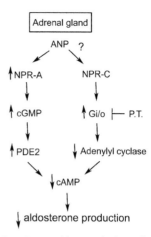

Fig. 5. Natriuretic peptide regulation of the adrenal gland: Natriuretic peptide-dependent decrease in aldosterone production is mediated via reduced cAMP concentrations. Potential mechanisms include: (1) Natriuretic peptide-dependent activation of NPR-A, with subsequent production of cGMP and stimulation of cAMP-hydrolyzing phospodieasterase (PDE) 2; and (2) NPR-C dependent inhibition of adelylyl cyclase via a pertussis toxin (PT) sensitive G-protein dependent pathway. (*From* Potter LR, Abbey-Hosch S, Dickey DM. Natriuretic peptides, their receptors, and cyclic guanosine monophosphate-dependent signaling functions. Endocr Rev 2006 February;27(1):47–2; with permission.)

Analytic Specifications

Assay description
Most available commercial assays for BNP and NT-proBNP are two-site immunometric (sandwich) methods. Sandwich assays are more specific and have lower detection limits than radioimmunoassays and competitive immunoassays. A sandwich assay includes two antibodies, one that is bound to a solid phase and one that is labelled with an enzyme catalyzing the reaction on which the detection is based. The immunometric assays for BNP use two monoclonal antibodies or a combination of monoclonal and omniclonal antibodies directed at the ring structure and the amino-terminus or carboxy-terminus of the peptide, whereas the assay for NT-proBNP is based on polyclonal antibodies directed against epitopes 1-21 and 39-50 of proBNP.[97] The most widely used principle of detection in the fully automated analytical systems is based on chemiluminescence (Roche, Abbott, Siemens, Biosite/Beckman-Coulter).

Cross-reactivity
The issue of cross-reactivity with other peptides is obviously important for the specificity of assays for natriuretic peptide determination. Assays for BNP

do not cross-react with ANP or the N-terminal fragments of proANP and proBNP. Conversely, assays for NT-proBNP do not cross-react with ANP, BNP, or NT-proANP. However, what is measured as NT-proBNP by commercial assays also includes variable amounts of proBNP 1-108, as well as fragments of NT-proBNP 1-76, such as NT-proBNP 1-22 and NT-proBNP 10-29.[30] Assays for BNP 1-32 probably also detect intact proBNP 1-108,[98] as well as various degradation products of BNP 1-32, such as BNP 3-32.

Turnaround time

The fully automated assays for BNP and NT-proBNP can provide test results in only 18–20 minutes; however, because of various logistic factors in the hospital, the time from blood sampling to the result is available to clinicians may be considerably longer in clinical practice. The point-of-care whole blood assays for BNP and NT-proBNP also require 15–20 minutes to measure the analyte, but, in general, the analytic performance of the point-of-care systems is somewhat inferior to the large central laboratory-based platforms.

Calibration and standardization

Synthetic BNP is used as a calibrator for BNP assays. Comparable to the situation for cardiac troponin I assays, there is currently no standardization of the BNP assays from the various manufacturers.[99] Reference intervals and decision limits must therefore be determined for each individual assay. It has been suggested that the BNP assays should be harmonized around the cut-off limit for heart failure (100 pg/mL).[99]

Synthetic NT-proBNP 1-76 is used to calibrate the NT-proBNP assay. There is no official standardization of the NT-proBNP assay, but because all major assays are using the same antibodies and calibrators (from Roche), the variation between assays is presumably small and the agreement between the reference intervals of these assays is acceptable.[99]

Specification of individual assays

The point-of-care instrument (Triage BNP) from Biosite was the first BNP assay to be approved by the Food and Drug Administration. Fully automated analyzers for BNP determination on large central laboratory-based platforms are available from several manufacturers. In general, the BNP assays have a measuring range of approximately 1–5000 pg/mL. Samples with levels of BNP greater than 5000 pg/mL must be diluted and retested to obtain accurate results.

As mentioned above, all available major commercial assays for NT-proBNP employ the same antibodies and calibrators supplied by Roche. Consequently, the harmonization of the NT-proBNP assays is less problematic than for BNP.[99] Technical specifications of selected individual assays for BNP and NT-proBNP, which are derived from the official documentation of assays given by the manufacturers, are summarized in **Table 4**.

Pre-analytic Factors

The pre-analytic phase is of importance for natriuretic peptide, and in particular ANP and BNP, test results. Incorrect pre-analytic handling of samples, including the use of an incorrect specimen type and prolonged storage at room temperature, may cause significant degradation of BNP, with a misleading test result as a consequence. In contrast to ANP, BNP and NT-proBNP are less prone to rapid fluctuations in circulating levels because of their longer half-lives and subsequent lower signal-noise ratios. Accordingly, factors like postural change and exercise only affect BNP levels to a minor degree, and because of the even longer in vivo half-life of NT-proBNP, this peptide may probably be drawn without consideration of these factors.

Administration of cardioactive drugs may affect circulating levels of both BNP and NT-proBNP significantly. For instance, drugs used for the treatment of heart failure, including diuretics and vasodilators, will cause a reduction in circulating BNP and NT-proBNP levels.[100] Following the initiation of such therapy, the drop in BNP may occur more rapidly than the drop in NT-proBNP because of the shorter half-life of BNP. Recombinant BNP (nesiritide) administered to patients who have acute heart failure will be recognized as BNP by immunoassays and give a misleading test result. Accordingly, BNP measurement for diagnosis or monitoring of acute heart failure is not recommended during or within the first 2 hours following nesiritide infusion. In contrast, nesiritide will usually result in a modest decrease in circulating levels of NT-proBNP.[101]

Specimen

Specimen requirements for the analysis of BNP differ significantly from those for the determination of NT-proBNP. EDTA-plasma (or, alternatively, EDTA whole blood for point-of-care instruments) is a requirement for the BNP assay; one reason is that EDTA significantly inhibits the activity of plasma proteases that may participate in the degradation of BNP. Other specimen types, including serum, citrate plasma, and heparin

Table 4
Analytic characteristics of selected assays for BNP and NT-proBNP

	NT-proBNP				BNP			
	Roche (Modular, Cobas, Elecsys)	Siemens (Immulite)	Roche, POC (Cardiac Reader)	Siemens, POC (Stratus CS)	Abbott (Architect)	Siemens (Advia Centaur)	Biosite (Beckman-Coulter)	Biosite, POC (triage BNP)
Sample type	Serum Plasma (EDTA, heparin)	Plasma (heparin)	Whole blood (heparin)	Whole blood (heparin)	Plasma (EDTA)	Plasma (EDTA)	Plasma (EDTA)	Whole blood or plasma (EDTA)
Sample storage								
20–25°C	3 days	Not recommended	8 hrs	3 days	4 hrs	Not recommended	4 hrs	4 hrs
2–8°C	6 days	3 days	Not recommended	3 days	24 hrs	24 hrs	—	—
<–20°C	24 mos	6 mos	Not recommended	12 mos	3 mos	9 mos	—	—
Range (pg/mL)	5–35.000	20–35.000	60–3000	15–20.000	10–5000	2–5000	1–5000	5–5000
Precision (%). In parenthesis, level (pg/mL)	2.6 (126)	4.4 (146)	< 14 (all range)	4.4 (97)	4.4 (92)	2.8 (119)	4.1 (77)	8.8 (71)
Analytical sensitivity (pg/mL)	5	10	—	15	10	2	1	5
Functional sensitivity	50	—	—	50	—	2.5	—	—

plasma, may cause suboptimal results. The samples should preferably be drawn into plastic tubes because the BNP molecule may adhere to glass surfaces or, via activation of kallekrein, may degrade in glass tubes, with incomplete recovery of BNP and lower test results as a consequence.[102] In contrast, serum, heparin plasma, and EDTA plasma may be used for the automated measurement of NT-proBNP.[97] However, EDTA plasma results in a consistent negative bias of approximately 10% compared with serum and heparin plasma.[99] For NT-proBNP point-of-care instruments, whole blood (heparin, EDTA) samples can be used.[103] Glass and plastic tubes may be used for the sampling and storage for measurements of NT-proBNP.

Both BNP and NT-proBNP may be detected in urine using the assays originally designed for measurements in serum or plasma. However, the concentrations in urine are substantially lower than circulating levels.[63] Measurements in urine are subject to high variability, and the results should also be interpreted with caution because of matrix differences, eg, the low protein content in urine. BNP production by tubular cells during pathophysiological conditions and the different degrees of dilution in urine are additional potential problems. BNP or NT-proBNP levels in urine may, therefore, not adequately reflect the concentration in the blood; the prevailing view is that BNP analysis in urine alone performs poorly compared with measurement in blood.[104]

Storage

Although both the in vivo and in vitro half-life is substantially longer for NT-proBNP than for BNP, the in vitro stability of both peptides is sufficient for use in clinical routine. However, in vitro stability of BNP reported by the different manufacturers of automatic analytical systems varies according to the assay and instrument used.[105] In contrast to BNP, NT-proBNP appears to be stable in plasma (EDTA, heparin) and whole blood for up to 3 days in room temperature, depending on the instrument used.[97] Repeated thawing–refreezing cycles do not seem to affect the measured level of NT-proBNP significantly.[106]

Biologic Variation

The intra-individual biologic variation of BNP and NT-proBNP is on the order of 20% to 40%.[107,108] The biologic variation has to be taken into account when differences in serial measurements from the same subject are evaluated. Based on the analytical imprecision of the assay and the intra-individual variation, changes of more than 85% for increases and 46% for decreases may,

at a minimum, signify clinically relevant changes in BNP and NT-proBNP levels.[99]

Potential Confounding Factors

Demographic factors influence circulating levels of natriuretic peptides. The concentrations of circulating BNP and NT-proBNP increase with age, and within each age group women have higher natriuretic peptide levels than men.[109,110] The age-related differences have been ascribed to various factors, including mild impairment of kidney function[61] and the increase in blood pressure and left ventricular relaxation abnormalities that occur with aging. However, differences persist to some extent after adjustment for such factors. Recent studies indicate that circulating free testosterone may contribute to the observed sex-related differences.[111] Although age and gender clearly affects circulating levels of BNP and NT-proBNP, both peptides perform well as diagnostic tools for heart failure in all age groups.[112] However, whereas the Food and Drug Administration has approved a flat BNP decision limit of 100 pg/mL for the diagnosis of heart failure, an age-adjusted decision limit is recommended for NT-proBNP (ie, 125 pg/mL for patients younger than 75 years; 450 pg/mL for those older than 75 years). Recent studies have suggested that the use of a flat exclusionary ("rule-out") cutoff and a more graded age-adjusted inclusionary ("rule-in") cutoff for heart failure may provide optimal discrimination for NT-proBNP.[113] Based on findings in epidemiologic studies,[109] it is likely that the same is true for BNP. All manufacturers provide data on reference intervals as a part of the official documentation of their assay (ie, insert sheet). It is however important that each laboratory validate the provided data in relation to its equipment and population, or establish their own reference intervals.

Several studies have studied the natriuretic peptide response to physical exercise in healthy subjects and patients who have heart failure. Taken together the results suggest that physical exercise induces a rapid and marked increase in plasma ANP,[114] but only a modest increase in circulating BNP and NT-proBNP,[115] both in healthy subjects and in patients with heart failure. Although it is unlikely that physical exercise will result in a BNP or NT-proBNP increase of sufficient magnitude to cause diagnostic misclassification, it has been recommended that the subject rests for 10–15 minutes before blood sampling for B-type natriuretic peptides analyses.

Other factors known to increase circulating levels of BNP and NT-proBNP include impaired renal function,[61] cardiac arrhythmias,[116] myocardial ischemia,[117] pulmonary embolism,[118] chronic pulmonary hypertension,[119] anemia,[120] hyperthyroidism,[121] and sepsis,[122] whereas obesity is associated with lower BNP and NT-proBNP levels.[65] Decision limits for the diagnosis of heart failure may have to be modified in the presence of such factors.

For the clinician, it is important to distinguish between elevated BNP levels caused by factors other than heart failure and analytic false positive test results. Analytic false positive test results should be suspected if elevated levels are reported in the absence of heart failure or known confounding factors. False negative BNP and NT-proBNP test results are rare but may be caused by extreme obesity, flash pulmonary edema, in medically optimized heart failure of mild to moderate severity, and in end-stage heart failure, where other molecular forms of natriuretic peptides may be produced. In very rare cases, false negative BNP and NT-proBNP results occur without any evident explanation.

SUMMARY

The advance in the understanding of the physiology of the natriuretic peptide during the past 27 years has been truly remarkable. It has become clear that the pleiotropic physiologic actions of these substances transcend the original paradigm of natriuretic peptides as hormonal factors with natriuretic and vasodilatory properties. Recent discoveries of significance include enhanced understanding of how natriuretic peptides modulate the growth and transformation of cells and the potential of a long-term beneficial effect of natriuretic peptide gene therapy for the treatment of arterial hypertension. B-type natriuretic peptides have also been documented to be reliable and accurate tools for the diagnosis of heart failure and fully automated analyses of these peptides have been implemented in clinical practice in hospitals worldwide.

REFERENCES

1. Chidsey CA, Kaiser GA, Braunwald E. Biosynthesis of norepinephrine in isolated canine heart. Science 1963;139:828–9.
2. Braunwald E, Harrison DC, Chidsey CA. The heart as an endocrine organ. Am J Med 1964;36:1–4.
3. Kisch B. Electron microscopy of the atrium of the heart. I. Guinea pig. Exp Med Surg 1956;14(2–3): 99–112.
4. Henry JP, Gauer OH, Reeves JL. Evidence of the atrial location of receptors influencing urine flow. Circ Res 1956;4(1):85–90.
5. De Bold AJ. Heart atria granularity effects of changes in water-electrolyte balance. Proc Soc Exp Biol Med 1979;161(4):508–11.
6. De Bold AJ, Borenstein HB, Veress AT, et al. A rapid and potent natriuretic response to intravenous injection of atrial myocardial extract in rats. Life Sci 1981;28(1):89–94.
7. Atlas SA, Kleinert HD, Camargo MJ, et al. Purification, sequencing and synthesis of natriuretic and vasoactive rat atrial peptide. Nature 1984; 309(5970):717–9.
8. Sudoh T, Kangawa K, Minamino N, et al. A new natriuretic peptide in porcine brain. Nature 1988; 332(6159):78–81.
9. Mukoyama M, Nakao K, Hosoda K, et al. Brain natriuretic peptide as a novel cardiac hormone in humans. Evidence for an exquisite dual natriuretic peptide system, atrial natriuretic peptide and brain natriuretic peptide. J Clin Invest 1991;87(4): 1402–12.
10. Sudoh T, Minamino N, Kangawa K, et al. C-type natriuretic peptide (CNP): a new member of natriuretic peptide family identified in porcine brain. Biochem Biophys Res Commun 1990;168(2):863–70.
11. Sundsfjord JA, Thibault G, Larochelle P, et al. Identification and plasma concentrations of the N-terminal fragment of proatrial natriuretic factor in man. J Clin Endocrinol Metab 1988;66(3):605–10.
12. Hunt PJ, Yandle TG, Nicholls MG, et al. The amino-terminal portion of pro-brain natriuretic peptide (Pro-BNP) circulates in human plasma. Biochem Biophys Res Commun 1995;214(3):1175–83.
13. Brunner-La Rocca HP, Kaye DM, Woods RL, et al. Effects of intravenous brain natriuretic peptide on regional sympathetic activity in patients with chronic heart failure as compared with healthy control subjects. J Am Coll Cardiol 2001;37(5):1221–7.
14. Schirger JA, Grantham JA, Kullo IJ, et al. Vascular actions of brain natriuretic peptide: modulation by atherosclerosis and neutral endopeptidase inhibition. J Am Coll Cardiol 2000;35(3):796–801.
15. Li P, Wang D, Lucas J, et al. Atrial natriuretic peptide inhibits transforming growth factor beta-induced Smad signaling and myofibroblast transformation in mouse cardiac fibroblasts. Circ Res 2008;102(2):185–92.
16. Levin ER, Gardner DG, Samson WK. Natriuretic peptides. N Engl J Med 1998;339(5):321–8.
17. Minamino N, Makino Y, Tateyama H, et al. Characterization of immunoreactive human C-type natriuretic peptide in brain and heart. Biochem Biophys Res Commun 1991;179(1):535–42.
18. Schweitz H, Vigne P, Moinier D, et al. A new member of the natriuretic peptide family is present

in the venom of the green mamba (Dendroaspis angusticeps). J Biol Chem 1992;267(20):13928–32.

19. Gunning M, Brenner BM. Urodilatin: a potent natriuretic peptide of renal origin. Curr Opin Nephrol Hypertens 1993;2(6):857–62.

20. Forte LR, Currie MG. Guanylin: a peptide regulator of epithelial transport. FASEB J 1995;9(8):643–50.

21. Tamura N, Ogawa Y, Yasoda A, et al. Two cardiac natriuretic peptide genes (atrial natriuretic peptide and brain natriuretic peptide) are organized in tandem in the mouse and human genomes. J Mol Cell Cardiol 1996;28(8):1811–5.

22. Martinez-Rumayor A, Richards AM, Burnett JC, et al. Biology of the natriuretic peptides. Am J Cardiol 2008;101(3A):3–8.

23. Richards AM. Natriuretic peptides: update on peptide release, bioactivity, and clinical use. Hypertension 2007;50(1):25–30.

24. Sawada Y, Suda M, Yokoyama H, et al. Stretch-induced hypertrophic growth of cardiocytes and processing of brain-type natriuretic peptide are controlled by proprotein-processing endoprotease furin. J Biol Chem 1997;272(33):20545–54.

25. Yan W, Wu F, Morser J, et al. Corin, a transmembrane cardiac serine protease, acts as a pro-atrial natriuretic peptide-converting enzyme. Proc Natl Acad Sci U S A 2000;97(15):8525–9.

26. Tateyama H, Hino J, Minamino N, et al. Concentrations and molecular forms of human brain natriuretic peptide in plasma. Biochem Biophys Res Commun 1992;185(2):760–7.

27. Liang F, O'Rear J, Schellenberger U, et al. Evidence for functional heterogeneity of circulating B-type natriuretic peptide. J Am Coll Cardiol 2007; 49(10):1071–8.

28. Lam CS, Burnett JC Jr, Costello-Boerrigter L, et al. Alternate circulating pro-B-type natriuretic peptide and B-type natriuretic peptide forms in the general population. J Am Coll Cardiol 2007;49(11): 1193–202.

29. Hawkridge AM, Heublein DM, Bergen HR III, et al. Quantitative mass spectral evidence for the absence of circulating brain natriuretic peptide (BNP-32) in severe human heart failure. Proc Natl Acad Sci U S A 2005;102(48):17442–7.

30. la-Kopsala M, Magga J, Peuhkurinen K, et al. Molecular heterogeneity has a major impact on the measurement of circulating N-terminal fragments of A- and B-type natriuretic peptides. Clin Chem 2004;50(9):1576–88.

31. Seidler T, Pemberton C, Yandle T, et al. The amino terminal regions of proBNP and proANP oligomerise through leucine zipper-like coiled-coil motifs. Biochem Biophys Res Commun 1999;255(2): 495–501.

32. Schellenberger U, O'Rear J, Guzzetta A, et al. The precursor to B-type natriuretic peptide is an O-linked glycoprotein. Arch Biochem Biophys 2006;451(2):160–6.

33. Yasue H, Yoshimura M, Sumida H, et al. Localization and mechanism of secretion of B-type natriuretic peptide in comparison with those of A-type natriuretic peptide in normal subjects and patients with heart failure. Circulation 1994;90(1): 195–203.

34. Kinnunen P, Vuolteenaho O, Ruskoaho H. Mechanisms of atrial and brain natriuretic peptide release from rat ventricular myocardium: effect of stretching. Endocrinology 1993;132(5):1961–70.

35. Murakami Y, Shimada T, Inoue S, et al. New insights into the mechanism of the elevation of plasma brain natriuretic polypeptide levels in patients with left ventricular hypertrophy. Can J Cardiol 2002; 18(12):1294–300.

36. Liang F, Atakilit A, Gardner DG. Integrin dependence of brain natriuretic peptide gene promoter activation by mechanical strain. J Biol Chem 2000;275(27):20355–60.

37. Tsuruda T, Boerrigter G, Huntley BK, et al. Brain natriuretic Peptide is produced in cardiac fibroblasts and induces matrix metalloproteinases. Circ Res 2002;91(12):1127–34.

38. Bruneau BG, Piazza LA, De Bold AJ. Alpha 1-adrenergic stimulation of isolated rat atria results in discoordinate increases in natriuretic peptide secretion and gene expression and enhances Egr-1 and c-Myc expression. Endocrinology 1996; 137(1):137–43.

39. Leskinen H, Vuolteenaho O, Ruskoaho H. Combined inhibition of endothelin and angiotensin II receptors blocks volume load-induced cardiac hormone release. Circ Res 1997;80(1):114–23.

40. Bianciotti LG, De Bold AJ. Modulation of cardiac natriuretic peptide gene expression following endothelin type A receptor blockade in renovascular hypertension. Cardiovasc Res 2001;49(4): 808–16.

41. Yuan K, Cao C, Han JH, et al. Adenosine-stimulated atrial natriuretic peptide release through A1 receptor subtype. Hypertension 2005;46(6):1381–7.

42. Han JH, Cao C, Kim SM, et al. Attenuation of lysophosphatidylcholine-induced suppression of ANP release from hypertrophied atria. Hypertension 2004;43(2):243–8.

43. Magga J, Marttila M, Mantymaa P, et al. Brain natriuretic peptide in plasma, atria, and ventricles of vasopressin- and phenylephrine-infused conscious rats. Endocrinology 1994;134(6):2505–15.

44. Hama N, Itoh H, Shirakami G, et al. Rapid ventricular induction of brain natriuretic peptide gene expression in experimental acute myocardial infarction. Circulation 1995;92(6):1558–64.

45. Lang CC, Choy AM, Turner K, et al. The effect of intravenous saline loading on plasma levels of

brain natriuretic peptide in man. J Hypertens 1993; 11(7):737–41.

46. Nakao K, Itoh H, Kambayashi Y, et al. Rat brain natriuretic peptide. Isolation from rat heart and tissue distribution. Hypertension 1990;15(6 Pt 2):774–8.

47. Ogawa Y, Nakao K, Nakagawa O, et al. Human C-type natriuretic peptide. Characterization of the gene and peptide. Hypertension 1992;19(6 Pt 2): 809–13.

48. Koller KJ, Goeddel DV. Molecular biology of the natriuretic peptides and their receptors. Circulation 1992;86(4):1081–8.

49. Gutkowska J, Nemer M. Structure, expression, and function of atrial natriuretic factor in extraatrial tissues. Endocr Rev 1989;10(4):519–36.

50. Misono KS. Natriuretic peptide receptor: structure and signaling. Mol Cell Biochem 2002;230(1–2): 49–60.

51. Feil R, Lohmann SM, de JH, et al. Cyclic GMP-dependent protein kinases and the cardiovascular system: insights from genetically modified mice. Circ Res 2003;93(10):907–16.

52. Hum D, Besnard S, Sanchez R, et al. Characterization of a cGMP-response element in the guanylyl cyclase/natriuretic peptide receptor A gene promoter. Hypertension 2004;43(6):1270–8.

53. Chen ZJ, Vetter M, Chang GD, et al. Cyclophilin A functions as an endogenous inhibitor for membrane-bound guanylate cyclase-A. Hypertension 2004;44(6):963–8.

54. Singh G, Kuc RE, Maguire JJ, et al. Novel snake venom ligand dendroaspis natriuretic peptide is selective for natriuretic peptide receptor-A in human heart: downregulation of natriuretic peptide receptor-A in heart failure. Circ Res 2006;99(2): 183–90.

55. Matsukawa N, Grzesik WJ, Takahashi N, et al. The natriuretic peptide clearance receptor locally modulates the physiological effects of the natriuretic peptide system. Proc Natl Acad Sci U S A 1999;96(13):7403–8.

56. Woodard GE, Rosado JA. Natriuretic peptides in vascular physiology and pathology. Int Rev Cell Mol Biol 2008;268:59–93.

57. Maack T, Okolicany J, Koh GY, et al. Functional properties of atrial natriuretic factor receptors. Semin Nephrol 1993;13(1):50–60.

58. Suga S, Nakao K, Hosoda K, et al. Receptor selectivity of natriuretic peptide family, atrial natriuretic peptide, brain natriuretic peptide, and C-type natriuretic peptide. Endocrinology 1992;130(1):229–39.

59. Pemberton CJ, Johnson ML, Yandle TG, et al. Deconvolution analysis of cardiac natriuretic peptides during acute volume overload. Hypertension 2000; 36(3):355–9.

60. Nakao K, Ogawa Y, Suga S, et al. Molecular biology and biochemistry of the natriuretic peptide system. II: Natriuretic peptide receptors. J Hypertens 1992;10(10):1111–4.

61. Das SR, Abdullah SM, Leonard D, et al. Association between renal function and circulating levels of natriuretic peptides (from the Dallas Heart Study). Am J Cardiol 2008;102(10):1394–8.

62. Schou M, Dalsgaard MK, Clemmesen O, et al. Kidneys extract BNP and NT-proBNP in healthy young men. J Appl Phys 2005;99(5):1676–80.

63. Ng LL, Geeranavar S, Jennings SC, et al. Diagnosis of heart failure using urinary natriuretic peptides. Clin Sci (Lond) 2004;106(2):129–33.

64. Wang TJ, Larson MG, Levy D, et al. Impact of obesity on plasma natriuretic peptide levels. Circulation 2004;109(5):594–600.

65. Das SR, Drazner MH, Dries DL, et al. Impact of body mass and body composition on circulating levels of natriuretic peptides: results from the Dallas Heart Study. Circulation 2005;112(14): 2163–8.

66. Richards AM, Tonolo G, Montorsi P, et al. Low dose infusions of 26- and 28-amino acid human atrial natriuretic peptides in normal man. J Clin Endocrinol Metab 1988;66(3):465–72.

67. Lin KF, Chao J, Chao L. Human atrial natriuretic peptide gene delivery reduces blood pressure in hypertensive rats. Hypertension 1995;26(6 Pt 1): 847–53.

68. Schillinger KJ, Tsai SY, Taffet GE, et al. Regulatable atrial natriuretic peptide gene therapy for hypertension. Proc Natl Acad Sci U S A 2005;102(39): 13789–94.

69. Cody RJ, Covit AB, Schaer GL, et al. Sodium and water balance in chronic congestive heart failure. J Clin Invest 1986;77(5):1441–52.

70. Olsen MH, Hansen TW, Christensen MK, et al. N-terminal pro brain natriuretic peptide is inversely related to metabolic cardiovascular risk factors and the metabolic syndrome. Hypertension 2005;46(4): 660–6.

71. Rubattu S, Sciarretta S, Ciavarella GM, et al. Reduced levels of N-terminal-proatrial natriuretic peptide in hypertensive patients with metabolic syndrome and their relationship with left ventricular mass. J Hypertens 2007;25(4):833–9.

72. Clarkson PB, Wheeldon NM, Macleod C, et al. Brain natriuretic peptide: effect on left ventricular filling patterns in healthy subjects. Clin Sci (Lond) 1995;88(2):159–64.

73. Kishimoto I, Rossi K, Garbers DL. A genetic model provides evidence that the receptor for atrial natriuretic peptide (guanylyl cyclase-A) inhibits cardiac ventricular myocyte hypertrophy. Proc Natl Acad Sci U S A 2001;98(5):2703–6.

74. John SW, Krege JH, Oliver PM, et al. Genetic decreases in atrial natriuretic peptide and salt-sensitive hypertension. Science 1995;267(5198):679–81.

75. Tamura N, Ogawa Y, Chusho H, et al. Cardiac fibrosis in mice lacking brain natriuretic peptide. Proc Natl Acad Sci U S A 2000;97(8):4239–44.

76. Oliver PM, Fox JE, Kim R, et al. Hypertension, cardiac hypertrophy, and sudden death in mice lacking natriuretic peptide receptor A. Proc Natl Acad Sci U S A 1997;94(26):14730–5.

77. Nakanishi M, Saito Y, Kishimoto I, et al. Role of natriuretic peptide receptor guanylyl cyclase-A in myocardial infarction evaluated using genetically engineered mice. Hypertension 2005;46(2):441–7.

78. Buxton IL, Duan D. Cyclic GMP/protein kinase G phosphorylation of Smad3 blocks transforming growth factor-beta-induced nuclear Smad translocation: a key antifibrogenic mechanism of atrial natriuretic peptide. Circ Res 2008;102(2):151–3.

79. Nakayama T, Soma M, Takahashi Y, et al. Functional deletion mutation of the 5'-flanking region of type A human natriuretic peptide receptor gene and its association with essential hypertension and left ventricular hypertrophy in the Japanese. Circ Res 2000;86(8):841–5.

80. Rubattu S, Bigatti G, Evangelista A, et al. Association of atrial natriuretic peptide and type a natriuretic peptide receptor gene polymorphisms with left ventricular mass in human essential hypertension. J Am Coll Cardiol 2006;48(3):499–505.

81. Tokudome T, Horio T, Soeki T, et al. Inhibitory effect of C-type natriuretic peptide (CNP) on cultured cardiac myocyte hypertrophy: interference between CNP and endothelin-1 signaling pathways. Endocrinology 2004;145(5):2131–40.

82. Langenickel TH, Buttgereit J, Pagel-Langenickel I, et al. Cardiac hypertrophy in transgenic rats expressing a dominant-negative mutant of the natriuretic peptide receptor B. Proc Natl Acad Sci U S A 2006;103(12):4735–40.

83. Soeki T, Kishimoto I, Okumura H, et al. C-type natriuretic peptide, a novel antifibrotic and antihypertrophic agent, prevents cardiac remodeling after myocardial infarction. J Am Coll Cardiol 2005;45(4):608–16.

84. Komatsu Y, Itoh H, Suga S, et al. Regulation of endothelial production of C-type natriuretic peptide in coculture with vascular smooth muscle cells. Role of the vascular natriuretic peptide system in vascular growth inhibition. Circ Res 1996;78(4):606–14.

85. Furuya M, Aisaka K, Miyazaki T, et al. C-type natriuretic peptide inhibits intimal thickening after vascular injury. Biochem Biophys Res Commun 1993;193(1):248–53.

86. Naruko T, Ueda M, van der Wal AC, et al. C-type natriuretic peptide in human coronary atherosclerotic lesions. Circulation 1996;94(12):3103–8.

87. Marin-Grez M, Fleming JT, Steinhausen M. Atrial natriuretic peptide causes pre-glomerular vasodilatation and post-glomerular vasoconstriction in rat kidney. Nature 1986;324(6096):473–6.

88. Grantham JA, Borgeson DD, Burnett JC Jr. BNP: pathophysiological and potential therapeutic roles in acute congestive heart failure. Am J Phys 1997;272(4 Pt 2):R1077–83.

89. Fried TA, McCoy RN, Osgood RW, et al. Effect of atriopeptin II on determinants of glomerular filtration rate in the in vitro perfused dog glomerulus. Am J Phys 1986;250(6 Pt 2):F1119–22.

90. Harris PJ, Thomas D, Morgan TO. Atrial natriuretic peptide inhibits angiotensin-stimulated proximal tubular sodium and water reabsorption. Nature 1987;326(6114):697–8.

91. Dillingham MA, Anderson RJ. Inhibition of vasopressin action by atrial natriuretic factor. Science 1986;231(4745):1572–3.

92. Zeidel ML, Kikeri D, Silva P, et al. Atrial natriuretic peptides inhibit conductive sodium uptake by rabbit inner medullary collecting duct cells. J Clin Invest 1988;82(3):1067–74.

93. Hunt PJ, Richards AM, Espiner EA, et al. Bioactivity and metabolism of C-type natriuretic peptide in normal man. J Clin Endocrinol Metab 1994;78(6):1428–35.

94. Floras JS. Sympathoinhibitory effects of atrial natriuretic factor in normal humans. Circulation 1990;81(6):1860–73.

95. Uemasu J, Matsumoto H, Kitano M, et al. Suppression of plasma endothelin-1 level by alpha-human atrial natriuretic peptide and angiotensin converting enzyme inhibition in normal men. Life Sci 1993;53(11):969–74.

96. Moro C, Klimcakova E, Lolmede K, et al. Atrial natriuretic peptide inhibits the production of adipokines and cytokines linked to inflammation and insulin resistance in human subcutaneous adipose tissue. Diabetologia 2007;50(5):1038–47.

97. Yeo KT, Wu AH, Apple FS, et al. Multicenter evaluation of the Roche NT-proBNP assay and comparison to the Biosite Triage BNP assay. Clin Chim Acta 2003;338(1–2):107–15.

98. Seferian KR, Tamm NN, Semenov AG, et al. The brain natriuretic peptide (BNP) precursor is the major immunoreactive form of BNP in patients with heart failure. Clin Chem 2007;53(5):866–73.

99. Apple FS, Wu AH, Jaffe AS, et al. National Academy of Clinical Biochemistry and IFCC Committee for Standardization of Markers of Cardiac Damage Laboratory Medicine practice guidelines: analytical issues for biomarkers of heart failure. Circulation 2007;116(5):e95–8.

100. Johnson W, Omland T, Hall C, et al. Neurohormonal activation rapidly decreases after intravenous therapy with diuretics and vasodilators for class IV heart failure. J Am Coll Cardiol 2002;39(10):1623–9.

101. Miller WL, Hartman KA, Burritt MF, et al. Biomarker responses during and after treatment with nesiritide infusion in patients with decompensated chronic heart failure. Clin Chem 2005;51(3):569–77.

102. Shimizu H, Aono K, Masuta K, et al. Degradation of human brain natriuretic peptide (BNP) by contact activation of blood coagulation system. Clin Chim Acta 2001;305(1–2):181–6.

103. Zugck C, Nelles M, Katus HA, et al. Multicentre evaluation of a new point-of-care test for the determination of NT-proBNP in whole blood. Clin Chem Lab Med 2006;44(10):1269–77.

104. Michielsen EC, Bakker JA, Kimmenade RR, et al. The diagnostic value of serum and urinary NT-proBNP for heart failure. Ann Clin Biochem 2008; 45(Pt 4):389–94.

105. Azzazy HM, Christenson RH, Duh SH. Stability of B-type natriuretic peptide (BNP) in whole blood and plasma stored under different conditions when measured with the Biosite Triage or Beckman-Coulter Access systems. Clin Chim Acta 2007;384(1–2):176–8.

106. Sokoll LJ, Baum H, Collinson PO, et al. Multicenter analytical performance evaluation of the Elecsys proBNP assay. Clin Chem Lab Med 2004;42(8): 965–72.

107. Schou M, Gustafsson F, Kjaer A, et al. Long-term clinical variation of NT-proBNP in stable chronic heart failure patients. Eur Heart J 2007;28(2):177–82.

108. Wu AH, Smith A, Wieczorek S, et al. Biological variation for N-terminal pro- and B-type natriuretic peptides and implications for therapeutic monitoring of patients with congestive heart failure. Am J Cardiol 2003;92(5):628–31.

109. Wang TJ, Larson MG, Levy D, et al. Impact of age and sex on plasma natriuretic peptide levels in healthy adults. Am J Cardiol 2002;90(3):254–8.

110. Raymond I, Groenning BA, Hildebrandt PR, et al. The influence of age, sex and other variables on the plasma level of N-terminal pro brain natriuretic peptide in a large sample of the general population. Heart 2003;89(7):745–51.

111. Chang AY, Abdullah SM, Jain T, et al. Associations among androgens, estrogens, and natriuretic peptides in young women: observations from the Dallas Heart Study. J Am Coll Cardiol 2007;49(1): 109–16.

112. Maisel AS, Clopton P, Krishnaswamy P, et al. Impact of age, race, and sex on the ability of B-type natriuretic peptide to aid in the emergency diagnosis of heart failure: results from the breathing not properly (BNP) multinational study. Am Heart J 2004;147(6):1078–84.

113. Januzzi JL, van KR, Lainchbury J, et al. NT-proBNP testing for diagnosis and short-term prognosis in acute destabilized heart failure: an international pooled analysis of 1256 patients: the International Collaborative of NT-proBNP Study. Eur Heart J 2006;27(3):330–7.

114. Omland T, Barvik S, Aakvaag A, et al. Plasma atrial natriuretic factor concentration during maximal cardiopulmonary exercise in men with mild heart failure. Int J Cardiol 1990;29(2):179–84.

115. McNairy M, Gardetto N, Clopton P, et al. Stability of B-type natriuretic peptide levels during exercise in patients with congestive heart failure: implications for outpatient monitoring with B-type natriuretic peptide. Am Heart J 2002;143(3):406–11.

116. Knudsen CW, Omland T, Clopton P, et al. Impact of atrial fibrillation on the diagnostic performance of B-type natriuretic peptide concentration in dyspneic patients: an analysis from the breathing not properly multinational study. J Am Coll Cardiol 2005;46(5):838–44.

117. Sabatine MS, Morrow DA, de Lemos JA, et al. Acute changes in circulating natriuretic peptide levels in relation to myocardial ischemia. J Am Coll Cardiol 2004;44(10):1988–95.

118. Kucher N, Printzen G, Goldhaber SZ. Prognostic role of brain natriuretic peptide in acute pulmonary embolism. Circulation 2003;107(20):2545–7.

119. Reesink HJ, Tulevski II, Marcus JT, et al. Brain natriuretic peptide as noninvasive marker of the severity of right ventricular dysfunction in chronic thromboembolic pulmonary hypertension. Ann Thorac Surg 2007;84(2):537–43.

120. Wold KC, Vik-Mo H, Omland T. Blood haemoglobin is an independent predictor of B-type natriuretic peptide (BNP). Clin Sci (Lond) 2005; 109(1):69–74.

121. Schultz M, Faber J, Kistorp C, et al. N-terminal-pro-B-type natriuretic peptide (NT-pro-BNP) in different thyroid function states. Clin Endocrinol (Oxf) 2004; 60(1):54–9.

122. Omland T. Advances in congestive heart failure management in the intensive care unit: B-type natriuretic peptides in evaluation of acute heart failure. Crit Care Med 2008;36(Suppl 1):S17–27.

Natriuretic Peptides in the Diagnosis and Management of Acute Heart Failure

Asim A. Mohammed, MD, James L. Januzzi, Jr, MD*

KEYWORDS

- Natriuretic peptides • Heart failure • Age
- Chronic kidney disease • Multi-marking panels

Heart failure (HF) is one of the major health problems in modern medicine. It is the most common cause of hospitalization in people older than 65 years. Despite advances in pharmacotherapy for treating HF, the incidence and the morbidity and mortality associated with HF continue to rise. This rise in incidence is in part because of the aging of the population and age-related prevalence of risk factors such as hypertension, and the improved survival of patients who have acute coronary syndromes, a group at especially high risk for developing HF. A recent study, which showed that in the last 25 years, the incidence of HF has tripled,[1] confirmed the magnitude of economic burden faced by the modern health system.

Traditionally, HF diagnosis has been challenging because of a broad differential diagnosis; this leads to high mortality, morbidity, and hospitalization rates in this patient population. Fortunately, since the discovery of atrial natriuretic factor, which draws attention to the endocrine function of the heart,[2] there has been remarkable advancement in the understanding of natriuretic peptides (NPs) and the potential role they may play in evaluating, prognosticating, and managing HF.

The NP assays commonly used clinically are B-type NP (BNP) and its amino-terminal cleavage equivalent (NT-proBNP); both are used worldwide for diagnosing and managing HF cost-effectively.

NATRIURETIC PEPTIDE BIOLOGY

After BNP gene transcription and translation occurs, a 108-amino acid intracellular precursor molecule, pro-BNP$_{108}$ is produced within the myocyte; this precursor subsequently is cleaved by furin- or coriin-like endoprotease to produce the 76-amino acid NT-proBNP and the biologically active C-terminal fragment BNP. The BNP gene is located on the chromosome 1. The nuclear transcription factor, GATA 4, is responsible for regulating the BNP gene transcription. The BNP gene is expressed in the atria and ventricles. The synthesis and release of BNP and NT-proBNP are caused by changes in the wall strain of cardiomyocyte in all chambers of heart. Aside from the wall tension, however, other triggers for NP release exist, including hormones such as norepinephrine, proinflamatory cytokines, glucocorticoids, and myocardial ischemia.

After release, NT-proBNP circulates with various degrees of glycosylation. With respect to BNP, the secreted 3- amino acid protein, BNP$_{1-32}$, is degraded rapidly to BNP$_{3-32}$ by neutral endopeptidases, and BNP$_{6-32}$ by meprin-A. Lastly, a significant amount of biologically inactive pro-BNP$_{108}$ also is released, which is cross-identified by commercial assays for detection of BNP and NT-proBNP.

Dr. Mohammed is supported by the Dennis and Marilyn Barry Fellowship in Cardiology, while Dr. Januzzi is supported in part by the Balson Fund for Cardiovascular Research.
Harvard Medical School, Boston, MA, USA
* Corresponding author. Division of Cardiology, Department of Medicine, Massachusetts General Hospital, Harvard Medical School, 32 Fruit Street, Yawkey 5984, Boston, MA 02114.
E-mail address: jjanuzzi@partners.org (J.L. Januzzi Jr.).

Heart Failure Clin 5 (2009) 489–500
doi:10.1016/j.hfc.2009.04.007
1551-7136/09/$ – see front matter

From the HF perspective, NPs may be viewed loosely as the body's response to the volume overload, neurohormonal derangement, and activation of the renin–angiotensin system. The principal actions of BNP are natriuresis, reduction in peripheral vascular resistance, hypotension, and diuresis. These effects are mediated by binding to NP receptors (NPRs), which are expressed in the cardiovascular system, lungs, kidneys, skin, platelets, and central nervous system. There are three types of NPRs: NPR-A, NPR-B, and NPR-C. The NPR-A and NPR-B receptors are distributed widely in the myocardium and blood vessels, while the NPR-C is a clearance receptor. The activation of NPR-A receptor activates guanylyl cyclase, leading to rise in cyclic guanylyl monophosphate, leading to the mentioned actions of BNP.

Half-Life and Clearance

The half-life of BNP is estimated as 21 minutes, and the half-life of NT-proBNP is estimated as 70 minutes. BNP is degraded after it binds to NPR-C by endopeptidases and other enzymes. BNP also is cleared passively by the kidneys. On the other hand, NT-proBNP is cleared passively by organs with high blood flows. This is responsible for its longer half-life.

ANALYTICAL CONSIDERATIONS

Assays for measuring BNP and NT-proBNP are widely available, and the choice of which assay clinicians should use depends partially on analyzers installed in their hospitals, as both NPs provide valuable information.

Preanalytical Factors

Blood collection in plastic tubes is essential for BNP, while either glass or plastic tubes are adequate for NT-proBNP. NT-proBNP is a relatively stable molecule that is not affected by temperature changes, making it a more convenient molecule to work with, whereas with BNP, rapidity of testing is very important, as it is unstable at room temperature.

Analytical Factors

Previously, methods to measure BNP and NT-proBNP were cumbersome radioimmunoassays, which have been replaced by point-of-care (POC) and automated solutions. Choosing POC, as opposed to automated testing mandates careful consideration, as both options have their strengths and weaknesses. The main advantage of POC testing is the proximity to the patient but at the cost of lower accuracy when compared with automated assays, which are considerably more accurate, less expensive, and allow for high-volume throughput, but take longer to provide the result. POC options for BNP and NT-proBNP are available, as are automated solutions. Automated versions of the NT-proBNP assay may provide superior harmony with their POC counterparts, compared with corresponding BNP methods.

Postanalytical Factors

It is critical to understand the importance of certain postanalytical factors such as age, gender, and ethnicity, to optimally appreciate the results of NP testing. Galasko and colleagues[3] identified that older age and female gender were associated with higher concentrations of NT-proBNP in apparently healthy subjects. The latter finding was investigated more comprehensively in the Dallas Heart Study,[4] where Chang and colleagues demonstrated that the higher levels of NPs in women were associated inversely with androgenic hormones, suggesting that in fact the observation is framed better, as men have lower levels of NPs because of the effects of androgenic hormones.

It has been reported that African Americans may have higher NP levels compared with non-African Americans, although these differences may not be significant when taking into consideration other relevant covariants, such as age, body mass index (BMI), and renal function. Notably, although these findings are apparent in healthy subjects, among those who have acute dyspnea with or without HF, the effects of age are manageable, and sex and race do not affect the diagnostic value of BNP or NT-proBNP.

Important variables to consider when interpreting BNP and NT-proBNP are renal function and BMI. Given that both peptides are low-molecular weight proteins, both BNP and NT-proBNP depend partially on renal function for their clearance, but the relationship is more complex than simple renal clearance. Patients who have chronic kidney disease (CKD) almost universally have elevated BNP or NT-proBNP values. These are prognostic across the spectrum of presentations from asymptomatic to acute dyspnea, suggesting that rather than being considered false positives, values of NPs in CKD are true elevations, reflecting the parallel increase in heart disease occurring with CKD.

The curious inverse association between BMI and NP values has been studied. It has been shown unequivocally that NP levels are lower in overweight and obese patients, in spite of their having higher left ventricular (LV) mass and higher intracardiac pressures when compared with subjects who have normal BMI. Although the mechanism remains unclear, several studies have reported an inverse association between NPs and BMI,[5–7] presumably on the basis of decreased release.

Biological Variability

Biologic variability refers to the daily or weekly alterations in NP concentrations in the absence of obvious clinical changes. It reflects the temporal changes in BNP or NT-proBNP production by each patient, and most probably is caused by shifts in cardiac filling pressures and hemodynamics. Although biological variability when expressed as a percentage of baseline value may be very high in healthy subjects, this is in the context of low absolute values of the NPs, where 100% changes in value may be meaningless. In the setting of HF, however, Schou and colleagues[8] demonstrated a biological variability of 23% for NT-proBNP and 43% for BNP in a population of well-controlled HF. Hence, in the context of measuring NP levels in a patient who has prior HF, it is of particular importance to have a baseline or dry NP level, which is defined as NP measured when the patient is most stable. Any change more than approximately 25% for NT-proBNP and 40% for BNP should be regarded as a significant change.[9,10]

NATRIURETIC PEPTIDE IN ACUTE HEART FAILURE

As noted, acute HF is often a difficult diagnosis to establish in the emergency department (ED), mainly because of the various conditions that may present with dyspnea. Also, HF may present with nonspecific symptoms such as fatigue and dizziness, making it a challenging diagnosis to secure. Hence, delays in HF diagnosis are not uncommon, which result not only in increased morbidity and mortality, but also increased cost of health care. Thoughtful application of NP testing has been shown to be helpful in this setting, and as such NP testing is incorporated into existing clinical guidelines for the diagnostic evaluation of HF.[11–13]

Role of Natriuretic Peptides in Diagnosis and Exclusion of Heart Failure

The Breathing Not Properly Multinational Study,[14] a landmark study of NP testing, highlighted the value of BNP testing in patients presenting to the ED with acute dyspnea. In this multicenter trial involving 1586 dyspneic patients, Maisel and colleagues[14] showed that a BNP concentration greater than 100 pg/mL had 83% accuracy for the clinical diagnosis of HF (**Fig. 1**), superior to existing The National Health and Nutrition Examination Survey criteria (67% accuracy) and the Framingham criteria (73% accuracy). Results of BNP testing were better than clinical judgment alone,

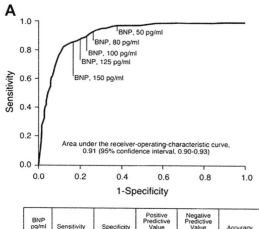

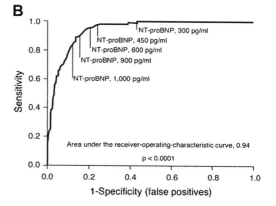

BNP pg/ml	Sensitivity	Specificity	Positive Predictive Value	Negative Predictive Value	Accuracy
50	97%	62%	71%	96%	79%
80	93%	74%	77%	92%	83%
100	90%	76%	79%	89%	83%
125	87%	79%	80%	87%	83%
150	85%	83%	83%	87%	84%

Cut Point pg/ml	Sensitivity	Specificity	Positive Predictive Value	Negative Predictive Value	Accuracy
300	99%	68%	62%	99%	79%
450	98%	76%	68%	99%	83%
600	96%	81%	73%	97%	86%
900	90%	85%	86%	94%	87%
1000	87%	86%	78%	91%	87%

Fig. 1. Receiver operating characteristic curve for various cutoff levels of (*A*) B-type natriuretic peptide (BNP) and (*B*) NT-proBNP. Both peptides are highly sensitive and specific for the diagnosing acute HF, with a highly significant area under the ROC (receiver operated curve). (*Adapted from* Maisel AS, Krishnswamy P, Nowak RM, et al. Rapid measurement of B-type natriuretic peptide in the emergency diagnosis of heart failure. N Engl J Med 2002;347(3):165; with permission; and Januzzi JL, Camargo CA, Anwaruddin S, et al. The N-terminal Pro-BNP investigation of dyspnea in the emergency department (PRIDE) study. Am J Cardiol 2005;95(8):951; with permission.)

but more importantly, the additive value of BNP plus clinical judgment was superior to either alone.

Although a BNP less than 100 pg/mL had a reasonable negative predictive value (NPV) of 88%, the value of BNP to confidently exclude acute HF (ie, a NPV greater than 95%) was considerably lower, at 30 pg/mL. Indeed, Cowie and colleagues[15] showed that a cut-off value of 22 pg/mL for BNP could rule out the diagnosis of HF with high NPV of 98%. The positive predictive value (PPV) of BNP for HF at 100 pg/mL was 79%. This relatively less robust PPV is expected, as several other conditions can cause a BNP in this range, even in the absence of HF (Table 1). Nonetheless, BNP testing in the Breathing Not Properly Multinational Study was valuable across a range of patients, including those who had prior HF[14] and CKD;[16] BNP was more important than chest radiography for diagnosing HF.[14] Bayes-Genis and colleagues[17] suggested the importance of NT-proBNP for diagnosing acute HF and proposed values to rule in and rule out this diagnosis. Later, data from Christchurch, New Zealand,[18] showed that the NT-proBNP levels were elevated greatly in acute HF and its utility was comparable to BNP for this indication. Likewise, Mueller and colleagues[19] evaluated both NPs in 251 dyspneic patients and found no difference between them for diagnostic evaluation. Most definitive data supporting NT-proBNP testing came from the ProBNP Investigation of Dyspnea in the Emergency Department (PRIDE) study,[20] a prospective study of 599 acutely dyspneic patients, of whom 209 had HF. The PRIDE study confirmed the value of NT-proBNP in the acute HF setting by demonstrating significant increases in NT-proBNP among those who had acute HF compared to those without (4435 pg/mL versus 131 pg/mL). Also, an NT-proBNP concentration greater than 900 pg/mL had a PPV of 76% for diagnosing acute HF, similar to the findings for a BNP greater than 100 pg/mL in the Breathing Not Properly Multinational Study. In the PRIDE study, NT-proBNP levels correlated with the severity of HF symptoms, and multivariable analysis showed that an elevation of NT-proBNP level was the strongest predictor of HF in acutely dyspneic patients in the ED. Furthermore, the PRIDE study also showed that, similar to BNP, the NT-proBNP was superior to clinical judgment for diagnosing HF in this setting, and NT-proBNP plus clinical judgment were superior to either alone (Fig. 2).

NPs received further support from the Brain Natriuretic Peptide for Acute Shortness of Breath Evaluation (BASEL)[21] and Improved Management of Patients with Congestive Heart Failure (IMPROVE

Table 1
Differential diagnosis for increased and decreased natriuretic peptides levels
Increased natriuretic peptides
Physiologic
Age
Female gender
Cardiovascular disease
Heart failure
Ischemia
Arrhythmia
Valvular heart disease
Hypertension with left ventricular hypertrophy
Asymptomatic left ventricular dysfunction
Noncardiac causes
Pulmonary embolism
Cor pulmonale
Sepsis
Pulmonary hypertension
Hyperthyroidism
Kidney failure
Tumors
Intracerebral hemorrhage
Advanced liver disease
Excessive cortisol levels
Decreased natriuretic peptides
Obesity
Cardiac medicine
Angiotensin-converting enzyme inhibitors
Angiotensin II receptor blockers
Diuretics
Spironolactone
Beta-blocker[a]
Nonpharmacological factors
Exercise
Cardiac resynchronization therapy
LV assist devices

[a] Beta-blockers may raise natriuretic peptide levels initially.

CHF)[22] studies, which were randomized, prospective decision-making trials. In the BASEL study, Mueller and colleagues[21] showed that the use of BNP levels significantly reduced the need for hospital admission (75% versus 85%) or to intensive care (15% versus 24%). Time to discharge also was reduced in the BNP group compared with the control group (8 days versus 11 days), without the trade-off of increased rehospitalization, resulting in

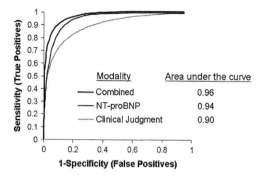

Fig. 2. Receiver operating characteristic curve comparison of results from NT-proBNP testing relative to clinical judgment. (*Adapted from* Januzzi JL, Camargo CA, Anwaruddin S, et al. The N-terminal Pro-BNP investigation of dyspnea in the emergency department (PRIDE) study. Am J Cardiol 2005;95(8):952; with permission.)

a significant cost reduction of 26%. Similarly, the IMPROVE CHF study[22] validated this point for NT-proBNP. In this randomized, controlled, blinded, prospective multicenter study, 500 patients presenting with shortness of breath to an ED were randomized to management strategy either guided by NT-proBNP results or standard clinical care. NT-proBNP guidance resulted in reduced duration of ED visits by 21% (6.3 to 5.6 hours; P = .031), rehospitalization over 60 days by 35% (51 to 33 days; P =. 046), and direct medical costs of all ED visits, hospitalizations, and subsequent outpatient services over 60 days from enrollment ($6129 to $5180 per patient; P= .023). These results were predicted by a decision-analytic framework analysis data obtained in the PRIDE study.[23]

The reductions in clinician indecision, common in dyspneic patients most likely explain the cost-effectiveness resulting from the use of NPs. Clinician indecision also is associated with more resource utilization, longer lengths of stay and worse outcomes. Routine earlier measurements of NPs have been related with better outcomes by reducing the clinician indecision about the correct diagnosis. This, along with more secure and early treatment, probably is linked to these differences in outcome.

Cut Points

NPs are continuously distributed variables, with some degree of overlap between patients with and without HF. The degree of this overlap is not fixed, with influence by numerous variables in the absence of HF, including normative processes such as age, but also relevant structural heart disease including abnormalities in heart rhythm, ischemic heart disease, valvular disease, and pulmonary hypertension. Accordingly, it should

not be surprising that a single cut point for either peptide is less helpful than considering the markers as continuous variables, where higher concentrations are more likely to be associated with HF and the converse.

For both BNP and NT-proBNP to exclude acute HF in symptomatic patients, very low values are necessary. For BNP, the value is approximately 20 to 30 pg/mL,[15] while for NT-proBNP, a cut point that has a NPV of 98% to 99% is 300 pg/mL.[20] Values above these levels, whether or not they are below the rule in cut point, may be associated with HF.

To identify acute HF, it has been argued that an advantage of BNP is the use of a single cut point of 100 pg/mL across all patient types. This overly simplistic approach ignores the foregoing discussion about the inability of this cut point to rule out HF, and the fact that several conditions, including advanced age, may lead to a BNP greater than 100 pg/mL in the absence of HF. Indeed, there is no manifest advantage of BNP over NT-proBNP when using a single cut point. The PRIDE investigators found that an NT-proBNP greater than 900 pg/mL provides an equal diagnostic value as a BNP greater than 100 pg/mL;[20] yet superior diagnostic accuracy could be had by simply adjusting for age, a significant confounder when interpreting both BNP and NT-proBNP. Accordingly, an age-stratified approach of 450/900/1800 pg/mL for ages less than 50/50 to 75/greater than 75 years was found to be superior to a single cut point.[24] Age-appropriate cut points for BNP are not known.

Gray Zone

When evaluating cut points of NPs in the diagnosis of HF, an intermediate or gray zone must be appreciated. For BNP, these values are between 100 pg/mL and 500 pg/mL, while for NT-proBNP, the value is between 300 pg/mL and the age-adjusted cut point (450 pg/mL, 900 pg/mL and 1800 pg/mL).[25,26]

Gray zone values of NPs are found in mild HF with normal systolic function, from other cardiac disorders such as myocardial ischemia or atrial fibrillation (AF), or from pulmonary embolism and infections. According to a subanalysis of the International Collaborative of NT-proBNP (ICON) study, clinical parameters including the absence of cough, a prior history of HF, presence of paroxysmal nocturnal dyspnea, jugular venous distention, and use of loop diuretics on presentation predict a diagnosis of HF.[26] Hence the clinical judgment assumes extra importance when the NP levels are in the gray zone.

ELEVATED NATRIURETIC PEPTIDE LEVELS WITHOUT HEART FAILURE

Chronic Kidney Disease

It has been reported that 33% to 56% of patients with HF have CKD, while conversely, patients with CKD have relevant structural heart disease that is equivalent to the loss of renal function. As noted previously, both NPs are cleared partially by the kidneys. Hence, patients who have CKD are expected to have elevated levels of BNP or NT-proBNP. Although this finding originally was considered a false positive, it now is known that elevated NPs in patients who have CKD predict structural heart disease and poor outcome.[27]

When used for diagnosing HF in patients who have CKD, BNP and NT-proBNP appear to be affected equally by loss of renal function. Both markers retain utility for diagnosing HF if adjusted for renal function. Subanalyses from the Breathing Not Properly Multicenter Study and the PRIDE study demonstrated that the accuracy of both NPs is impaired only modestly in patients who have renal dysfunction when compared with patients who have normal renal function with slightly higher cut points (200 pg/mL for BNP and 1200 pg/mL for NT-proBNP).[14,16,20] Using the age-adjusted cut points recommended by the ICON study, there was no need for changing the cut points to diagnose HF in patients who had CKD.[24]

Chronic Heart Failure

Among patients who have prior HF, elevation of NPs is anticipated, as they are sensitive measures of HF presence and severity, and these elevations are correlated directly with outcomes. When a dyspneic patient who has prior HF is evaluated with BNP and NT-proBNP, however, it may be challenging to differentiate acute or chronic HF from other causes of dyspnea. In this situation, it is important to compare the NP level with previous available NP values, or ideally with the dry NP value. As described previously, with the knowledge that the biological variation in stable chronic HF is 25%, a change in NP of greater than 25% is supportive of acute destabilization.

Coronary Artery Disease

Expression of the cardiac BNP gene is increased in myocardial ischemia, resulting in elevation of BNP and NT-proBNP. It is uncertain how ischemia triggers BNP release, but it may be related in part to ischemia-mediated wall stress or tissue-level hypoxia. Indeed, based on basic and clinical observations, such tissue-level hypoxia/ischemia has

been noted as an independent trigger for BNP release.[28–30] NPs may not be diagnostic of acute coronary syndrome, but are excellent predictors of mortality and morbidity in this condition.

Atrial Fibrillation

Both BNP and NT-proBNP levels are elevated in patients who have acute and chronic AF. NT-proBNP levels are higher in HF patients who have AF than in HF patients with sinus rhythm and have an independent prognostic value despite the presence of AF. Moreover, NP levels decrease after restoration of sinus rhythm by cardioversion. Furthermore, the NP levels also have been shown to predict the recurrence of AF following cardioversion and predict development of AF following pacemaker placement for sick sinus syndrome and postcardiac surgery.

Valvular Heart Disease

Diseases of cardiac valves may cause chronic pressure and volume overload, which leads to increase in myocardial wall stress; hence, there is increased secretion of NPs, even in the absence of HF. Among patients who have aortic stenosis, NP levels correlate directly with the mean transaortic valve pressure gradient, LV wall stress, and symptom status and inversely with valve area. Furthermore, NP levels have been shown to be predictive of the development of symptoms in asymptomatic patients with aortic stenosis and with outcomes after valve replacement surgery. Similar data exist for aortic regurgitation.

With respect to the mitral valve, BNP and NT-proBNP rise in parallel with the severity of regurgitation, even in the absence of symptoms and predict clinical outcomes. Similarly, among patients who have mitral stenosis, it has been reported that NP levels rise in proportion to the severity of the stenosis, which runs counter to the concept that they are LV markers. Lastly, right-sided valvular heart disease also may lead to elevations of BNP or NT-proBNP, but such elevations are typically lower than those associated with left-sided lesions; nonetheless, right-sided valvular heart disease should be considered when interpreting concentrations of these markers.

Pulmonary Diseases

Both BNP and NT-proBNP have been shown to be of value in sorting out the cause of dyspnea among patients who have both chronic obstructive airway disease and concomitant HF, and they may be able to identify a significant percentage of patients with chronic lung disease who have unexpected or masked HF. Having said this, NPs have been shown to be elevated in non-HF disorders that cause chronic right ventricular (RV) dysfunction, such as primary pulmonary hypertension, chronic obstructive pulmonary disease, thromboembolic pulmonary hypertension, and left-to-right cardiac shunts. In patients who have chronic pulmonary hypertension, an increase in NPs not only correlates with the degree of RV dysfunction but also with the risk for mortality.

With respect to pulmonary thromboembolism, a low NP level is useful for ruling out an adverse outcome, and elevated NP levels in patients who have acute pulmonary embolism suggest RV dysfunction and warrant further evaluation. A persistent elevation of NT-proBNP levels within 24 hours after an acute pulmonary embolism suggests severe right ventricular dysfunction and hence a poor prognosis, which warrants aggressive management. Based on this correlation, investigators have incorporated NT-proBNP in a risk stratification algorithm for patients who have acute pulmonary embolism.[31]

Critical Illness

Sepsis, major trauma, complicated major surgery, or other critical illness can impair cardiac function directly, leading to poor outcomes. Elevations of BNP and NT-proBNP levels occur in these settings and are directly predictive of adverse outcomes including death, independent of HF, LV mass, or intracardiac filling pressures, possibly reflecting myocardial depression from direct toxic effect of inflammatory mediators. Both BNP and NT-proBNP are independent predictors of outcome in unselected patients who are critically ill.

LOW NATRIURETIC PEPTIDE LEVELS IN HEART FAILURE
Nonsystolic Heart Failure

HF with preserved systolic function affects up to 50% of patients who have HF and is an important consideration when applying NP testing. Maisel and O'Donoghue and their colleagues[32,33] demonstrated that the presence of nonsystolic HF is associated with lower values for BNP and NT-proBNP, respectively, than those in patients who have systolic HF. This may lead, in patients who have nonsystolic HF, to an NP value below the rule in threshold, but rarely does it lead to a result below the rule out cut-point of 30 pg/mL and 300 pg/mL for BNP and NT-proBNP, respectively.

Body Mass Index

Levels of both NPs are significantly lower in overweight and obese patients in a manner parallel to BMI, and independent of the elevated filling pressures in these patients. The effects of BMI-mediated NP suppression include a change in optimal cut points for BNP, but not NT-proBNP. The authors of the Breathing Not Properly Multinational Study proposed a cut point of BNP 54 pg/mL in obese patients to improve sensitivity in this population. Although the level of NT-proBNP is also lower in obese patients, a subanalysis of the ICON study demonstrated no need for cut point adjustment for BMI when using the age-adjusted cut points, and NT-proBNP retained its prognostic ramification across all weight categories.

NATRIURETIC PEPTIDES IN THE MANAGEMENT OF ACUTE HEART FAILURE

A prerequisite for adequate management of HF is the correct and timely recognition of its presence and severity. As already discussed, NPs are not only important in evaluating patients for acute dyspnea in the ED but also, their use for managing acute HF in the ED is associated with less resource utilization, shorter hospitalization stay, and significant reduction in rehospitalization.

The standard approach for managing patients who have acutely decompensated HF is based on clinical assessment (including history, physical examination, vital signs, daily weights, and urinary output) and simple laboratory evaluations, including assessment of renal function. These approaches, however, have relatively poor sensitivity and specificity in decompensated HF patients, leading to high short-, medium-, and long-term mortality and readmission rates. Using simple parameters such as renal function, blood pressure, and some other variables, patients who have HF can be stratified as low-risk and high-risk. These parameters are less helpful, however, in treating and monitoring patients. In this regard, there is increasing interest in the use of NPs to monitor adequacy of therapy for acute HF, from presentation to outpatient follow-up.

It is accepted that NP levels at presentation offer significant prognostic information. A follow-up measure after treatment may be of even more value, however. More favorable outcomes are observed in patients who have considerable reductions in NP concentration during acute HF therapy, which argues for an association between adequacy of therapy for HF and NP values. Fall in the NP level after treatment for HF reflects reduction of the acutely raised filling pressures in patients who have acutely destabilized HF. Kazanegra and colleagues[34] first showed that among patients who responded to HF treatment, BNP levels fell in parallel with pulmonary capillary wedge pressure. Knebel and colleagues[35] also showed similar reductions in NT-proBNP, with a drop in pulmonary capillary wedge pressure following treatment. In contrast, those patients who did not have a significant improvement in filling pressures or hemodynamics did not have a significant decline in NT-proBNP values. Cioffi and colleagues[36] showed that the lack of response of NPs after treatment was not necessarily always associated with a fall in filling pressures, but was associated with reduction in adverse outcome.

The clinical significance of the response of NT-proBNP to therapeutic intervention in terms of clinical events has been assessed. Among 100 patients presenting with acute dyspnea, Bayes-Genis and colleagues[17] showed that the transhospital (day 1 to day 7) change in levels of NT-proBNP was 15% or less in patients who developed complications, when compared with patients who survived, who usually showed a 50% or greater fall in NT-proBNP levels from day 1 to day 7. In this study, the percentage reduction in NT-proBNP during admission for acute HF had an area under the receiver operating characteristic curve of 0.78 ($P = .002$), better than the presenting NT-proBNP concentration. Di Somma and colleagues[37] also showed a reduction of 58% in NT-proBNP concentrations over a 7-day period following successful treatment for acutely destabilized HF. Logeart and colleagues[38] showed that high predischarge BNP levels were a strong,

independent predictor of death or readmission, stronger than the commonly used clinical and echocardiographic parameters, following an episode of decompensated HF. These investigators also showed that patients who achieved a predischarge BNP level under 350 pg/mL had the most favorable longer-term outcomes.

Bettencourt and colleagues[39] demonstrated the importance of the transhospital gradient of NT-proBNP concentrations for predicting outcomes. Even though an NT-proBNP greater than 6779 pg/mL at presentation predicted a trend towards hazard for readmission or death, the post-treatment NT-proBNP value greater 4137 pg/mL was a more powerful predictor of hazard and a 8% increase in the odds for death or readmission over 6 months per 1000 pg/mL of NT-proBNP over this threshold ($P<.0001$). Furthermore, patients who had exhibited a greater than 30% drop in their NT-proBNP concentrations had superior outcomes compared with patients who had less than 30% decline, and dramatically better than those who actually had a rise in their NT-proBNP despite being considered ready for discharge from the hospital. This latter group had a very poor event-free survival after discharge (**Fig. 3**). These data support the monitoring of the discharge NP levels to determine the adequacy of the HF therapy and to predict hazard.

In light of these findings, a possible algorithm for BNP or NT-proBNP based management of in-patients who have acute decompensated HF is to obtain a baseline measurement for diagnosis, triage, and in-hospital prognostication, then treat the patient using the usual guidelines for HF.

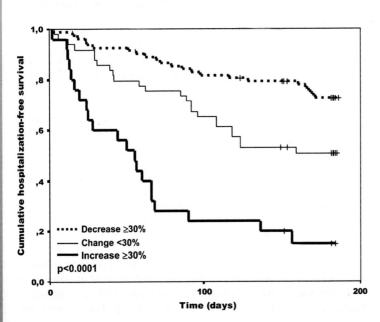

Fig. 3. Association between in-hospital change in NT-proBNP concentrations and subsequent outcomes among patients treated for acute heart failure. Among those with inadequate fall (or rise) in NT-proBNP concentrations, a significant risk for death or rehospitalization is noted. (*From* Bettencourt P, Azevedo A, Pimenta J, et al. N-terminal-pro-brain natriuretic peptide predicts outcome after hospital discharge in heart failure patients. Circulation 2004;110:2172; with permission.)

When the patient is viewed to be recompensated successfully on clinical grounds, obtain a BNP or NT-proBNP to evaluate for successful resolution (**Fig. 4**). Current data suggest that a fall of at least 30% during inpatient hospitalization would be desirable for either peptide, with absolute target values of less than 350 pg/mL for BNP and less than 4000 pg/mL for NT-proBNP.

FUTURE APPLICATIONS: MULTIMARKER PANELS

Now that it is established that BNP and NT-proBNP are powerful prognostic markers when used in isolation, there is considerable interest in the use of other biomarkers that complement risk stratification together with BNP or NT-proBNP, and which offer other targets for therapeutic intervention.

Natriuretic Peptides and Renal Function

The Acute Decompensated Heart Failure National Registry investigators demonstrated the importance of abnormal renal function for predicting death after an acute HF presentation,[40] but this analysis lacked NPs. As demonstrated by van Kimmenade and colleagues,[27,41] abnormalities in renal function are independently predictive of adverse outcome in patients who have acute decompensated HF, but only in those who present with very high NT-proBNP concentrations. Indeed, a proposal to redefine the concept of cardio–renal syndrome (previously defined as a change in serum creatinine greater than or equal to 0.3 mg/dL during acute HF treatment) was suggested by these investigators, who found that such a change in serum creatinine was of prognostic importance only in the context of a markedly elevated NT-proBNP. Furthermore, they showed that combining the two variables (ie, elevated NT-proBNP and a glomerular filtration rate (GFR) less than 60 mL/min/1.73 m^2) was superior for identifying patients with HF at highest risk for short-term death than either variable alone. In addition, they showed that HF subjects who had moderate or severe renal dysfunction but lower NT-proBNP concentrations had 60-day outcomes comparable to those without renal dysfunction.

Natriuretic Peptides and Troponins

Troponins frequently are elevated in HF without manifest myocardial ischemia. Despite the unclear nature of their mechanism of release, multiple studies have demonstrated a prognostic role for troponins in HF. As demonstrated by Sakhuja and colleagues,[42] the combined predictive value of an NP with a troponin in 209 patients who presented to the ED with acute HF was superior to either marker alone (see article by Latini in this issue).

Natriuretic Peptides and Anemia

Anemia is common in patients who have HF, and it has been related with poor outcomes in the acute HF setting. In addition, the deleterious effects of anemia on myocardial function may lead to elevated NP levels, even in the absence of HF. The ICON study[24] showed the serum hemoglobin level to be a significant independent predictor of short-term adverse outcome in acute HF. Baggish and colleagues[43] studied the combined predictive

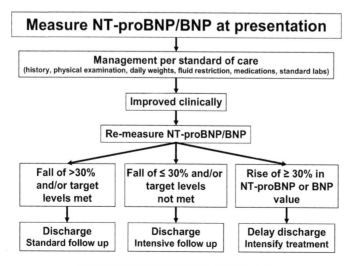

Fig. 4. A suggested algorithm for natriuretic peptide-based management of the inpatient with acutely destabilized heart failure.

power of hemoglobin as a function of NT-proBNP concentration in 690 patients who presented to an ED with acute HF, demonstrating higher 60-day mortality rates in anemic patients who had high NT-proBNP (23.5%) when compared to anemic patients with low NT-proBNP (9.2%) and nonanemic patients who had high NT-proBNP (13.9%). The investigators concluded that the combination of hemoglobin and NT-proBNP (greater than 5180 pg/mL) measurements provides powerful additive information and is superior to the use of either in isolation.

Natriuretic Peptides and Other Biomarkers

Apart from markers discussed previously, there are other markers that potentially can be used for risk stratification in acute HF. These include C-reactive protein (CRP), galectin-3 (a marker produced by activated cardiac macrophages), and ST2 (an interleukin receptor family member, produced by myocytes in response to stretch).

CRP was examined in the PRIDE study by Rehman and colleagues,[44] who demonstrated the importance of inflammation together with myocyte stretch (as reflected in NT-proBNP concentrations). In their analysis, hs (high sensitivity) CRP was independently and additively prognostic to NT-proBNP. This suggests that inflammation plays a pivotal role in the response to acute HF, and may be causative in negative remodeling after such an event. Indeed, the results from measuring markers of myocardial fibrosis, galectin-3 and ST2, support this concept.

Galectin-3, in combination with NT-proBNP has been shown to be a strong predictor of short-term mortality in acute HF.[45] An even more powerful predictor of death in acute HF is the marker ST2, a protein secreted by stretched cardiac myocytes and fibroblasts. ST2 has been examined in the PRIDE study[46] and in a larger pooled analysis.[47] In both, ST2 was a powerful prognostic marker, additive to NT-proBNP or BNP, and the combination provided superior risk stratification (see articles by Lee and de Lemos I in this issue).

Ultimately, a multimarker strategy such as that proposed by Rehman and colleagues[48] **(Fig. 5)** may provide such utility. Critical to this approach, however, is the recognition that expanded use of biomarkers for evaluating and managing acute HF will depend on the following four factors: (1) That the markers used provide independent (rather than redundant) physiologic information; (2) That the markers used provide independent prognostic value; (3) That the individual markers present a target for clinical decision making; and (4) That the markers used are robust, widely available, and cost-effective.

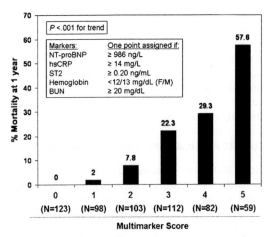

Fig. 5. Rates of mortality at 1 year among patients with dyspnea as a function of multimarker score. (*From* Rehman SU, Martinez-Rumayor A, Mueller T, et al. Independent and incremental prognostic value of multimarker testing in acute dyspnea: results from the ProBNP Investigation of Dyspnea in the Emergency Department (PRIDE) study. Clin Chim Acta 2008;392:43; with permission.)

SUMMARY

HF is a growing problem for the modern healthcare system, and the use of NP testing in patients who have known or suspected HF is useful in diagnosis and risk stratification. Such testing is being expanded to assess the efficacy of treatment of patients who have acute HF, and ultimately to the postdischarge care of such patients. The first steps into the biological era of HF care have been taken in acute HF. This era will expand, including biomarkers as an important component of the entire spectrum of management, from diagnosis through to chronic treatment.

REFERENCES

1. Fang J, Mensah GA, Croft JB, et al. Heart failure-related hospitalization in the U.S., 1979 to 2004. J Am Coll Cardiol 2008;52(6):428–34.
2. de Bold AJ, Borenstein HB, Veress AT, et al. A rapid and potent natriuretic response to intravenous injection of atrial myocardial extracts in rats. Life Sci 1981;28:89–94.
3. Galasko GI, Lahiri A, Barnes SC, et al. What is the normal range for N-terminal probrain natriuretic peptide? How well does this normal range screen for cardiovascular disease? Eur Heart J 2005; 26(21):2269–76.
4. Chang AY, Abdullah SM, Jain T, et al. Associations among androgens, estrogens, and natriuretic

peptides in young women: observations from the Dallas Heart Study. J Am Coll Cardiol 2007;49(1):109–16.

5. Das SR, Drazner MH, Dries DL, et al. Impact of body mass and body composition on circulating levels of natriuretic peptides: results from the Dallas Heart Study. Circulation 2005;112(14):2163–8.

6. Krauser DG, Lloyd-Jones DM, Chae CU, et al. Effect of body mass index on natriuretic peptide levels in patients with acute congestive heart failure: a ProBNP Investigation of Dyspnea in the Emergency Department (PRIDE) substudy. Am Heart J 2005;149(4):744–50.

7. McCord J, Mundy BJ, Hudson MP, et al. Relationship between obesity and B-type natriuretic peptide levels. Arch Intern Med 2004;164(20):2247–52.

8. Schou M, Gustafsson F, Kjaer A, et al. Long-term clinical variation of NT pro-BNP in stable chronic heart failure patients. Eur Heart J 2007;28(2):177–82.

9. Wu AH, Smith A, Wieczorek S, et al. Biological variation for N-terminal pro- and B-type natriuretic peptides and implications for therapeutic monitoring of patients with congestive heart failure. Am J Cardiol 2003;92(5):628–31.

10. Bruins S, Fokkema MR, Romer JW, et al. High intra-individual variation of B-type natriuretic peptide (BNP) and amino-terminal pro-BNP in patients with stable chronic heart failure. Clin Chem 2004; 50(11):2052–8.

11. Hunt SA, Abraham WT, Chin MH, et al. ACC/AHA 2005 guideline update for the diagnosis and management of chronic heart failure in the adult: a report of the American College of Cardiology/ American Heart Association Task Force on Practice Guidelines (Writing Committee to Update the 2001 guidelines for the evaluation and management of heart failure): developed in collaboration with the American College of Chest Physicians and the International Society for Heart and Lung Transplantation: endorsed by the Heart Rhythm Society. Circulation 2005;112(12):e154–235.

12. Arnold JM, Liu P, Demers C, et al. Canadian Cardiovascular Society consensus conference recommendations on heart failure 2006: diagnosis and management. Can J Cardiol 2006;22(1):23–45.

13. Tang WH, Francis GS, Morrow DA, et al. National Academy of Clinical Biochemistry Laboratory Medicine practice guidelines: Clinical utilization of cardiac biomarker testing in heart failure. Circulation 2007;116(5):e99–109.

14. Maisel AS, Krishnaswamy P, Nowak RM, et al. Rapid measurement of B-type natriuretic peptide in the emergency diagnosis of heart failure. N Engl J Med 2002;347(3):161–7.

15. Cowie MR, Struthers AD, Wood DA, et al. Value of natriuretic peptides in assessment of patients with possible new heart failure in primary care. Lancet 1997;350(9088):1349–53.

16. McCullough PA, Duc P, Omland T, et al. B-type natriuretic peptide and renal function in the diagnosis of heart failure: an analysis from the Breathing Not Properly Multinational Study. Am J Kidney Dis 2003;41(3):571–9.

17. Bayes-Genis A, Santalo-Bel M, Zapico-Muniz E, et al. N-terminal probrain natriuretic peptide (NT pro-BNP) in the emergency diagnosis and in-hospital monitoring of patients with dyspnoea and ventricular dysfunction. Eur J Heart Fail 2004;6(3):301–8.

18. Lainchbury JG, Campbell E, Frampton CM, et al. Brain natriuretic peptide and N-terminal brain natriuretic peptide in the diagnosis of heart failure in patients with acute shortness of breath. J Am Coll Cardiol 2003;42(4):728–35.

19. Mueller T, Gegenhuber A, Poelz W, et al. Head-to-head comparison of the diagnostic utility of BNP and NT pro-BNP in symptomatic and asymptomatic structural heart disease. Clin Chim Acta 2004;341: 41–8.

20. Januzzi JL Jr, Camargo CA, Anwaruddin S, et al. The N-terminal Pro-BNP Investigation of Dyspnea in the emergency department (PRIDE) study. Am J Cardiol 2005;95(8):948–54.

21. Mueller C, Laule-Kilian K, Schindler C, et al. Cost-effectiveness of B-type natriuretic peptide testing in patients with acute dyspnea. Arch Intern Med 2006;166(10):1081–7.

22. Moe GW, Howlett J, Januzzi JL, et al. N-terminal pro-B-type natriuretic peptide testing improves the management of patients with suspected acute heart failure: primary results of the Canadian prospective randomized multicenter IMPROVE-CHF study. Circulation 2007;115(24):3103–10.

23. Siebert U, Januzzi JL Jr, Beinfeld MT, et al. Cost-effectiveness of using N-terminal probrain natriuretic peptide to guide the diagnostic assessment and management of dyspneic patients in the emergency department. Am J Cardiol 2006;98(6):800–5.

24. Januzzi JL, van Kimmenade R, Lainchbury J, et al. NT pro-BNP testing for diagnosis and short-term prognosis in acute destabilized heart failure: an international pooled analysis of 1256 patients: the International Collaborative of NT-proBNP Study. Eur Heart J 2006;27(3):330–7.

25. Maisel AS, McCord J, Nowak RM, et al. Bedside B-type natriuretic peptide in the emergency diagnosis of heart failure with reduced or preserved ejection fraction. Results from the Breathing Not Properly Multinational Study. J Am Coll Cardiol 2003;41(11):2010–7.

26. van Kimmenade RRJ, Pinto YM, Bayes-Genis A, et al. Usefulness of intermediate amino–terminal probrain natriuretic peptide concentrations for diagnosis and prognosis of acute heart failure. Am J Cardiol 2006; 98(3):386–90.

27. van Kimmenade R, Januzzi JL Jr, Baggish AL, et al. Amino-terminal pro-brain natriuretic peptide, renal

function and outcomes in acute heart failure; redefining the cardio–renal interaction? J Am Coll Cardiol 2006;48(8):1621–7.

28. Toth M, Vuorinen KH, Vuolteenaho O, et al. Hypoxia stimulates release of ANP and BNP from perfused rat ventricular myocardium. Am J Physiol 1994; 266:H1572–80.

29. Marumoto K, Hamada M, Hiwada K. Increased secretion of atrial and brain natriuretic peptides during acute myocardial ischaemia induced by dynamic exercise in patients with angina pectoris. Clin Sci (Lond) 1995;88(5):551–6.

30. Kyriakides ZS, Markianos M, Michalis L, et al. Brain natriuretic peptide increases acutely and much more prominently than atrial natriuretic peptide during coronary angioplasty. Clin Cardiol 2000; 23(4):285–8.

31. Binder L, Pieske B, Olschewski M, et al. N-terminal probrain natriuretic peptide or troponin testing followed by echocardiography for risk stratification of acute pulmonary embolism. Circulation 2005; 112(11):1573–9.

32. Maisel A, Hollander JE, Guss D, et al. Primary results of the Rapid Emergency Department Heart Failure Outpatient Trial (REDHOT). A multicenter study of B-type natriuretic peptide levels, emergency department decision making, and outcomes in patients presenting with shortness of breath. J Am Coll Cardiol 2004;44(6):1328–33.

33. O'Donoghue M, Chen A, Baggish AL, et al. The effects of ejection fraction on N-terminal pro-BNP and BNP levels in patients with acute CHF: analysis from the ProBNP Investigation of Dyspnea in the Emergency Department (PRIDE) study. J Card Fail 2005;11(Suppl 5):S9–14.

34. Kazanegra R, Cheng V, Garcia A, et al. A rapid test for B-type natriuretic peptide correlates with falling wedge pressures in patients treated for decompensated heart failure: a pilot study. J Card Fail 2001; 7(1):21–9.

35. Knebel F, Schimke I, Pliet K, et al. NT-ProBNP in acute heart failure: correlation with invasively measured hemodynamic parameters during recompensation. J Card Fail 2005;11(Suppl 5):S38–41.

36. Cioffi G, Tarantini L, Stefenelli C, et al. Changes in plasma N-terminal proBNP levels and ventricular filling pressures during intensive unloading therapy in elderly with decompensated congestive heart failure and preserved left ventricular systolic function. J Card Fail 2006;12(8):608–15.

37. Di Somma S, Magrini L, Mazzone M, et al. Decrease in NTproBNP plasma levels indicates clinical improvement of acute decompensated heart failure. Am J Emerg Med 2007;25(3):335–9.

38. Logeart D, Thabut G, Jourdain P, et al. Predischarge B-type natriuretic peptide assay for identifying patients at high risk of re-admission after decompensated heart failure. J Am Coll Cardiol 2004; 43(4):635–41.

39. Bettencourt P, Azevedo A, Pimenta J, et al. N-terminal probrain natriuretic peptide predicts outcome after hospital discharge in heart failure patients. Circulation 2004;110(15):2168–74.

40. Heywood JT, Fonarow GC, Costanzo MR, et al. High prevalence of renal dysfunction and its impact on outcome in 118,465 patients hospitalized with acute decompensated heart failure: a report from the ADHERE database. J Card Fail 2007;13(6):422–30.

41. van Kimmenade RR, Pinto Y, Januzzi JL Jr. When renal and cardiac insufficiencies intersect: is there a role for natriuretic peptide testing in the cardio–renal syndrome? Eur Heart J 2007;28(24):2960–1.

42. Sakhuja R, Green S, Oestreicher EM, et al. Amino terminal probrain natriuretic peptide, brain natriuretic peptide, and troponin T for prediction of mortality in acute heart failure. Clin Chem 2007; 53(3):412–20.

43. Baggish AL, van Kimmenade R, Bayes-Genis A, et al. Hemoglobin and N-terminal probrain natriuretic peptide: independent and synergistic predictors of mortality in patients with acute heart failure Results from the International Collaborative of NT-proBNP (ICON) study. Clin Chim Acta 2007;381(2):145–50.

44. Rehman S, Lloyd-Jones DM, Martinez-Rumayor A, et al. Inflammatory markers, amino terminal probrain natriuretic peptide, and mortality risk in dyspneic patients. Am J Clin Pathol 2008;130(2):305–11.

45. van Kimmenade RR, Januzzi JL Jr, Ellinor PT, et al. Utility of amino terminal probrain natriuretic peptide, galectin-3, and apelin for the evaluation of patients with acute heart failure. J Am Coll Cardiol 2006; 48(6):1217–24.

46. Januzzi JL Jr, Peacock WF, Maisel AS, et al. Measurement of the interleukin family member ST2 in patients with acute dyspnea: results from the PRIDE (ProBrain Natriuretic Peptide Investigation of Dyspnea in the Emergency Department) study. J Am Coll Cardiol 2007;50(7):607–13.

47. Rehman SU, Mueller T, Januzzi JL Jr. Characteristics of the novel interleukin family biomarker ST2 in patients with acute heart failure. J Am Coll Cardiol 2008;52(18):1458–65.

48. Rehman SU, Martinez-Rumayor A, Mueller T, et al. Independent and incremental prognostic value of multimarker testing in acute dyspnea: results from the ProBNP Investigation of Dyspnea in the Emergency Department (PRIDE) study. Clin Chim Acta 2008;392:41–5.

Natriuretic Peptides in the Diagnosis and Management of Chronic Heart Failure

Guido Boerrigter, MD*, Lisa C. Costello-Boerrigter, MD, PhD, John C. Burnett, Jr, MD

KEYWORDS
- Natriuretic peptides • Biomarker • Heart failure
- Diagnosis • Prognosis

The concept of the heart as an endocrine organ was advanced 3 decades ago with the discovery that the heart synthesized and secreted atrial natriuretic peptide (ANP).[1,2] The authors[3] and other investigators[4] demonstrated the production and release of ANP and B-type natriuretic peptide (BNP) from models of experimental heart failure (HF) and from humans who had HF. These hormones have emerged as cardiac biomarkers that can aid in the diagnosis, prognosis, and management of HF. This article reviews the important clinical applications of these cardiac peptides, with a special focus on BNP.

B-TYPE NATRIURETIC PEPTIDE: A CARDIAC HORMONE ACTIVATED IN HEART FAILURE

Within the heart, the BNP gene (*NPPB*) produces a 134–amino acid pre-proBNP precursor peptide, which after removal of a 26–amino acid signal peptide, results in the 108–amino acid prohormone, proBNP (**Fig. 1**). Subsequently, the enzyme corin cleaves ProBNP into the biologically active mature 32–amino acid, BNP (BNP 1–32), containing the critical 17–amino acid disulfide ring. A second cleavage product is the linear 76–amino acid N-terminal peptide, NTproBNP 1–76. All studies suggest that mature BNP 1–32 binds to the natriuretic peptide A receptor, NPR-A;

activates the production of the second messenger cyclic GMP (cGMP); and mediates the biologic actions of BNP. These actions include natriuresis, vasodilatation, enhancement of ventricular relaxation, inhibition of fibroblast activation, and suppression of the renin-angiotensin-aldosterone system. The authors[5] and other investigators[6] reported that NTproBNP has no ability to activate NPR-A and generate cGMP and that the ability of proBNP to do so is markedly reduced. This reduced activation of NPR-A by proBNP and NTproBNP is highly relevant to the pathophysiology of HF because increasing evidence demonstrates that proBNP, not BNP 1–32, is the predominant circulating form. Thus, chronic HF may be considered a state of relative BNP deficiency.

Recent investigations have also documented that BNP 1–32 undergoes further processing by dipeptidyl peptidase IV, which removes the two N-terminal amino acids (Ser and Pro), producing BNP 3–32.[7] It is important to note that BNP 3–32 circulates, and its concentrations are increased in human HF.[8] Its physiologic significance is high because BNP 3–32 compared with BNP 1–32 has reduced natriuretic and diuretic properties and lacks renal vasodilatation.[9]

Treatment of HF can be challenging, especially when common symptoms and signs have only

---

This research was supported by PO1 HL76611 and RO1 HL36634 (JCB), and by T32 HL07111 (GB). JCB also has research support from BioRad.

Mayo Clinic College of Medicine, Rochester, MN, USA

* Corresponding author. Cardiorenal Research Laboratory, Division of Cardiovascular Diseases, Mayo Clinic College of Medicine, 200 First Street SW, Rochester, MN 55905.

E-mail address: boerrigter.guido@mayo.edu (G. Boerrigter).

Heart Failure Clin 5 (2009) 501–514
doi:10.1016/j.hfc.2009.04.002
1551-7136/09/$ – see front matter © 2009 Elsevier Inc. All rights reserved.

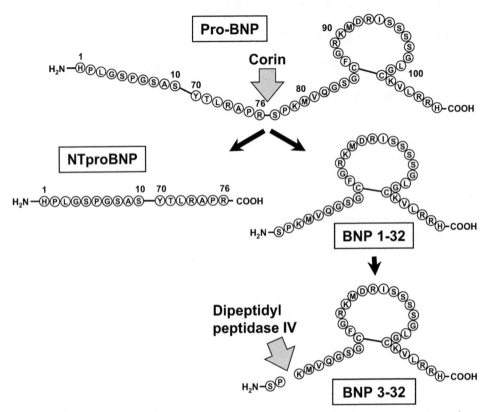

Fig. 1. Schematic of proBNP and its processing to NTproBNP and BNP 1–32 by the protease corin, and processing of BNP 1–32 to BNP 3–32 by dipeptidyl peptidase IV.

limited specificity. For that reason, a sensitive, objective, and cost-effective measure of patient status is highly desirable. The cardiac-derived natriuretic peptide BNP and its related peptides may be such markers. Given that myocardial stretch stimulates BNP production and release, that the heart is the major source of BNP, and that BNP can easily be measured in plasma, there is a straightforward rationale for evaluating circulating BNP as a biomarker for cardiac overload.[10,11] The following issues should be considered when interpreting data on BNP and its forms:

- Although BNP and NTproBNP have important biologic differences, many studies yield qualitatively similar results for these two proBNP products.[12,13]
- Although most BNP and NTproBNP assays were developed using antibodies directed against epitopes of these specific peptides, the forms ultimately detected in a sample can be expected to have considerable heterogeneity.[5,8]
- Many studies discussed in this article treated BNP as a stand-alone test; however, in practice, clinical assessment and other test results would also be considered (eg,

accounting for conventional risk factors can reduce the additional prognostic information gained from novel biomarkers).[14]
- Rather than using BNP with a single cut point, it may be better in many clinical applications to interpret BNP as a continuous variable; the use of two cut points with an intermediate gray zone has also been suggested.[12,15]
- BNP levels are affected not only by age, sex, cardiac load and clearance but also by genotype. For instance, a common single nucleotide polymorphism in the promoter region of the BNP gene (rs198389; also referred to as T-381C) was associated with 30% higher BNP levels per C-allele.[16–21] Not only may this genetic BNP elevation confound the interpretation of assay results, it may, given BNP's unloading actions, even paradoxically be associated with improved outcomes.
- Results observed in a specific population during a specific period of time cannot necessarily be extrapolated to other populations at other times with potentially different treatment standards.

The usefulness of BNP in the diagnosis of acute HF is described in an article by Januzzi found elsewhere in this issue, so the present review focuses on the following potential applications of BNP assays in chronic HF: (1) diagnostic and prognostic significance, (2) prognostic value of changes over time, (3) prediction of therapy benefit, (4) BNP-guided therapy, and (5) what is on the horizon.

DIAGNOSTIC AND PROGNOSTIC SIGNIFICANCE OF B-TYPE NATRIURETIC PEPTIDE

Given its association with cardiac load, it is not surprising that BNP has been found to convey diagnostic and prognostic information in acute HF and in other settings. Of note, BNP levels are affected not only by cardiac overload but also by factors such as age, sex, renal function, obesity, and genetic factors.[16–21] In the setting of acute HF, the contribution of these factors is small compared with the impact of cardiac overload so that even single, unadjusted BNP values can provide very good diagnostic yield. In the setting of asymptomatic disease, however, the contribution of these other factors is more relevant, and adjusting them may significantly improve test characteristics.[21,22]

The guidelines promulgated by the European Society of Cardiology[23] indicate that evidence supports the use of natriuretic peptides for diagnosing, staging, making hospitalization/discharge decisions, and identifying patients at risk for clinical events. The evidence for their use in monitoring and adjusting drug therapy is less clearly established.[23]

Wang and colleagues[24] showed in the Framingham Offspring Study that in asymptomatic individuals, BNP elevations well below levels used in the diagnosis of acute HF were associated with increased risk of death, first cardiovascular event, HF, atrial fibrillation, and stroke or transient ischemic attack after adjustment for cardiovascular risk factors. McKie and colleagues[25] confirmed in a large random sample of the general population in Olmsted County, Minnesota, that higher BNP and NTproBNP levels are associated with increased mortality even after adjusting for risk factors and echocardiographic parameters including systolic and diastolic dysfunction, left ventricular (LV) hypertrophy, and left atrial enlargement. This suggests that BNP can provide prognostic information beyond not only standard risk factors but also echocardiographic parameters. The investigators also reported that individuals in the highest tertiles of BNP had a higher prevalence of cardiovascular drug use, hypertension, coronary artery disease, and history of myocardial infarction. Of note, a small number of subjects who had BNP levels in the highest tertile did not have risk factors or echocardiographic abnormalities and did not show higher mortality (P.M. McKie, unpublished data, 2006). This finding might be explained by the impact of the genetic contribution mentioned earlier;[17–19] indeed, it would be worthwhile to formally evaluate the impact of genotype on outcomes.

In the Prevention of Events With Angiotensin-Converting Enzyme Inhibition (PEACE) trial, angiotensin-converting enzyme (ACE) inhibition with trandolapril compared with placebo in patients who had established coronary artery disease and an LV ejection fraction (LVEF) greater than 40% did not improve the primary end point, which was death from cardiovascular causes, myocardial infarction, or coronary revascularization, but it reduced the number of patients requiring hospitalization for or dying of HF. Omland and colleagues[26] evaluated 3761 study participants who had coronary artery disease but preserved LV function to determine whether baseline BNP and NTproBNP levels provided prognostic information in this patient population. After adjusting for relevant parameters, the hazard ratio per standard deviation of log-transformed NTproBNP was significantly increased for cardiovascular mortality (1.69), fatal/nonfatal HF (2.35), fatal/nonfatal stroke (1.63), but not fatal/nonfatal myocardial infarction (1.02). The corresponding hazard ratios for BNP were 1.06, 1.62, 1.15, and 0.91, with only fatal/nonfatal HF being significant. The inability of BNPs to predict fatal/nonfatal myocardial infarction may reflect the complex pathophysiology of acute coronary syndromes, which includes vascular and rheologic factors unlikely to be reflected by BNPs. Using the c-statistic as a measure of overall prognostic accuracy, NTproBNP in multivariate analysis performed significantly better than BNP in prediction of cardiovascular mortality, fatal/nonfatal HF, and fatal/nonfatal stroke. The addition of NTproBNP to the best multivariable model significantly improved the c-statistic for prediction of cardiovascular mortality (from 0.74 to 0.77) and HF (from 0.82 to 0.85); for BNP, this was only the case for prediction of HF (from 0.82 to 0.84). It would be interesting to know to what extent these findings would be affected if analyses were further adjusted for the rs198389 genotype, which as is discussed later, can influence circulating BNP. Also, it is unclear what therapeutic consequences, if any, elevated BNPs would have.

Epidemiologic studies have shown that about 50% of individuals who have LV systolic dysfunction are asymptomatic.[27,28] It has also been demonstrated that these patients who have acute

LV dysfunction are at increased risk of developing overt HF.[29] These patients have been shown to benefit from treatment, providing a powerful rationale to screen for asymptomatic LV dysfunction, and BNP has been evaluated for this purpose.[21,22,30–32] Reviews and meta-analyses are also available.[13,33,34]

Given that BNP can be elevated in a variety of conditions, a positive BNP test should be followed by an imaging study to confirm a cardiac pathology. Thus, choosing a BNP cutoff value with good sensitivity to keep the false-negative test results low may lead to a considerable number of false-positive test results; that is, a relatively large number of individuals will have normal imaging studies. Although these individuals would be considered "false positive" from the perspective of screening for LV dysfunction, given the risk associated with elevated BNP levels in the general population discussed earlier, it should be evaluated whether these false positives have a worse prognosis than subjects who have true-negative test results and would benefit from intervention.

The cost-effectiveness of BNP screening will be affected by the test characteristics of the BNP test, the costs of the assay and the imaging study, and the disease prevalence in the population. Therefore, screening in specific populations at higher risk (ie, patients who have coronary artery disease, hypertension, or diabetes, or are elderly) may be more cost-effective than screening the general population.

Fig. 2 shows receiver operating characteristic analyses and area-under-the-curve data for BNP (Biosite Triage assay, Biosite Inc., San Diego, CA) and NTproBNP (Roche assay, Roche Diagnostics, Indianapolis, IN) in the total population and in some subgroups of a random sample of the general population in Olmsted County, Minnesota. As mentioned previously, the common rs198389 single nucleotide polymorphism in the promoter region of the BNP gene has been shown to increase BNP values by about 30% per allele; this impact is comparable to that of sex, so accounting for it can be expected to improve test characteristics. Genotyping, however, would also affect the cost of the screening strategy.

In patients hospitalized for acute HF, higher BNP values at admission or discharge, in addition to percentage change, have been associated with worse outcomes. Logeart and colleagues[35] evaluated predictors of postdischarge outcomes of patients hospitalized for acute HF. The main outcome variable, which was death or rehospitalization for HF, was significantly predicted in univariate analysis by inotropic drug use; Doppler mitral inflow pattern; BNP values (Biosite Triage assay) measured at admission, at discharge, and during the hospitalization; and percentage decrease of BNP. In multivariate analysis, only predischarge BNP levels remained significant (hazard ratio: 1.14 [1.02–1.28] per 100-ng/L increment). Further analysis showed that a BNP level of 350 ng/L best discriminated between patients who had and did not have an event, and that the range from 350 to 700 ng/L represented an intermediate risk (**Fig. 3**). Prospective studies are required to assess whether strategies that decrease predischarge BNP levels will lead to improved outcomes.

CHANGES OF B-TYPE NATRIURETIC PEPTIDE OVER TIME

If cardiac overload negatively impacts prognosis and if BNP reflects cardiac overload, then

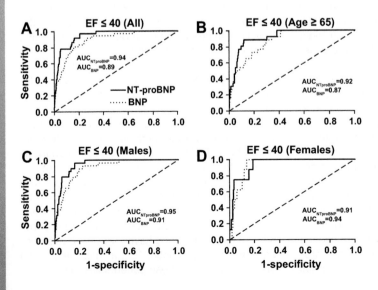

Fig. 2. Receiver operating characteristic curves of NTproBNP and BNP for detecting an ejection fraction of 40% or less in a random sample of the general population aged 45 years or older from Olmsted County, Minnesota, for the entire population (*A*), for patients aged 65 years or older (*B*), for male subjects (*C*), and for female subjects (*D*). AUC, area under the curve; EF, ejection fraction. (*From* Costello-Boerrigter LC, Boerrigter G, Redfield MM, et al. Amino-terminal pro-B-type natriuretic peptide and B-type natriuretic peptide in the general community: determinants and detection of left ventricular dysfunction. J Am Coll Cardiol 2006;47(2):349; with permission.)

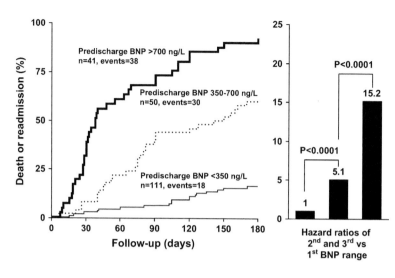

Fig. 3. Kaplan-Meier curves showing the cumulative incidence of death or hospital readmission according to predischarge BNP ranges in patients hospitalized for decompensated HF; $P<.001$ for trend among BNP ranges. Hazard ratios are shown on the right. (*From* Logeart D, Thabut G, Jourdain P, et al. Predischarge B-type natriuretic peptide assay for identifying patients at high risk of readmission after decompensated heart failure. J Am Coll Cardiol 2004;43(4):639; with permission.)

reductions in BNP would be expected to indicate an improved prognosis. If this were so, BNP could be used to help assess the efficacy of a therapeutic intervention in normal clinical practice and in clinical trials. Elevated levels could indicate impending clinical deterioration not yet apparent from symptoms and signs and trigger an earlier intervention, which could result in improved outcomes. With regard to BNP changes over time, there are important questions for clinical practice. How often should BNP values be determined? What constitutes a significant change that should trigger an intervention such as medication change or hospitalization?

Anand and colleagues[36] evaluated the prognostic information of BNP (Shionogi assay, Shionogi Co. Ltd., Tokyo, Japan) and norepinephrine in terms of baseline values and for changes from baseline at 4 and 12 months in the Valsartan Heart Failure Trial, which evaluated valsartan versus placebo in patients who had stable symptomatic HF and an LVEF less than 40% (mean age 63 years, mean LVEF 27%). Higher quartiles of baseline BNP were associated with a higher likelihood of the composite of mortality and first morbid event, defined as death, sudden death with resuscitation, hospitalization for HF, or intravenous inotropic or vasodilator therapy for at least 4 hours. Mortality rates in the four BNP quartiles (<41 pg/mL, 41–96 pg/mL, 97–237 pg/mL, and ≥238 pg/mL) were 9.7%, 14.3%, 20.7%, and 32.4%, respectively; relative risks for all-cause mortality were 1.47, 2.27, and 4.0 for quartiles 2,3,4, respectively, versus quartile 1; the corresponding values for relative risk of first morbid event were 1.50, 2.46, and 4.10. When change from baseline was expressed in absolute values, the highest mortality rates were found in the quartiles with the lowest and with the highest change.

Because marked reductions of BNP can occur only in patients who have high baseline values, which confer a higher risk, these results should not be surprising. Indeed, average baseline BNP was highest in the quartile that had the largest reductions. When changes from baseline were expressed as percentage change, however, the baseline values in the quartiles of percentage change were similar and mortality increased from the lowest to highest quartile (ie, patients who had larger percentage decreases fared better). The relative risk of adverse outcome was also significantly increased when quartiles of percentage change of BNP were adjusted for baseline BNP (1.30, 1.36, and 1.92 for quartiles 2, 3, 4, respectively, versus quartile 1; the corresponding values for relative risk of first morbid event were 1.41, 1.67, and 2.2). The investigators mentioned that the prognostic information of BNP was similar at different time points and in both randomization groups individually. To summarize, in this study, baseline BNP and percentage change over time were able to reflect risk of adverse outcomes, with the baseline data providing more robust information.

More recently, Miller and colleagues[37] investigated whether baseline cardiac troponin T (cTnT) and BNP (Shionogi assay) and changes over time were predictive of outcome (death, cardiac transplantation, hospitalization) in stable HF patients in an outpatient setting (n = 190, average age 71 years, median baseline BNP 305 pg/mL). Blood samples were collected every 3 months and physicians were blinded to the results. For the analyses, cTnT levels were divided into three categories (<0.01 ng/mL, ≥0.01–0.03 ng/mL, and >0.03 ng/mL). BNP values were dichotomized, with an elevation being defined as greater than 95th percentile of a normal, age- and sex-matched population. Elevated baseline cTnT and elevated BNP were associated with worse outcomes. An increase in cTnT over time increased risk, whereas a decrease reduced risk. In contrast, a change from normal to elevated BNP indicated an increase in risk, but after being elevated, this increased risk persisted regardless of subsequent changes. Combination of the two markers further refined risk prediction (**Fig. 4**). Of note, this study did not assess whether monitoring the two biomarkers added information that was not already obvious from the clinical assessment.

In a second report, Miller and colleagues[38] used the same dataset to better define what degrees of change in BNP are associated with outcomes. For this analysis, the investigators also measured NTproBNP. Changes were defined on a percentage basis (>80% decrease, 20%–80% decrease, no change, 20%–80% increase, >80% increase) and on whether there was a movement from below to above a cut point or vice versa (500 pg/mL for BNP, 1000 pg/mL for NTproBNP). The impact of changes on outcomes is shown in **Fig. 5**. With regard to BNP, only a BNP reduction of greater than 80% was associated with a risk reduction, whereas an increase from below to above 500 pg/mL was associated with an increased risk. With regard to NTproBNP, only a reduction from above to below the 500 pg/mL cut point was associated with a reduced risk of death. The investigators indicated that this analysis was meant to be hypothesis generating and did not correct for multiple comparisons. These findings are consistent with the high biologic variability reported in other studies. They also noted that although there was considerable overlap in category changes of BNP and NTproBNP, there was

also substantial variability. It remains to be established whether one assay is superior for monitoring HF patients or whether combining the information from both assays would be worthwhile.

B-TYPE NATRIURETIC PEPTIDE–GUIDED THERAPY

As discussed earlier, higher BNP levels are related to cardiac overload and have been associated with worse outcomes. This association provides the rationale for the hypothesis that intensifying treatment so as to reduce BNP levels below a certain threshold could improve outcomes. Important study characteristics to consider are the treatment goal (ie, target BNP value) and the treatment algorithm to be followed. Some of the study characteristics discussed in the following paragraphs are shown in **Table 1**.

Murdoch and colleagues[39] in 1999 published a small pilot study (n = 20) in which ACE-inhibitor dose was increased in stable, well-compensated HF patients according to target dose based on clinical trial data or so as to achieve a reduction of plasma BNP below 50 pg/mL. During the 8-week study, drug dose was increased significantly more in the BNP-guided group. BNP levels were significantly lower between groups only at 4 weeks. Hemodynamic function including right atrial pressure and systemic and pulmonary vascular resistance assessed at baseline and at 8 weeks was not different, with the exception of heart rate, which was lower in the BNP-guided group. The major limitation of this study was the small number of patients and the corresponding limited statistical power. Of importance, only 3 of 10 patients in the control group and 4 of 10 in the BNP-guided group achieved BNP levels below

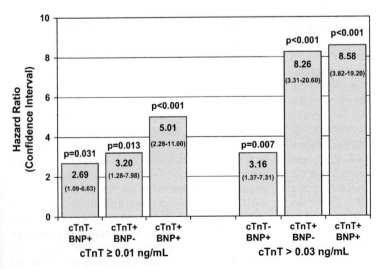

Fig. 4. Hazard ratios for risk of death/cardiac transplantation in ambulatory patients who have HF. Time-dependent multivariate model with serial follow-up cTnT and BNP values (every 3 months). + indicates elevated BNP or cTnT ≥0.01 ng/mL or >0.03 ng/mL; − indicates not elevated (hazard ratio 1.0 for no elevation of BNP or cTnT). (*From* Miller WL, Hartman KA, Burritt MF, et al. Serial biomarker measurements in ambulatory patients with chronic heart failure: the importance of change over time. Circulation 2007;116(3):254; with permission.)

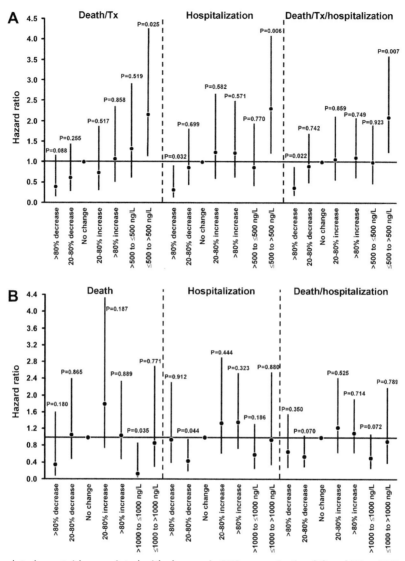

Fig. 5. Cardiac-related event risks associated with changes in BNP concentration (*A*) and NTproBNP concentrations (*B*) in ambulatory patients who have HF. Hazard ratios (95% confidence interval) from Cox models relative to no changes in BNP or NTproBNP or to no crossing over from more than to less than the BNP (500 ng/L) or NTproBNP (1000 ng/L) cut point values. Tx, transplantation. (*From* Miller WL, Hartman KA, Grill DE, et al. Only large reductions in concentrations of natriuretic peptides (BNP and NT-proBNP) are associated with improved outcome in ambulatory patients with chronic heart failure. Clin Chem 2008(1):81; with permission.)

the goal of 50 pg/mL. Therefore, although one expectation before the study was that BNP guidance might demonstrate that lower doses of ACE inhibitors would be sufficient to improve hemodynamic function and achieve "normal" BNP levels, the hormone guidance essentially forced maximization of therapy in most patients without necessarily achieving target BNP levels.

Troughton and colleagues[40] were the first to assess the impact of NTproBNP-guided therapy on long-term outcome in a study conducted from 1998 to 1999 (**Fig. 6**). Patients who had an LVEF

less than 40%, New York Heart Association (NYHA) class II through IV HF, and a plasma creatinine level 200 μmol/L or less were randomized to a control group (n = 36) or an NTproBNP-guided group (n = 33). The control group received standard care, which was up-titrated when clinical status as expressed by an HF score based on Framingham criteria indicated decompensation. In the NTproBNP-guided group, an additional aim was to reduce NTproBNP levels to less than 200 pmol/mL (about 1700 pg/mL). Of note, less than 15% of patients received β-blockers during this

Table 1
Baseline parameters in studies evaluating natriuretic peptide–guided therapy

Study	N	Age (y)	NYHA Class (Mean)	NYHA Class ≥ III (%)	LVEF (%)	Baseline NP (pg/mL)	Treatment Goal (pg/mL)
BNP							
Murdoch et al[39]	20	64/62	2.4/2.5	NA	25/25	139/111 pg/mL (mean)	<50
STARS-BNP[41]	220	66/65	2.2/2.3	21/29	32/30	NA/352 (mean)	<100
NTproBNP							
Troughton et al[40]	69	68/72	2.3/2.3	28/33	28/26	1835/2122	<1700
TIME-CHF[42,43]	499	77/76	NA	75/74	30/30	4657/3998 (median)	<400 (60–74 y) <800 (≥75 y)
BATTLESCARRED[44]	364	76–77 (median)	~2.2	24	37	1997–2021 (median)	<1300

Values are given for control group/hormone-guided group or for groups combined. The BATTLESCARRED trial consisted of three groups.
Abbreviations: BATTLESCARRED, NTproBNP-AssisTed Treatment to LEssen Serial CARdiac REadmissions and Death; NA, not assessed; NP, natriuretic peptide; NYHA, New York Heart Association; STARS-BNP, Systolic Heart Failure Treatment Supported by BNP; TIME-CHF, Trial of Intensified Versus Standard Medical Therapy in Elderly Patients with Congestive Heart Failure.

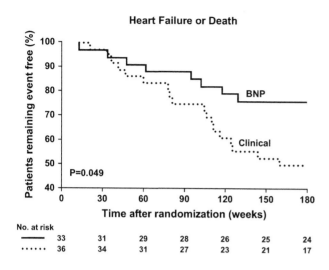

Heart Failure or Death

No. at risk

—— 33	31	29	28	26	25	24
······ 36	34	31	27	23	21	17

Fig. 6. Kaplan-Meier event curves for time to HF event or death in HF patients randomized to an NTproBNP-guided group (BNP) or a control group (Clinical). (*From* Troughton RW, Frampton CM, Yandle TG, et al. Treatment of heart failure guided by plasma aminoterminal brain natriuretic peptide (N-BNP) concentrations. Lancet 2000;355(9210):1128; with permission.)

study. During a median follow-up of about 9.5 months, the primary combined clinical end point (cardiovascular death, hospital admission, and outpatient HF) was significantly lower in the hormone-guided group compared with the control group (19 versus 54 events), whereas changes in symptomatic and functional status did not differ between groups. NTproBNP levels decreased in the hormone-guided group (−79 pmol/L) but remained unchanged in the control group (−3 pmol/L, P = .16 between groups). ACE inhibitor doses were increased significantly more, and more patients were started on spironolactone in the hormone-guided group. The average number of extra visits per patient was 1.7 in the BNP group and 0.8 in the clinical group (P = .19). Of note, in this study, a relatively high NTproBNP target was chosen compared with the other studies discussed in this section, and the average baseline NTproBNP value was only slightly above these levels, so achieving the treatment goal in the hormone-guided group was possible to a substantial degree.

The Systolic Heart Failure Treatment Supported by BNP trial enrolled 220 patients who had stable HF (no hospital stay in the previous month), NYHA class II through III HF, an LVEF less than 45%, stable (≥1 month) HF medication, including diuretic and guideline-recommended doses of ACE inhibitors/angiotensin II receptor blockers and β-blockers unless not tolerated.[41] Patients who had plasma creatinine levels greater than 250 μmol/L were excluded. Patients were randomized to standard medical therapy or to a BNP-guided group, in which the goal was to reduce BNP to below 100 pg/mL. Adjustment of therapy in both groups was at the discretion of the investigator. Patients were seen every month in the first 3 months (titration phase) and every 3 months

thereafter (follow-up phase). During the titration period, there were significantly more medication changes in the BNP-guided group compared with the control group (134 versus 66), and 79% of changes in the BNP-guided group were triggered by elevated BNP values. At the end of the titration phase, dosages of ACE inhibitors and β-blocker were significantly higher in the BNP-guided group. Although there were no differences in event rates between groups in the first 3 months, in the follow-up period, the primary end point, which consisted of unplanned hospital stays for HF or death related to HF, occurred significantly less often in the BNP group than in the control group (24% versus 52%). Event-free survival was also significantly better (84% versus 73%). All-cause mortality (7 versus 11) and all-cause hospital stays (52 versus 60 days) were not statistically different between the BNP group and the control group. Hospital stays for HF, however, were lower in the BNP-guided group (22 versus 48 patients), as were repeat HF hospitalizations (2 versus 10 patients). Mean BNP levels decreased from 352 to 284 pg/mL, with the proportion of patients who had BNP values less than 100 pg/mL increasing from 16% at baseline to 33% at 3 months.

The Trial of Intensified Versus Standard Medical Therapy in Elderly Patients with Congestive Heart Failure (TIME-CHF) was designed to assess BNP-guided therapy in younger (60–74 years, n = 210) and in older (≥75 years, n = 289) HF patients, the latter a group that is frequently underrepresented in HF trials.[42,43] Patients were included if they had an LVEF less than 45%, had been hospitalized for HF in the previous year, were in NYHA class II or higher, and had an NTproBNP value greater than 400 or 800 pg/mL for the younger or older patients, respectively.

Among the exclusion criteria were a body mass index over 35 kg/m^2 to reduce the impact of weight on symptoms and a plasma creatinine level greater than 220 μmol/L. The control group received standard medical therapy, and the aim was to reduce NYHA functional class to class II or lower. In the intensified treatment group, an additional treatment aim was to reduce NTproBNP levels to less than 400 pg/mL and 800 pg/mL for younger and older patients, respectively. The older patient group was, on average, not only older but also more symptomatic, had worse renal function, had more comorbidites, included a higher proportion of women and patients who had coronary artery disease, and had higher NTproBNP values compared with the younger group (5063 versus 2998 pg/mL).

The primary end points were quality of life and survival free of any hospitalizations; overall they did not reach significance. The secondary end points were survival and survival without hospitalization for HF. Mortality was reduced with BNP guidance in the younger group but not in the older group. Of interest, there was no difference in change in quality-of-life measures with intensified treatment in the younger group; however, patients in the older group who had NTproBNP guidance improved significantly less than those randomized to standard therapy. NTproBNP-guided patients received significantly higher doses of ACE inhibitors (or angiotensin II receptor blockers) and β-blockers, although there was no difference with respect to diuretics, nitrates, and digoxin. NTproBNP levels decreased in all treatment groups, but the decrease tended to be greater with intensified treatment in the younger ($P = .056$) but not the older patients ($P = .30$). It is important to note that even in the hormone-guided group, most patients did not achieve levels below the target NTproBNP levels.

The findings in the TIME-CHF show promising signals for NTproBNP guidance in younger patients and have provocative implications for the treatment of older patients. The major effect of BNP guidance was a dose increase of ACE inhibitors and β-blockers and the addition of mineralocorticoid receptor antagonists. All these interventions would generally have been assumed to improve outcomes on the basis of clinical trials (which were frequently conducted in younger patients who had fewer comorbidities). That this medication increase was not associated with a survival benefit but rather with less improvement in quality of life poses the question of whether medication target doses should be lower in at least some older patients. It should be noted that the lack of benefit in older

patients may be due to their poorer health rather than their age.

As mentioned earlier, NTproBNP levels decreased in both treatment groups in both age categories. It is important to note, however, that NTproBNP tended to decrease more in the NTproBNP-guided group than in the control group in younger individuals ($P = .056$), whereas this was not the case in the older patients ($P = .30$). If one accepts that NTproBNP truly reflects cardiac load, then one could draw the conclusion that NTproBNP-guided therapy did not improve outcomes because the therapeutic strategy used was not able to reduce cardiac load compared with the control group. In other words, the lack of benefit seen in older patients does not disprove the concept of a hormone-guided treatment approach but rather questions the efficacy of the treatment.

The NTproBNP-AssisTed Treatment to LEssen Serial CARdiac REadmissions and Death (BAT-TLESCARRED) trial was conducted at the Christchurch Hospital in New Zealand and enrolled patients within 2 weeks of an HF hospitalization.[44] Patients who had a reduced and preserved ejection fraction were eligible, but they needed to have prerandomization NTproBNP levels greater than 50 pmol/L (approximately 400 pg/mL) and a serum creatinine level less than or equal to 250 μmol/L. The trial was designed to compare three treatment strategies: usual care, intensive standardized clinical assessment, and intensive standardized clinical assessment plus NTproBNP guidance. In contrast to usual care, the two other treatments included a visit to the Christchurch Hospital research outpatient clinic at least once every 3 months with a thorough clinical assessment and, if appropriate, titration of medication according to a treatment algorithm. Intensification of drug therapy was triggered when a clinical HF score increased above a certain threshold indicating decompensation and, in the hormone-guided group, when the NTproBNP level was above 150 pmol/L (about 1300 pg/mL). Preliminary results were recently reported.[45]

Compared with the TIME-CHF trial, this study was conducted in a healthier patient population and had a less aggressive treatment goal. At 12 months after randomization, all-cause mortality was significantly lower with intensive follow-up compared with usual care, but without additional benefit from NTproBNP guidance (18.9% with usual care, 9.1% with intensive follow-up, and 9.1% with additional hormone guidance). At 2 and 3 years, there were no significant differences between treatments overall. In patients aged 75 years or younger, however, cumulative all-cause mortality was significantly reduced by NTproBNP guidance compared with (1) usual care throughout follow-up (cumulative mortality rates at 1, 2, and 3 years were 1.7%, 7.3%, and 15.5% versus 20.3%, 23.4%, and 31.3%, respectively) and (2) intensive follow-up by 3 years (cumulative mortality rates at 1, 2, and 3 years were 7.3%, 20.1%, and 30.9%; which was only significant compared with usual care at 1 year). The composite end point of death or hospital admission with HF was reduced with hormone-guided therapy compared with usual care only in patients younger than 75 years. No benefits were seen in patients older than 75 years.

The TIME-CHF and the BATTLESCARRED trial are very interesting studies. Important questions remain: Should there be individualized target NP values (eg, considering age, sex, renal function, body mass index, and genotype)? How many patients were able to reach the target range and what was their outcome? Is trying to lower the natriuretic peptide levels below the prespecified targets for most patients an exercise in futility that cannot be achieved by treatment algorithm and that consequently leads to maximal tolerated therapy? What was the number of physician visits in the treatment groups? What were the changes in medication (eg, diuretic dose)? Is further up-titration not required when patients have values below the target level? To what degree are cardiac status and comorbidities rather than age responsible for the differential results in younger versus older patients? One of the major conclusions may be that maximization of therapy beneficial in younger patients may be of less or no benefit in older individuals who have more comorbidities.

HF therapies come not only with a financial cost but also with a risk of complications and side effects. For that reason, it would be desirable to have a biomarker that could indicate in which patients the treatment is not required because of low risk or which patients are unlikely to benefit from a risky intervention. For instance, cardiac resynchronization therapy (CRT) significantly improves symptomatic status and survival, but a substantial percentage of patients appear to be nonresponders. In the Cardiac Resynchronization in Heart Failure trial, elevated NTproBNP was a significant predictor of adverse outcome, but patients below and above the median derived benefit from CRT relative to the control subjects who did not receive CRT.[46] Thus, NTproBNP levels do not seem to help in deciding for or against CRT.

In the PEACE trial, ACE inhibition with trandolapril compared with placebo in patients who had established coronary artery disease and an LVEF greater than 40% did not improve the primary end point, which was death from cardiovascular causes, myocardial infarction, or coronary revascularization, but it reduced the number of patients requiring hospitalization for or dying of HF. Given the association of BNPs with outcomes, it was hypothesized that patients who had higher baseline natriuretic peptide levels would have been more likely to benefit from ACE inhibition; however, no such interaction was found.[26]

ON THE HORIZON
What Exactly Are We Measuring?

As mentioned previously, most current assay systems use antibodies directed against epitopes of BNP 1–32 or NTproBNP. This approach can have only limited specificity, and indeed, several conventional assays also detect circulating proBNP.[5,6] Because proBNP has reduced biologic activity compared with BNP 1–32, nonspecific assays may not accurately reflect biologic activity.[5,6] Recently, a proBNP assay was developed that uses an antibody directed against the hinge region of proBNP so that better differentiation between prohormone and cleavage products is possible.[47] The capability to specifically measure proBNP may be important as it could reveal impaired processing of proBNP to BNP due to, for example, peptide glycosylation or decreased enzymatic activity.[48,49] Also, when a BNP assay uses antibodies directed against the ring structure and the carboxy terminus, it will not be able to differentiate between BNP forms that have a full compared with a cleaved amino terminus. BNP 3–32, which at least in vivo is produced when BNP 1–32 is cleaved by the ubiquitous aminopeptidase dipeptidyl peptidase IV, can be detected in plasma by specific assays, biochemically, or by mass spectrometry.[7,8,50,51] Although BNP 3–32 and BNP 1–32 have similar cGMP-activating properties in vitro in canine cardiac fibroblasts, the bioactivity of BNP 3–32 in vivo in healthy canines is reduced, presumably due to a shorter half-life.[9]

Other cleavage products of BNP 1–32 have been described by mass spectrometry, but their biologic activity and significance remains undefined.[8] It should be noted that in general, peptide cleavage may not only mean a quantitative reduction in bioactivity but may also qualitatively change the activity profile of a hormone.[52] At this time it is unclear whether more specific characterization of BNP immunoreactivity will yield higher diagnostic and prognostic information for the clinician than currently available assays that seem to provide a composite of different molecular forms. Tools such as mass spectrometry, however, will most certainly improve our understanding of the biology of the natriuretic peptide system and may provide the rationale for more specific assay developments and innovative therapies.[8,53]

Personalized Medicine with B-type Natriuretic Peptide

As mentioned earlier, BNP is a good example of how diagnostic tests can be affected by genetic variation. Accounting for genotype may improve test characteristics and thus improve patient management/prevention strategies. It can be expected that similar test-modifying genetic variants will be found in the future, as has been seen with prostate-specific antigen,[54] so that it may become worthwhile to develop a chip with a multitude of genetic markers that will help to individualize and refine the interpretation of diagnostic tests and the approach to prevention and treatment. In addition, it would be worthwhile to investigate whether genetically elevated BNP values have a protective effect regarding cardiovascular disease and especially HF. Such findings could provide a rationale for supplementing BNP or similar NPR-A agonists in subjects who have relatively reduced endogenous levels.

REFERENCES

1. de Bold AJ, Borenstein HB, Veress AT, et al. A rapid and potent natriuretic response to intravenous injection of atrial myocardial extract in rats. Life Sci 1981; 28(1):89–94.
2. Kangawa K, Matsuo H. Purification and complete amino acid sequence of alpha-human atrial natriuretic polypeptide (alpha-hANP). Biochem Biophys Res Commun 1984;118(1):131–9.
3. Burnett JC Jr, Kao PC, Hu DC, et al. Atrial natriuretic peptide elevation in congestive heart failure in the human. Science 1986;231(4742):1145–7.
4. Mukoyama M, Nakao K, Hosoda K, et al. Brain natriuretic peptide as a novel cardiac hormone in humans. Evidence for an exquisite dual natriuretic peptide system, atrial natriuretic peptide and brain natriuretic peptide. J Clin Invest 1991;87(4): 1402–12.
5. Heublein DM, Huntley BK, Boerrigter G, et al. Immunoreactivity and guanosine 3′,5′-cyclic monophosphate activating actions of various molecular forms of human B-type natriuretic peptide. Hypertension 2007;49(5):1114–9.
6. Liang F, O'Rear J, Schellenberger U, et al. Evidence for functional heterogeneity of circulating B-type natriuretic peptide. J Am Coll Cardiol 2007;49(10):1071–8.
7. Brandt I, Lambeir AM, Ketelslegers JM, et al. Dipeptidyl-peptidase IV converts intact B-type natriuretic peptide into its des-SerPro form. Clin Chem 2006; 52(1):82–7.
8. Niederkofler E, Kiernan U, O'Rear J, et al. Detection of endogenous B-type natriuretic peptide at very low concentrations in patients with heart failure. Circ Heart Fail 2008;1:258–64.
9. Boerrigter G, Costello-Boerrigter LC, Harty GJ, et al. Des-serine-proline brain natriuretic peptide 3-32 in cardiorenal regulation. Am J Physiol Regul Integr Comp Physiol 2007;292(2):R897–901.
10. Nakagawa O, Ogawa Y, Itoh H, et al. Rapid transcriptional activation and early mRNA turnover of brain natriuretic peptide in cardiocyte hypertrophy. Evidence for brain natriuretic peptide as an "emergency" cardiac hormone against ventricular overload. J Clin Invest 1995;96(3):1280–7.
11. Maeda K, Tsutamoto T, Wada A, et al. Plasma brain natriuretic peptide as a biochemical marker of high left ventricular end-diastolic pressure in patients with symptomatic left ventricular dysfunction. Am Heart J 1998;135(5 Pt 1):825–32.
12. Maisel A, Mueller C, Adams K Jr, et al. State of the art: using natriuretic peptide levels in clinical practice. Eur J Heart Fail 2008;10(9):824–39.
13. Clerico A, Fontana M, Zyw L, et al. Comparison of the diagnostic accuracy of brain natriuretic peptide (BNP) and the N-terminal part of the propeptide of BNP immunoassays in chronic and acute heart failure: a systematic review. Clin Chem 2007;53(5):813–22.
14. Wang TJ, Gona P, Larson MG, et al. Multiple biomarkers for the prediction of first major cardiovascular events and death. N Engl J Med 2006; 355(25):2631–9.
15. Coste J, Jourdain P, Pouchot J. A gray zone assigned to inconclusive results of quantitative diagnostic tests: application to the use of brain natriuretic peptide for diagnosis of heart failure in acute dyspneic patients. Clin Chem 2006;52(12): 2229–35.
16. Wang TJ, Larson MG, Levy D, et al. Heritability and genetic linkage of plasma natriuretic peptide levels. Circulation 2003;108(1):13–6.
17. Meirhaeghe A, Sandhu MS, McCarthy MI, et al. Association between the T-381C polymorphism of the brain natriuretic peptide gene and risk of type 2 diabetes in human populations. Hum Mol Genet 2007;16(11):1343–50.
18. Lanfear DE, Stolker JM, Marsh S, et al. Genetic variation in the B-type natriuretic peptide pathway affects BNP levels. Cardiovasc Drugs Ther 2007; 21(1):55–62.
19. Costello-Boerrigter LC, Boerrigter G, Ameenuddin S, et al. The B-type natriuretic peptide T-381C polymorphism is associated with increased BNP plasma immunoreactivity and higher prevalence of type 2 diabetes mellitus and atrial fibrillation. Eur Heart J 2008; 29(Abstract Supplement):766.
20. Redfield MM, Rodeheffer RJ, Jacobsen SJ, et al. Plasma brain natriuretic peptide concentration: impact

of age and gender. J Am Coll Cardiol 2002;40(5): 976–82.

21. Costello-Boerrigter LC, Boerrigter G, Redfield MM, et al. Amino-terminal pro-B-type natriuretic peptide and B-type natriuretic peptide in the general community: determinants and detection of left ventricular dysfunction. J Am Coll Cardiol 2006; 47(2):345–53.

22. Redfield MM, Rodeheffer RJ, Jacobsen SJ, et al. Plasma brain natriuretic peptide to detect preclinical ventricular systolic or diastolic dysfunction: a community-based study. Circulation 2004; 109(25):3176–81.

23. Dickstein K, Cohen-Solal A, Filippatos G, et al. ESC guidelines for the diagnosis and treatment of acute and chronic heart failure 2008: the Task Force for the Diagnosis and Treatment of Acute and Chronic Heart Failure 2008 of the European Society of Cardiology. Developed in collaboration with the Heart Failure Association of the ESC (HFA) and endorsed by the European Society of Intensive Care Medicine (ESICM). Eur Heart J 2008;29(19):2388–442.

24. Wang TJ, Larson MG, Levy D, et al. Plasma natriuretic peptide levels and the risk of cardiovascular events and death. N Engl J Med 2004;350(7):655–63.

25. McKie PM, Rodeheffer RJ, Cataliotti A, et al. Amino-terminal pro-B-type natriuretic peptide and B-type natriuretic peptide: biomarkers for mortality in a large community-based cohort free of heart failure. Hypertension 2006;47(5):874–80.

26. Omland T, Sabatine MS, Jablonski KA, et al. Prognostic value of B-type natriuretic peptides in patients with stable coronary artery disease: the PEACE Trial. J Am Coll Cardiol 2007;50(3):205–14.

27. Redfield MM, Jacobsen SJ, Burnett JC Jr, et al. Burden of systolic and diastolic ventricular dysfunction in the community: appreciating the scope of the heart failure epidemic. JAMA 2003;289(2):194–202.

28. McDonagh TA, Morrison CE, Lawrence A, et al. Symptomatic and asymptomatic left-ventricular systolic dysfunction in an urban population. Lancet 1997;350(9081):829–33.

29. Wang TJ, Evans JC, Benjamin EJ, et al. Natural history of asymptomatic left ventricular systolic dysfunction in the community. Circulation 2003; 108(8):977–82.

30. McDonagh TA, Robb SD, Murdoch DR, et al. Biochemical detection of left-ventricular systolic dysfunction. Lancet 1998;351(9095):9–13.

31. Vasan RS, Benjamin EJ, Larson MG, et al. Plasma natriuretic peptides for community screening for left ventricular hypertrophy and systolic dysfunction: the Framingham Heart Study. JAMA 2002;288(10): 1252–9.

32. Hedberg P, Lonnberg I, Jonason T, et al. Electrocardiogram and B-type natriuretic peptide as screening tools for left ventricular systolic dysfunction in

a population-based sample of 75-year-old men and women. Am Heart J 2004;148(3):524–9.

33. Ewald B, Ewald D, Thakkinstian A, et al. Meta-analysis of B type natriuretic peptide and N-terminal pro B natriuretic peptide in the diagnosis of clinical heart failure and population screening for left ventricular systolic dysfunction. Intern Med J 2008; 38(2):101–13.

34. Battaglia M, Pewsner D, Juni P, et al. Accuracy of B-type natriuretic peptide tests to exclude congestive heart failure: systematic review of test accuracy studies. Arch Intern Med 2006;166(10):1073–80.

35. Logeart D, Thabut G, Jourdain P, et al. Predischarge B-type natriuretic peptide assay for identifying patients at high risk of re-admission after decompensated heart failure. J Am Coll Cardiol 2004; 43(4):635–41.

36. Anand IS, Fisher LD, Chiang YT, et al. Changes in brain natriuretic peptide and norepinephrine over time and mortality and morbidity in the Valsartan Heart Failure Trial (Val-HeFT). Circulation 2003; 107(9):1278–83.

37. Miller WL, Hartman KA, Burritt MF, et al. Serial biomarker measurements in ambulatory patients with chronic heart failure: the importance of change over time. Circulation 2007;116(3):249–57.

38. Miller WL, Hartman KA, Grill DE, et al. Only large reductions in concentrations of natriuretic peptides (BNP and NT-proBNP) are associated with improved outcome in ambulatory patients with chronic heart failure. Clin Chem 2009;55(1):78–84.

39. Murdoch DR, McDonagh TA, Byrne J, et al. Titration of vasodilator therapy in chronic heart failure according to plasma brain natriuretic peptide concentration: randomized comparison of the hemodynamic and neuroendocrine effects of tailored versus empirical therapy. Am Heart J 1999;138(6 Pt 1):1126–32.

40. Troughton RW, Frampton CM, Yandle TG, et al. Treatment of heart failure guided by plasma aminoterminal brain natriuretic peptide (N-BNP) concentrations. Lancet 2000;355(9210):1126–30.

41. Jourdain P, Jondeau G, Funck F, et al. Plasma brain natriuretic peptide-guided therapy to improve outcome in heart failure: the STARS-BNP Multicenter Study. J Am Coll Cardiol 2007;49(16):1733–9.

42. Brunner-La Rocca HP, Buser PT, Schindler R, et al. Management of elderly patients with congestive heart failure–design of the Trial of Intensified versus standard Medical Therapy in Elderly patients with Congestive Heart Failure (TIME-CHF). Am Heart J 2006;151(5):949–55.

43. Pfisterer M, Buser P, Rickli H, et al. TIME-CHF Investigators. BNP-guided vs symptom-guided heart failure therapy: the Trial of Intensified vs Standard Medical Therapy in Elderly Patients With Congestive Heart Failure (TIME-CHF) randomized trial. JAMA 2009;301(4):383–92.

44. Lainchbury JG, Troughton RW, Frampton CM, et al. NTproBNP-guided drug treatment for chronic heart failure: design and methods in the "BATTLE-SCARRED" trial. Eur J Heart Fail 2006;8(5):532–8.

45. Richards AM, Lainchbury JG, Troughton RW, et al. NTproBNP guided treatment for chronic heart failure: results from the BATTLESCARRED trial. Circulation 2008;118(18):S1035, 5946.

46. Cleland J, Freemantle N, Ghio S, et al. Predicting the long-term effects of cardiac resynchronization therapy on mortality from baseline variables and the early response: a report from the CARE-HF (Cardiac Resynchronization in Heart Failure) trial. J Am Coll Cardiol 2008;52(6):438–45.

47. Giuliani I, Rieunier F, Larue C, et al. Assay for measurement of intact B-type natriuretic peptide pro-hormone in blood. Clin Chem 2006;52(6):1054–61.

48. Schellenberger U, O'Rear J, Guzzetta A, et al. The precursor to B-type natriuretic peptide is an O-linked glycoprotein. Arch Biochem Biophys 2006;451(2):160–6.

49. Wang W, Liao X, Fukuda K, et al. Corin variant associated with hypertension and cardiac hypertrophy exhibits impaired zymogen activation and natriuretic peptide processing activity. Circ Res 2008;103(5):502–8.

50. Lam CS, Burnett JC Jr, Costello-Boerrigter L, et al. Alternate circulating pro-B-type natriuretic peptide and B-type natriuretic peptide forms in the general population. J Am Coll Cardiol 2007;49(11):1193–202.

51. Shimizu H, Masuta K, Aono K, et al. Molecular forms of human brain natriuretic peptide in plasma. Clin Chim Acta 2002;316(1–2):129–35.

52. Ban K, Noyan-Ashraf MH, Hoefer J, et al. Cardioprotective and vasodilatory actions of glucagon-like peptide 1 receptor are mediated through both glucagon-like peptide 1 receptor-dependent and -independent pathways. Circulation 2008;117(18):2340–50.

53. Hawkridge AM, Heublein DM, Bergen HR 3rd, et al. Quantitative mass spectral evidence for the absence of circulating brain natriuretic peptide (BNP-32) in severe human heart failure. Proc Natl Acad Sci U S A 2005;102(48):17442–7.

54. Cramer SD, Chang BL, Rao A, et al. Association between genetic polymorphisms in the prostate-specific antigen gene promoter and serum prostate-specific antigen levels. J Natl Cancer Inst 2003;95(14):1044–53.

ST2 and Adrenomedullin in Heart Failure

Rahul Kakkar, MD[a],*, Richard T. Lee, MD[b]

KEYWORDS

- Adrenomedullin • ST2 • Heart failure • Biomarker
- Systolic dysfunction

The assessment of congestive heart failure is based primarily on clinical history, physical examination, and hemodynamic assessment that are rooted in the observations and writings of humanity's first physicians. In contrast, our knowledge of the systemic perturbations, organ-based adaptations, and cellular and molecular alterations of advanced heart failure has exploded over the past half century. As the power of molecular biology has been brought to bear on this devastating disease, novel ways of diagnosing and monitoring heart failure are beginning to emerge. One new approach is centered on the biomarkers that are induced by mechanically overloaded myocardium. One of the most conspicuous examples of this is that of the natriuretic peptides, which were characterized and introduced into routine clinical practice over the past two decades. Further work has identified numerous potential biomarkers that are currently undergoing evaluation.[1,2] Two of these proteins, ST2 and adrenomedullin, are discussed in this article.

ST2, which was originally described in the context of CD4+ T-cell function in inflammatory conditions such as asthma, has recently emerged as a cardiovascular biomarker for the presence of ventricular mechanical overload. Serum ST2 levels help dichotomize patients who presented with acute dyspnea of unclear etiology into those who are and those who are not suffering from an acute heart failure exacerbation, and serum ST2 concentrations also offer prognostic value complementary to that afforded by the natriuretic peptides.

Adrenomedullin, which was originally identified as a vasoactive compound able to activate platelets, appears to counteract the myriad known systemic derangements that typify the syndrome of heart failure, from alterations in systemic vascular resistance to control of renal fluid handling. Adrenomedullin appears to modulate ventricular remodeling in the face of altered loading conditions as well. In addition to these physiologic effects, the measurement of serum adrenomedullin concentrations can be used to predict mortality in patients with acute heart failure.

ST2
Biology

ST2 is a protein receptor classified as a member of the toll-like/IL-1-receptor superfamily. The gene for ST2 spans approximately 40 kilobases on human chromosome 2, which is part of the larger human IL-1 gene locus (**Fig. 1**). ST2 (also referred to in the literature as IL1RL1, DER4, T1, and FIT-1) displays marked conservation across species, with homologs in the genomes of the mouse, rat, and fruit fly. ST2 was initially discovered in 1989 at two laboratories by investigators working with *in vitro* growth-stimulated mouse fibroblasts. They independently described a secreted,

Brigham and Women's Hospital has filed for intellectual property rights on ST2, listing Richard T. Lee as an inventor.

[a] Massachusetts General Hospital, Boston, MA, USA
[b] Brigham and Women's Hospital Partners Research Facility, Cambridge, MA, USA
* Corresponding author. Division of Cardiology, Massachusetts General Hospital, 55 Fruit Street, GRB-804, Boston, MA 02114.
E-mail address: rkakkar@partners.org (R. Kakkar).

Heart Failure Clin 5 (2009) 515–527
doi:10.1016/j.hfc.2009.04.009
1551-7136/09/$ – see front matter © 2009 Published by Elsevier Inc.

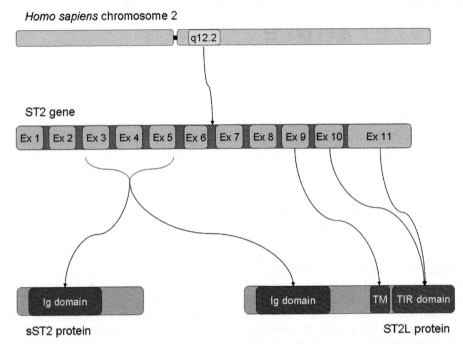

Fig. 1. Human ST2. A schematic representation of the ST2 gene on human chromosome 2 with its intron/exon structure and a depiction of the protein structure of soluble (sST2) and membrane-bound (ST2L) ST2 variants. Also depicted are the immunoglobulin (Ig) domains common to sST2 and ST2L and the transmembrane (TM) and the class-identifying toll/Interleukin-1 receptor domain domain unique to ST2L.

glycosylated protein that would come to be known as soluble ST2 (sST2).[3–7] In 1993, a related mRNA transcript, which encodes a transmembrane motif, was identified. This transcript would ultimately prove to be the cell-surface form of the ST2 receptor ST2L.[8] The overall structure of ST2L is similar to the structure of the type 1 IL-1 receptors, which are composed of an extracellular domain of three linked immunoglobulin-like motifs, a transmembrane segment, and a toll/Interleukin-1 receptor domain cytoplasmic domain that mediates intracellular signaling. The soluble isoform of ST2 lacks the transmembrane and cytoplasmic domains contained within the structure of ST2L.[9] Several splice variants of ST2 exist as well.[10]

Initial investigation into the expression pattern and biology of ST2 revealed that ST2L is constitutively expressed and restricted to the surface of type 2 helper T cells and mast cells, not expressed by type 1 helper T cells or other immune cells.[11–13] A role for ST2L in diseases attributed to T cell–mediated inflammation, such as asthma and rheumatoid arthritis, was subsequently documented.[14,15] In contrast, sST2 expression is largely inducible and initially appeared restricted to the integument (including fibroblasts).[16,17] Early work suggested that sST2 may serve as a biomarker for type 2 helper T cell–related inflammatory conditions, particularly for acute exacerbations of asthma.[18]

For more than a decade, the ligand for ST2L remained elusive, despite a search by investigators in many laboratories. In 2005, a protein was identified by mining the public genome database using a sequence common to IL-1 and fibroblast growth factor.[19] The 30-kDa protein, which was processed using caspase-1 to an 18-kDa form, was named IL-33 and has been classified as a member of the IL-1 interleukin family (designated IL-1F11). Members of this family of proteins are characterized by an array of 12 β strands (the IL-1/FGF "β-trefoil fold") and the absence of a classical secretory amino-terminus peptide sequence.

Relations to IL-33

IL-33 is synthesized by many cell types. After synthesis, secreted IL-33 probably binds either extracellular sST2, where it is sequestered from the biologically active pool, or ST2L on an effector cell's surface plasma membrane (**Fig. 2**). The IL-33 receptor is a complex of ST2L and the IL-1 receptor accessory protein. After binding with IL-33, this receptor complex associates with intracellular adaptor molecules to initiate a signal cascade that displays many features of the canonical

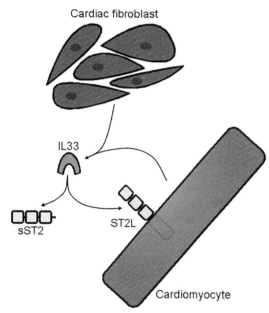

Cardiac fibroblast

IL33

sST2

ST2L

Cardiomyocyte

Fig. 2. A model for IL-33 and ST2 signaling in the heart. IL-33 released from cardiac fibroblasts and ventricular cardiomyocytes during episodes of increased biomechanical strain may bind to free sST2, thereby removing it from the bioactive pool. Alternatively, IL-33 may bind to its receptor on the cardiomyocyte plasma membrane, a complex that includes ST2L. Binding of IL-33 to its receptor elicits an intracellular signaling cascade that ultimately results in nuclear-factor kappaB–mediated transcription and the initiation of an antihypertrophic, prosurvival gene program.

toll-like receptor signaling pathway. Several protein kinases are activated, and concurrently, induction of nuclear-factor kappaB activity results in initiation of a nuclear transcription program.

In 2002, a microarray-based search for up-regulated transcripts in mechanically stimulated cardiomyocytes in vitro uncovered the first evidence of inducible ST2 expression in the cardiovascular system.[20] Because the components of the IL-33/ST2 system were classically known to exist in fibroblasts and immune cells, it was hypothesized that perhaps this ligand–receptor pair was involved in cross talk between cardiomyocytes and support cells of the cardiac ventricle under conditions of elevated biomechanical strain. Supporting this hypothesis, data published to date suggest that IL-33 and ST2 may compose a myocyte–fibroblast paracrine system that regulates responses of the ventricular myocardium to altered loading conditions, including myocyte hypertrophy and chamber fibrosis.[21,22]

In the face of exogenous prohypertrophic stimuli such as angiotensin II, IL-33 administration results

in attenuation of cellular hypertrophy. If sST2 is added to the cell culture media, the effects of IL-33 are inhibited, consistent with the hypothesis that sST2 functions as a "decoy" receptor. IL-33 itself is expressed robustly by cardiac fibroblasts, at levels greater than those seen in cardiac myocytes. Cardiac fibroblast expression levels increase in response to mechanical strain and angiotensin II exposure.[23] In animal experiments using mice with germ-line deletion of ST2 and therefore loss of the IL-33 receptor, partial transaortic constriction (as a model of increased afterload) resulted in a greater degree of ventricular fibrosis and myocyte hypertrophy than that seen in wild-type mice. Enhanced chamber hypertrophy and a reduced ejection fraction were observed in the ST2 null mice. In wild-type mice subjected to transaortic constriction that were exposed to exogenous IL-33, cardiac hypertrophy was attenuated, gene expression of brain natriuretic peptide (BNP) reduced, and survival improved in comparison with untreated controls.[23] Taken together, these data suggest that cardiac fibroblast–derived IL-33 may exert a beneficial antihypertrophic effect on overloaded cardiomyocytes and that the IL-33/ST2 system may be critical for preventing fibroblast-mediated myocardial fibrosis in the face of elevated biomechanical strain.

A less commonly discussed feature of heart failure is that of cellular inflammation, which is measurable using serum markers and on pathologic and histologic examination of the myocardium.[1,24,25] There is evidence for a CD4+ T-cell component to the myocardial inflammation of chronic heart failure,[26] and because ST2 was originally described in the context of T-cell functions, it is intriguing to consider how a T cell–based inflammatory process may represent leukocyte-fibroblast-myocyte cross talk within the injured or stressed ventricle. The specific role that the ST2 may be playing in this aspect of the heart failure phenotype is as of yet unstudied.

ST2 as a Biomarker

sST2 is believed to be a secreted protein in that it is measurable in serum. Although the precise tissue origin of serum ST2 is a subject of some debate,[27] its initial cardiovascular characterization suggested that serum concentrations increase transiently in the period after experimental myocardial infarction.[20] To determine the possible applicability of these findings to human biology, serum samples from a subset of patients who had an acute ST-segment elevation or Q-wave myocardial infarction and who were enrolled in the Healing and Early Afterload Reducing Therapy

(HEART) study were analyzed. Serum ST2 concentrations were elevated during the initial days after presentation, falling thereafter. Peak levels correlated with peak creatine kinase levels and correlated inversely with left ventricular ejection fraction.[20]

Whether these observations implied that serum ST2 reflected ventricular injury or ventricular strain (as its basic biology would suggest) was still unclear. To explore this, in 2004, Shimpo and colleagues[28] assayed serum ST2 concentrations in more than 800 patients who presented to a tertiary care hospital with an acute ST-elevation myocardial infarction. Levels of sST2 at the time of presentation were found to correlate with in-hospital and 30-day mortality. Multivariate analysis demonstrated that the serum ST2 level was independently associated with 30-day mortality, after controlling for established clinical factors such as age, heart rate, blood pressure, infarct territory, and Killip heart failure class (**Fig. 3**).

These data suggested that sST2 may be similar to the natriuretic peptides, representing a marker of ventricular biomechanical strain rather than cardiomyocyte plasma membrane disruption, the presumed mechanism of release of troponin and creatine kinase. To explore the role of sST2 in the absence of infarction, a subsequent study analyzed serum levels of ST2 in patients who had advanced, stable, nonischemic congestive heart failure that was defined as a reduced left ventricular ejection fraction and New York Heart Association (NYHA) functional class III and IV symptoms. In this context, serum levels of sST2 at the time of study entry correlated with serum norepinephrine and brain natriuretic peptide levels. Furthermore, an increase in serum ST2 levels (though not baseline levels) over a 2-week period was found to independently predict the risk for reaching a combined clinical endpoint of mortality and cardiac transplantation in a multivariate model inclusive of serum levels of the natriuretic peptides BNP and atrial natriuretic peptide.[29]

Clinical Value of ST2 Measurements

The potential clinical utility of sST2 was explored by examining serum levels in patients enrolled in the Pro-Brain Natriuretic Peptide Investigation of Dyspnea in the Emergency Department (PRIDE) study, which was a prospective study of patients who presented to an emergency department with dyspnea. The PRIDE study was designed to validate the use of amino-terminal pro-brain natriuretic peptide (NT-proBNP) in differentiating acute heart failure from other causes of shortness of breath.[30] In an analysis of blood samples from nearly 600 patients, serum concentrations of sST2 were significantly higher in those who presented with acute systolic heart failure in comparison with serum levels in patients who presented with noncardiac causes of dyspnea. Patients who had a serum sST2 level on presentation greater than the median of 0.20 ng/mL had an 11-fold increase in the risk for death at 1 year in comparison with patients who had lower serum sST2 concentrations (**Fig. 4A**). When stratified by decile, patients in the lowest decile concentration of serum sST2 had a 1-year mortality of less than 5%, whereas those in the highest decile had a 1-year mortality of nearly 45%. Of the patients who presented with acute heart failure and an elevated serum NT-proBNP concentration, a concurrent elevation of serum ST2 level conferred a marked increase in the risk for death over the ensuing year. Of those patients who presented with acute dyspnea who were determined to have heart failure on clinical grounds but who had a low serum NT-proBNP concentration, the measurement of serum ST2 levels did not provide additional prognostic information (see **Fig. 4B**).[31] A recent follow-up study that combined data from

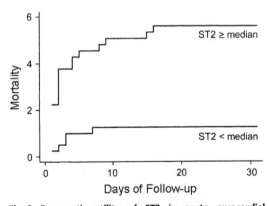

Fig. 3. Prognostic utility of ST2 in acute myocardial infarction. The prognostic utility of serum ST2 in the context of an acute coronary syndrome was evaluated in patients enrolled in the TIMI 14 and TIMI 38 clinical trials. In more than 800 patients who had an acute ST-elevation myocardial infarction, sST2 levels at the time of presentation were found to correlate with in-hospital and 30-day mortality. Multivariate analysis demonstrated that the serum ST2 level was independently associated with 30-day mortality, after controlling for established predictors of mortality such as age, heart rate, blood pressure, infarct territory, and Killip heart failure class. (*Adapted from* Shimpo M, Morrow DA, Weinberg EO, et al. Serum levels of the interleukin-1 receptor family member ST2 predict mortality and clinical outcome in acute myocardial infarction. Circulation 2004;109(18):2188; with permission.)

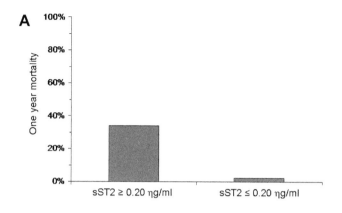

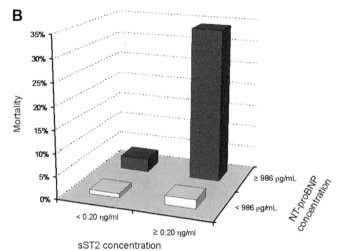

Fig. 4. Prognostic value of ST2 in patients with acute heart failure. (*A*) The prognostic utility of serum ST2 was evaluated in a study of patients who presented to a hospital emergency ward with dyspnea. Patients who had a serum sST2 concentration greater than the median of 0.2 ηg/mL conferred a mortality rate of approximately 35% over the ensuing year. This contrasted with that of patients who had a serum sST2 concentration of less than the median, who had 1-year mortality rate of less than 5%. (*B*) ST2 in combination with NT-proBNP in patients who had acute heart failure. In the same cohort of patients as **Fig. 4A**, those patients who had been determined to have heart failure on clinical grounds and were noted to have an elevated NT-proBNP concentration ($\geq$986 ρg/mL), an sST2 level greater than the median of 0.2 ηg/mL conferred an approximately 35% mortality rate over the ensuing year. For those who had clinical heart failure and NT-proBNP levels below 986 ρg/mL, the measurement of serum ST2 added little prognositc information. (*Data from* Januzzi JL. Jr, Peacock WF, Maisel AS, et al. Measurement of the interleukin family member ST2 in patients with acute dyspnea: results from the PRIDE (Pro-Brain Natriuretic Peptide Investigation of Dyspnea in the Emergency Department) study. J Am Coll Cardiol 2007;50(7):607–13.)

the PRIDE study and a second NT-proBNP trial suggested that ST2 concentrations are elevated in patients who have both ischemic and nonischemic heart failure. In this analysis, ST2 was determined to be a predictor of mortality independent of NT-proBNP and to add power to the prognostic utility of the natriuretic peptide in both subcategories of cardiomyopathy.[32]

Other studies bolstered the concept that sST2 provides prognostic information that is independent and complementary to more traditional methods of risk stratification. As reported by Sabatine and colleagues,[33] serum sST2 levels of 1200 patients in the Clopidogrel as Adjunctive Reperfusion Therapy - Thrombolysis in Myocardial Infarction 28 study, which enrolled patients who presented to a hospital with an acute ST-elevation myocardial infarction, correlated with impaired epicardial coronary flow and the subsequent risk for cardiovascular death or congestive heart failure. In a multivariate analysis, serum sST2 concentration was found to be independently predictive of cardiovascular death or heart failure

within 30 days of presentation. Patients who presented with an ST-elevation myocardial infarction and a baseline NT-proBNP level in the highest quartile displayed an odds ratio of 2.4 for the risk for cardiovascular death or heart failure at 30 days, whereas those with a baseline sST2 level in the highest quartile had an odds ratio of 3.6 (**Fig. 5**). In patients who presented with ST-elevation myocardial infarction but with a low TIMI risk score, those who had serum sST2 and NT-proBNP concentrations that were greater than the median demonstrated a 6.6-fold increase in the risk for cardiovascular death or heart failure at 30 days, which was equivalent to the risk afforded by a high TIMI risk score alone. Patients who had a high TIMI risk score and sST2 and NT-proBNP levels greater than the median had an approximately 25-fold increase in the risk for cardiovascular death or heart failure (**Fig. 6**).[33]

Morrow and de Lemos[2] set out three criteria by which potential biomarkers should be evaluated. They suggested that biomarkers seeking a place within the clinician's toolbox must be measurable

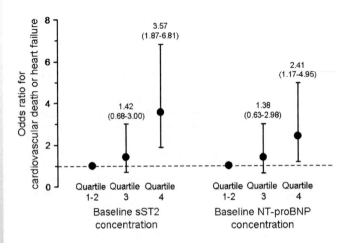

Fig. 5. Prognostic utility of ST2 in acute myocardial infarction. The prognostic utility of serum ST2 was evaluated in patients who presented to a hospital with an acute coronary syndrome as part of the Clopidogrel as Adjunctive Reperfusion Therapy - Thrombolysis in Myocardial Infarction 28 trial. In more than 1200 patients who had an acute ST-elevation myocardial infarction, the baseline serum ST2 level was correlated with the combined endpoint of cardiovascular death and heart failure through 30 days. Multivariable-adjusted odds ratios are shown, with vertical bars representing 95% confidence intervals. The variables that are adjusted for include age, gender, presence of hypertension, diabetes mellitus, prior myocardial infarction, prior congestive heart failure, creatinine clearance, infarct location, Killip class, time from symptom onset to thrombolytic delivery, type of thrombolytic, and peak creatine kinase. Patients are grouped based on the serum biomarker level quartile. (Adapted from Sabatine MS, Morrow DA, Higgins LJ, et al. Complementary roles for biomarkers of biomechanical strain ST2 and N-terminal prohormone B-type natriuretic peptide in patients with ST-elevation myocardial infarction. Circulation 2008;117(15):1936–44; with permission.)

in a fashion consistent with routine testing performed currently, must provide the clinician with information either unobtainable or more relevant than that gleaned from current testing modalities, and must provide clinically useful information such as earlier detection, prognostication, and monitoring, or assist in the triage of therapy. sST2 appears promising when evaluated by these standards. It is readily assayable using an enzyme-linked immunosorbant assay, although a rapid turnaround platform such as the point-of-care immunoassays used in clinical practice today for

troponin and NT-proBNP measurement has not been developed. sST2 has been shown to be a biomarker with prognostic power similar to NT-proBNP and adds prognostic information when included in an algorithm inclusive of clinical assessment and natriuretic peptide measurement.[33] It remains to be determined whether greater precision in risk stratification to identify patients at highest risk for death or heart failure after myocardial infarction or for death from progressive heart failure would help tailor therapy in a clinically meaningful way. Gross measures of

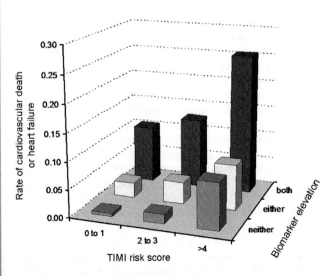

Fig. 6. Prognostic utility of ST2 in combination with established predictors. The prognostic power of serum ST2 in relation to NT-proBNP and traditional clinical determinants of adverse outcome was evaluated in patients who presented to a hospital with an acute ST-elevation myocardial infarction as part of the TIMI 28 trial. Event rates of cardiovascular death or heart failure at 30 days after presentation in patients who had an elevation of serum ST2 and NT-proBNP were equivalent to those of patients who had a TIMI risk score greater than 4. Patients who had elevations in both biomarkers and a TIMI risk score of greater than 4 had event rates that exceeded 25% at 30 days. (Adapted from Sabatine MS, Morrow DA, Higgins LJ, et al. Complementary roles for biomarkers of biomechanical strain ST2 and N-terminal prohormone B-type natriuretic peptide in patients with ST-elevation myocardial infarction. Circulation 2008;117(15):1936–44; with permission.)

risk such as clinical symptoms and left ventricular ejection fraction are currently used to tailor oral pharmacotherapy and to make the decision to implant cardiac defibrillators in patients who have advanced heart failure or who have had a myocardial infarction. More precise measures, such as multiple biomarker panels, may refine risk stratification and thereby identify patients who would most likely benefit from advanced therapies. Additionally, a multimarker approach may assist in designing future clinical trials by identifying the highest-risk patients for inclusion, thereby limiting the size and cost of initial studies to evaluate new therapies.

In summary, ST2 is the receptor component of a novel paracrine system that may mediate communication between cardiac fibroblasts and myocytes in response to ventricular mechanical strain. ST2 is rapidly being established as a possible diagnostic aid and as a novel biomarker that is able to add prognostic information to established measures of clinical risk in patients who have heart failure. How these discoveries translate into potential new diagnostic tests, disease-specific bioassays, and clinical tools to guide treatment strategies remains to be seen.

ADRENOMEDULLIN
Biology

Adrenomedullin was discovered in 1993 by Kitamura and colleagues,[34] from an extract of human pheochromocytoma tissue, as a protein that is able to activate platelets. The adrenomedullin gene is located on human chromosome 11, encoding an 185-amino-acid pre-protein, pre-pro-adrenomedullin (**Fig. 7**). Endopeptidase processing of pre-pro-adrenomedullin releases several vasoactive fragments and mature adrenomedullin.[35,36] This mature form is a 52-amino-acid protein that displays a six-membered ring structure and C-terminal amidation, placing it within the calcitonin protein superfamily. Adrenomedullin is highly conserved across animal species and is found within the genome of mammals, fish, birds, amphibians, and marsupials.

Physiology

In 1998, McLatchie and colleagues[37] identified the adrenomedullin receptor by uncovering the dual nature of the calcitonin-receptor-like-receptor, based on alternative usage of intracellular adaptor proteins. The receptor is a member of the G-protein-coupled receptor family, and after adrenomedullin binding, is internalized to the subcellular endo-lysosomal compartment to subsequently modulate cyclic adenosine monophosphate production, protein kinase A activity, and intracellular calcium flux.[38] Additionally, adrenomedullin stimulates nitric oxide production by increasing phospholipase C–mediated cyclic guanosine monophosphate signaling.[39]

The initial biologic function ascribed to adrenomedullin was that of a vasoactive peptide. Rats administered intravenous adrenomedullin displayed a marked dose-dependent decrease in mean arterial blood pressure.[34] Early studies in humans documented measurable adrenomedullin in blood plasma; interestingly, steady-state concentrations were higher in hypertensive individuals, particularly those who had renal dysfunction.[40–42] These findings suggested that adrenomedullin may act as a regulator of systemic vascular tone, a hypothesis that was further tested by evaluating the hemodynamic effects of an intravenous

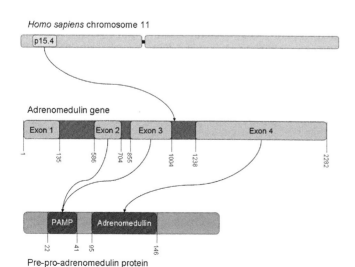

Fig. 7. Human adrenomedullin. A schematic representation of the adrenomedullin gene on human chromosome 11, with its intron/exon structure. Also depicted are the protein structure of pre-pro-adrenomedullin, with the location of pro-adrenomedullin N-terminal 20 peptide (PAMP) and mature adrenomedullin within the parent molecule indicated. (The nucleotide base pairs of the gene and numbered amino acid positions of the protein are as indicated.)

infusion of adrenomedullin in healthy human volunteers. The majority of these studies documented dose-dependent changes in blood pressure in response to adrenomedullin exposure,[42–46] a response that is partially dependent on nitric oxide signaling.[47] Despite the fact that it reduces mean arterial pressure, adrenomedullin infusion causes an increase in cardiac output.[48] This is likely the net result of a decrease in afterload, a reflexive increase in heart rate, and cAMP-dependent and cAMP-independent increases in myocardial inotropy.[49,50]

Adrenomedullin also has neurohormonal effects that may work in concert with its vasoactive properties to modulate tissue-level perfusion. Adrenomedullin increases plasma renin concentrations in human subjects without affecting in vivo aldosterone secretion.[43,48] Adrenomedullin also selectively attenuates the pressor effects of angiotensin II.[51,52] Infusion of adrenomedullin into healthy human subjects to mimic pathophysiologic serum concentrations produces mild alterations in systemic blood pressure but fails to produce natriuretic or diuretic effects.[42] Higher doses of adrenomedullin increase renal blood flow, urine output, and sodium excretion in a nitric oxide–dependent manner.[43,53,54] Overall, the doses of adrenomedullin required to affect renal physiology are larger than those required to modulate the renin/aldosterone neurohormonal axis, which are larger than those needed to alter vasomotor tone.[48]

Although adrenomedullin is produced by smooth muscle and endothelial cells of most vascular beds examined,[55,56] the tissue source of plasma adrenomedullin during periods of myocardial injury and pressure overload appears to include the myocardium itself. Adrenomedullin protein and messenger RNA are elevated to greater-than-basal levels in the atria and ventricles of failing myocardium.[57,58] Direct concurrent sampling of adrenomedullin concentrations in coronary sinus and aortic blood samples of patients who had heart failure revealed higher concentrations in the cardiac venous effluent.[59] Whether production of adrenomedullin by failing or injured cardiomyocytes has effects on vascular beds at a distance is unclear. However, local myocyte adrenomedullin production may exert antihypertrophic and antimitogenic effects on the ventricles. Adrenomedullin inhibits protein synthesis in stimulated rat neonatal cardiomyocytes.[60,61] This antihypertrophic effect may in part be due to direct interactions between the downstream intracellular signals of adrenomedullin, angiotensin, and adrenergic receptors.[62] Similarly, adrenomedullin inhibits cardiac fibroblast proliferation and protein synthesis,[63] and by way of stimulation of adenylate cyclase may inhibit the transformation of cardiac fibroblasts to myofibroblasts.[62,64] Collectively, these in vitro data have been corroborated by in vivo data documenting the attenuation of ventricular hypertrophy and fibrosis in rat models of hypertension and pressure overload.[65] Beyond limiting maladaptive ventricular remodeling, adrenomedullin may additionally exert prosurvival influences over cardiomyocytes. In a rat-infarct model, adrenomedullin gene transfer reduced infarct size, the degree of cellular apoptosis, and the rate of postinfarct ventricular fibrillation.[66,67] Although in vivo data are confounded by the potentially protective hemodynamic effects of adrenomedullin, there is some evidence that adrenomedullin's antihypertrophic and antifibrotic properties are greater than expected based on its degree of afterload reduction alone.[57]

Adrenomedullin as a Biomarker

The data discussed above support the concept that adrenomedullin is a hormone active in the syndrome of heart failure that exerts positive influences over vasomotor perturbations, cardio-renal interactions, and ventricular maladaptations. Given that serum adrenomedullin is measurable, the question emerges as to whether adrenomedullin may serve as a potential biomarker for disease activity. The first study to document such a relationship was conducted by Jougasaki and colleagues[57] in 1995. Serum adrenomedullin concentrations were assayed in 11 patients who had either ischemic or nonischemic cardiomyopathy, a mean left ventricular ejection fraction of 17%, and NYHA functional class III or greater. All patients were free of renal disease. Patients who had advanced heart failure had serum adrenomedullin concentrations of 47 ± 7 pg/mL, compared with 13 ± 2 in a cohort of matched controls. In a follow-up study published later that year by Nishikimi and colleagues,[68] 66 patients who had heart failure primarily attributed to coronary artery or valvular disease were enrolled along with 27 patients who did not have heart disease. Again, all patients were free of nephropathy. The patients who had heart failure showed a wide range in their left ventricular ejection fractions and their NYHA functional class. Plasma adrenomedullin levels were equivalent between patients who had NYHA functional class I symptoms and members of the control group, but rose stepwise with worsening functional classes, becoming statistically greater in patients who were in functional class III or higher. Significant correlations were noted between plasma adrenomedullin concentrations and levels of plasma norepinephrine, atrial natriuretic peptide, and brain natriuretic peptide, and an inverse correlation was documented between adrenomedullin and left ventricular ejection fraction. In a subset of patients who improved in their symptoms during the course of the study, serum adrenomedullin concentrations were noted to decrease in parallel.[69]

Hemodynamic assessment of 45 patients who had heart failure due to a variety of causes showed that adrenomedullin levels correlated significantly with pulmonary artery wedge pressure and mean pulmonary artery pressure.[70] In a subsequent study, plasma adrenomedullin levels were shown to be tightly correlated with the derivative of the pressure-time relationship (dP/dt) as assessed using Doppler echocardiography, and displayed a higher correlation coefficient than that for the natriuretic peptides.[71]

Adrenomedullin concentration is not simply a predictor of left ventricular ejection fraction. In a group of patients who had clinical heart failure

and symptoms consistent with NYHA functional class II or greater, plasma adrenomedullin concentrations were elevated in patients who had a restrictive left ventricular filling pattern, as assessed using Doppler echocardiography, with "restrictive" defined as an early- to late-diastolic filling-velocity ratio greater than 2 or an isovolumic relaxation time less than 140 milliseconds. This observation held regardless of the ejection fraction, with a subset of the cohort manifesting normal ejection fraction. Adrenomedullin concentrations did not correlate with NYHA functional class in this study.[71]

In addition to serving as a biomarker for heart failure severity, adrenomedullin may be a prognostic tool as well. In 1996, Kobayashi and colleagues[69] published the first data in this regard, assaying serum adrenomedullin in 15 patients during ST-elevation myocardial infarction. Plasma concentration was measured at admission and serially over a 3-week follow-up period. Adrenomedullin levels were highest for approximately 72 hours after presentation, displaying a downward

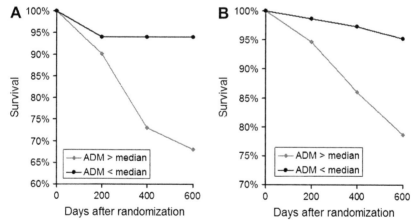

Fig. 8. (*A*) **Adrenomedullin (ADM) in patients after acute myocardial infarction.** In a prospective analysis of 121 patients who presented with an acute coronary syndrome, those with an initial serum concentration greater than the cohort median of 14 pmol/L had a statistically higher mortality rate over the follow-up period of 2 years. Adrenomedullin levels correlated with N-terminal brain natriuretic peptide levels and inversely correlated with left ventricular ejection fraction at 4 months. (*Adapted from* Richards AM, Nicholls MG, Yandle TG, et al. Plasma N-terminal pro-brain natriuretic peptide and adrenomedullin: prognostic utility and prediction of benefit from carvedilol in chronic ischemic left ventricular dysfunction. Australia-New Zealand Heart Failure Group. J Am Coll Cardiol 2001;37(7):1781–7; with permission.) (*B*) **Adrenomedullin (ADM) levels in patients who had ischemic cardiomyopathy.** In a prospective analysis of nearly 300 patients who had ischemic cardiomyopathy (average left ventricular ejection fraction of 29% and stable NYHA functional class II and III symptoms), those whose plasma adrenomedullin levels were greater or less than the median value for the cohort displayed divergent Kaplan-Meier curves for mortality. Furthermore, adrenomedullin levels measured at study inception correlated with rates of all-cause mortality, heart-failure mortality, hospital admission due to heart failure, and worsening heart failure over the 18-month follow-up period. The prognostic power of adrenomedullin was independent of age, NYHA functional class, left ventricular ejection fraction, presence of previous myocardial infarction, or previous admission with heart failure. (*Adapted from* Richards AM, Doughty R, Nicholls MG, et al. Plasma N-terminal pro-brain natriuretic peptide and adrenomedullin: new neurohormonal predictors of left ventricular function and prognosis after myocardial infarction. Circulation 1998;97(19):1921–9; with permission.)

trend thereafter. Throughout the follow-up period, plasma adrenomedullin levels were higher in the patients who subsequently developed heart failure.[72] In a larger series of 121 patients who presented to a hospital with hemodynamically stable ST-elevation or non-ST-elevation myocardial infarction, plasma adrenomedullin concentrations during the first 96 hours after symptom onset were elevated significantly in relation to those of an unmatched cohort of normal subjects. Patients who had serum concentrations greater than the cohort median of 14 pmol/L had a statistically higher mortality rate over a follow-up period of 2 years. Adrenomedullin levels correlated with N-terminal brain natriuretic peptide levels and inversely correlated with left ventricular ejection fraction at 4 months (**Fig. 8**A).[73]

In a subsequent analysis of nearly 300 patients who had ischemic cardiomyopathy (average left ventricular ejection fraction of 29%), the majority of whom manifested chronic, stable NYHA functional class II and III symptoms, adrenomedullin levels measured at study inception correlated with rates of all-cause mortality, heart-failure mortality, hospital admission due to heart failure, and worsening heart failure over an 18-month follow-up period. Specifically, patients whose plasma adrenomedullin concentrations were greater than the median value for the cohort displayed divergent Kaplan-Meier curves for mortality and event-free survival, but not for hospital admission due to acute coronary syndrome, versus those with adrenomedullin concentrations less than the median. The prognostic power of adrenomedullin was independent of age, NYHA functional class, left ventricular ejection fraction, presence of previous myocardial infarction, or previous admission for heart failure (see **Fig. 8**B).[74,75]

As previously discussed, mature adrenomedullin is processed from a precursor peptide. Most early work used nonstandardized radioimmunoassays to quantitate adrenomedullin levels in plasma. More recent studies have used a commercially available assay to specifically measure mid-regional pro-adrenomedullin. Similar to the results of early work with mature adrenomedullin, midregional pro-adrenomedullin has been shown to be an independent predictor of mortality in acute decompensated heart failure and after myocardial infarction, providing in some cases further risk stratification over and above that provided by N-terminal pro-BNP.[75]

In summary, adrenomedullin has emerged as a peptide with multifaceted properties. It was discovered and initially characterized as a secreted protein with vasodilatory effects,

acting on vascular smooth muscle and endothelium. Adrenomedullin displays neurohormonal effects, regulating the renin-angiotensin axis and renal fluid handling. It appears to limit cardiomyocyte hypertrophy and maladaptive ventricular fibrosis. All of these actions suggest that adrenomedullin may act as a counterbalance to the known cardiovascular and cardio-renal derangements of heart failure. As a biomarker, adrenomedullin tracks with many of the clinical and serologic parameters used for risk stratification and clinical monitoring of heart failure. Specifically, serum adrenomedullin concentrations correlate with NYHA functional class, with hemodynamic parameters such as pulmonary capillary wedge pressure, with other established biomarkers such as the natriuretic peptides, and inversely with left ventricular ejection fraction. Finally, adrenomedullin has proven itself as a prognostic marker for adverse outcomes after myocardial infarction and in patients who have heart failure.

SUMMARY

ST2 and adrenomedullin are two proteins that are members of novel hormonal systems and which appear to participate in the pathophysiology of heart failure. sST2 and adrenomedullin are readily measurable in human serum and may play roles in the new paradigm of biomarker-based monitoring and treatment of congestive heart failure.

REFERENCES

1. Braunwald E. Biomarkers in heart failure. N Engl J Med 2008;358(20):2148–59.
2. Morrow DA, de Lemos JA. Benchmarks for the assessment of novel cardiovascular biomarkers. Circulation 2007;115(8):949–52.
3. Tominaga S. A putative protein of a growth specific cDNA from BALB/c-3T3 cells is highly similar to the extracellular portion of mouse interleukin 1 receptor. FEBS Lett 1989;258(2):301–4.
4. Werenskiold AK, Hoffmann S, Klemenz R. Induction of a mitogen-responsive gene after expression of the Ha-ras oncogene in NIH 3T3 fibroblasts. Mol Cell Biol 1989;9(11):5207–14.
5. Klemenz R, Hoffmann S, Werenskiold AK. Serum- and oncoprotein-mediated induction of a gene with sequence similarity to the gene encoding carcinoembryonic antigen. Proc Natl Acad Sci U S A 1989;86(15):5708–12.
6. Werenskiold AK. Characterization of a secreted glycoprotein of the immunoglobulin superfamily inducible by mitogen and oncogene. Eur J Biochem 1992;204(3):1041–7.

7. Takagi T, Yanagisawa K, Tsukamoto T, et al. Identification of the product of the murine ST2 gene. Biochim Biophys Acta 1993;1178(2):194–200.

8. Yanagisawa K, Takagi T, Tsukamoto T, et al. Presence of a novel primary response gene ST2L, encoding a product highly similar to the interleukin 1 receptor type 1. FEBS Lett 1993;318(1):83–7.

9. Gachter T, Werenskiold AK, Klemenz R. Transcription of the interleukin-1 receptor-related T1 gene is initiated at different promoters in mast cells and fibroblasts. J Biol Chem 1996;271(1):124–9.

10. Kakkar R, Lee RT. The IL-33/ST2 pathway: therapeutic target and novel biomarker. Nat Rev Drug Discov 2008;7(10):827–40.

11. Lohning M, Stroehmann A, Coyle AJ, et al. T1/ST2 is preferentially expressed on murine Th2 cells, independent of interleukin 4, interleukin 5, and interleukin 10, and important for Th2 effector function. Proc Natl Acad Sci U S A 1998;95(12):6930–5.

12. Yanagisawa K, Naito Y, Kuroiwa K, et al. The expression of ST2 gene in helper T cells and the binding of ST2 protein to myeloma-derived RPMI8226 cells. J Biochem 1997;121(1):95–103.

13. Xu D, Chan WL, Leung BP, et al. Selective expression of a stable cell surface molecule on type 2 but not type 1 helper T cells. J Exp Med 1998; 187(5):787–94.

14. Trajkovic V, Sweet MJ, Xu D. T1/ST2—an IL-1 receptor-like modulator of immune responses. Cytokine Growth Factor Rev 2004;15(2–3):87–95.

15. Barksby HE, Lea SR, Preshaw PM, et al. The expanding family of interleukin-1 cytokines and their role in destructive inflammatory disorders. Clin Exp Immunol 2007;149(2):217–25.

16. Bergers G, Reikerstorfer A, Braselmann S, et al. Alternative promoter usage of the Fos-responsive gene Fit-1 generates mRNA isoforms coding for either secreted or membrane-bound proteins related to the IL-1 receptor. Embo J 1994;13(5):1176–88.

17. Rossler U, Thomassen E, Hultner L, et al. Secreted and membrane-bound isoforms of T1, an orphan receptor related to IL-1–binding proteins, are differently expressed in vivo. Dev Biol 1995;168(1):86–97.

18. Oshikawa K, Kuroiwa K, Tago K, et al. Elevated soluble ST2 protein levels in sera of patients with asthma with an acute exacerbation. Am J Respir Crit Care Med 2001;164(2):277–81.

19. Schmitz J, Owyang A, Oldham E, et al. IL-33, an interleukin-1–like cytokine that signals via the IL-1 receptor-related protein ST2 and induces T helper type 2–associated cytokines. Immunity 2005;23(5): 479–90.

20. Weinberg EO, Shimpo M, De Keulenaer GW, et al. Expression and regulation of ST2, an interleukin-1 receptor family member, in cardiomyocytes and myocardial infarction. Circulation 2002;106(23): 2961–6.

21. Hill JA, Olson EN. Cardiac plasticity. N Engl J Med 2008;358(13):1370–80.

22. Berk BC, Fujiwara K, Lehoux S. ECM remodeling in hypertensive heart disease. J Clin Invest 2007; 117(3):568–75.

23. Sanada S, Hakuno D, Higgins LJ, et al. IL-33 and ST2 comprise a critical biomechanically induced and cardioprotective signaling system. J Clin Invest 2007; 117(6):1538–49.

24. Deswal A, Petersen NJ, Feldman AM, et al. Cytokines and cytokine receptors in advanced heart failure: an analysis of the cytokine database from the Vesnarinone trial (VEST). Circulation 2001; 103(16):2055–9.

25. Torre-Amione G. Immune activation in chronic heart failure. Am J Cardiol 2005;95(11):3C–8C [discussion: 38C–40C].

26. Fukunaga T, Soejima H, Irie A, et al. Relation between CD4+ T-cell activation and severity of chronic heart failure secondary to ischemic or idiopathic dilated cardiomyopathy. Am J Cardiol 2007; 100(3):483–8.

27. Bartunek J, Delrue L, Van Durme F, et al. Nonmyocardial production of ST2 protein in human hypertrophy and failure is related to diastolic load. J Am Coll Cardiol 2008;52(25):2166–74.

28. Shimpo M, Morrow DA, Weinberg EO, et al. Serum levels of the interleukin-1 receptor family member ST2 predict mortality and clinical outcome in acute myocardial infarction. Circulation 2004;109(18): 2186–90.

29. Weinberg EO, Shimpo M, Hurwitz S, et al. Identification of serum soluble ST2 receptor as a novel heart failure biomarker. Circulation 2003;107(5):721–6.

30. Januzzi JL Jr, Camargo CA, Anwaruddin S, et al. The N-terminal Pro-BNP investigation of dyspnea in the emergency department (PRIDE) study. Am J Cardiol 2005;95(8):948–54.

31. Januzzi JL Jr, Peacock WF, Maisel AS, et al. Measurement of the interleukin family member ST2 in patients with acute dyspnea: results from the PRIDE (Pro-Brain Natriuretic Peptide Investigation of Dyspnea in the Emergency Department) study. J Am Coll Cardiol 2007;50(7):607–13.

32. Rehman SU, Mueller T, Januzzi JL Jr. Characteristics of the novel interleukin family biomarker ST2 in patients with acute heart failure. J Am Coll Cardiol 2008;52(18):1458–65.

33. Sabatine MS, Morrow DA, Higgins LJ, et al. Complementary roles for biomarkers of biomechanical strain ST2 and N-terminal prohormone B-type natriuretic peptide in patients with ST-elevation myocardial infarction. Circulation 2008;117(15):1936–44.

34. Kitamura K, Kangawa K, Kawamoto M, et al. Adrenomedullin: a novel hypotensive peptide isolated from human pheochromocytoma. Biochem Biophys Res Commun 1993;192(2):553–60.

35. Kitamura K, Kangawa K, Eto T. Adrenomedullin and PAMP: discovery, structures, and cardiovascular functions. Microsc Res Tech 2002;57(1):3–13.

36. Gumusel B, Chang JK, Hyman A, et al. Adrenotensin: an ADM gene product with the opposite effects of ADM. Life Sci 1995;57(8):PL87–90.

37. McLatchie LM, Fraser NJ, Main MJ, et al. RAMPs regulate the transport and ligand specificity of the calcitonin-receptor-like receptor. Nature 1998; 393(6683):333–9.

38. Kuwasako K, Shimekake Y, Masuda M, et al. Visualization of the calcitonin receptor–like receptor and its receptor activity–modifying proteins during internalization and recycling. J Biol Chem 2000; 275(38):29602–9.

39. Shimekake Y, Nagata K, Ohta S, et al. Adrenomedullin stimulates two signal transduction pathways, cAMP accumulation and Ca2+ mobilization, in bovine aortic endothelial cells. J Biol Chem 1995;270(9):4412–7.

40. Ishimitsu T, Nishikimi T, Saito Y, et al. Plasma levels of adrenomedullin, a newly identified hypotensive peptide, in patients with hypertension and renal failure. J Clin Invest 1994;94(5):2158–61.

41. Kohno M, Hanehira T, Kano H, et al. Plasma adrenomedullin concentrations in essential hypertension. Hypertension 1996;27(1):102–7.

42. Lainchbury JG, Cooper GJ, Coy DH, et al. Adrenomedullin: a hypotensive hormone in man. Clin Sci (Lond) 1997;92(5):467–72.

43. Lainchbury JG, Troughton RW, Lewis LK, et al. Hemodynamic, hormonal, and renal effects of short-term adrenomedullin infusion in healthy volunteers. J Clin Endocrinol Metab 2000;85(3):1016–20.

44. Meeran K, O'Shea D, Upton PD, et al. Circulating adrenomedullin does not regulate systemic blood pressure but increases plasma prolactin after intravenous infusion in humans: a pharmacokinetic study. J Clin Endocrinol Metab 1997;82(1):95–100.

45. Nagaya N, Satoh T, Nishikimi T, et al. Hemodynamic, renal, and hormonal effects of adrenomedullin infusion in patients with congestive heart failure. Circulation 2000;101(5):498–503.

46. Troughton RW, Lewis LK, Yandle TG, et al. Hemodynamic, hormone, and urinary effects of adrenomedullin infusion in essential hypertension. Hypertension 2000;36(4):588–93.

47. Nakamura M, Yoshida H, Makita S, et al. Potent and long-lasting vasodilatory effects of adrenomedullin in humans. Comparisons between normal subjects and patients with chronic heart failure. Circulation 1997;95(5):1214–21.

48. Nicholls MG. Hemodynamic and hormonal actions of adrenomedullin. Braz J Med Biol Res 2004; 37(8):1247–53.

49. Stangl V, Dschietzig T, Bramlage P, et al. Adrenomedullin and myocardial contractility in the rat. Eur J Pharmacol 2000;408(1):83–9.

50. Szokodi I, Kinnunen P, Tavi P, et al. Evidence for cAMP-independent mechanisms mediating the effects of adrenomedullin, a new inotropic peptide. Circulation 1998;97(11):1062–70.

51. Charles CJ, Nicholls MG, Rademaker MT, et al. Comparative actions of adrenomedullin and nitroprusside: interactions with ANG II and norepinephrine. Am J Physiol Regul Integr Comp Physiol 2001;281(6):R1887–94.

52. Troughton RW, Frampton CM, Lewis LK, et al. Differing thresholds for modulatory effects of adrenomedullin infusion on haemodynamic and hormone responses to angiotensin II and adrenocorticotrophic hormone in healthy volunteers. Clin Sci (Lond) 2001;101(1):103–9.

53. Hirata Y, Hayakawa H, Suzuki Y, et al. Mechanisms of adrenomedullin-induced vasodilation in the rat kidney. Hypertension 1995;25(4 Pt 2):790–5.

54. Miura K, Ebara T, Okumura M, et al. Attenuation of adrenomedullin-induced renal vasodilatation by NG-nitro L-arginine but not glibenclamide. Br J Pharmacol 1995;115(6):917–24.

55. Sugo S, Minamino N, Kangawa K, et al. Endothelial cells actively synthesize and secrete adrenomedullin. Biochem Biophys Res Commun 1994;201(3): 1160–6.

56. Sugo S, Minamino N, Shoji H, et al. Production and secretion of adrenomedullin from vascular smooth muscle cells: augmented production by tumor necrosis factor-alpha. Biochem Biophys Res Commun 1994;203(1):719–26.

57. Jougasaki M, Wei CM, McKinley LJ, et al. Elevation of circulating and ventricular adrenomedullin in human congestive heart failure. Circulation 1995; 92(3):286–9.

58. Perez-Villa F, Leivas A, Roig E, et al. Adrenomedullin messenger RNA expression is increased in myocardial tissue of patients with idiopathic dilated cardiomyopathy. J Heart Lung Transplant 2004;23(11): 1297–300.

59. Jougasaki M, Rodeheffer RJ, Redfield MM, et al. Cardiac secretion of adrenomedullin in human heart failure. J Clin Invest 1996;97(10):2370–6.

60. Tsuruda T, Kato J, Kitamura K, et al. Adrenomedullin: a possible autocrine or paracrine inhibitor of hypertrophy of cardiomyocytes. Hypertension 1998;31(1 Pt 2):505–10.

61. Autelitano DJ, Ridings R, Tang F. Adrenomedullin is a regulated modulator of neonatal cardiomyocyte hypertrophy in vitro. Cardiovasc Res 2001;51(2): 255–64.

62. Kato J, Tsuruda T, Kitamura K, et al. Adrenomedullin: a possible autocrine or paracrine hormone in the cardiac ventricles. Hypertens Res 2003;26(Suppl): S113–9.

63. Swaney JS, Roth DM, Olson ER, et al. Inhibition of cardiac myofibroblast formation and collagen

synthesis by activation and overexpression of adenylyl cyclase. Proc Natl Acad Sci U S A 2005; 102(2):437–42.

64. Nishikimi T, Yoshihara F, Mori Y, et al. Cardioprotective effect of adrenomedullin in heart failure. Hypertens Res 2003;26(Suppl):S121–7.

65. Kato K, Yin H, Agata J, et al. Adrenomedullin gene delivery attenuates myocardial infarction and apoptosis after ischemia and reperfusion. Am J Physiol Heart Circ Physiol 2003;285(4):H1506–14.

66. Nakamura R, Kata J, Kitamura K, et al. Beneficial effects of adrenomedullin on left ventricular remodeling after myocardial infarction in rats. Cardiovasc Res 2002;56(3):373–80.

67. Nakamura R, Kata J, Kitamura K, et al. Adrenomedullin administration immediately after myocardial infarction ameliorates progression of heart failure in rats. Circulation 2004;110(4):426–31.

68. Nishikimi T, Saito Y, Kitamura K, et al. Increased plasma levels of adrenomedullin in patients with heart failure. J Am Coll Cardiol 1995;26(6):1424–31.

69. Kobayashi K, Kitamura K, Hirayama N, et al. Increased plasma adrenomedullin in acute myocardial infarction. Am Heart J 1996;131(4):676–80.

70. Morales MA, Del Ry S, Startari U, et al. Plasma adrenomedullin relation with Doppler-derived dP/dt in patients with congestive heart failure. Clin Cardiol 2006;29(3):126–30.

71. Yu CM, Cheung BM, Leung R, et al. Increase in plasma adrenomedullin in patients with heart failure characterised by diastolic dysfunction. Heart 2001; 86(2):155–60.

72. Richards AM, Nicholls MG, Yandle TG, et al. Plasma N-terminal pro-brain natriuretic peptide and adrenomedullin: new neurohormonal predictors of left ventricular function and prognosis after myocardial infarction. Circulation 1998;97(19):1921–9.

73. Richards AM, Doughty R, Nicholls MG, et al. Plasma N-terminal pro-brain natriuretic peptide and adrenomedullin: prognostic utility and prediction of benefit from carvedilol in chronic ischemic left ventricular dysfunction. Australia-New Zealand Heart Failure Group. J Am Coll Cardiol 2001; 37(7):1781–7.

74. Khan SQ, O'Brien RJ, Struck J, et al. Prognostic value of midregional pro-adrenomedullin in patients with acute myocardial infarction: the LAMP (Leicester Acute Myocardial Infarction Peptide) study. J Am Coll Cardiol 2007;49(14):1525–32.

75. Gegenhuber A, Struck J, Dieplinger B, et al. Comparative evaluation of B-type natriuretic peptide, mid-regional pro-A-type natriuretic peptide, mid-regional pro-adrenomedullin, and Cope tin to predict 1-year mortality in patients with acute destabilized heart failure. J Card Fail 2007; 13(1):42–9.

Biomarkers of Myocyte Injury in Heart Failure

Roberto Latini, MD*, Serge Masson, PhD

KEYWORDS

- Heart failure • Troponin • Myocyte • Injury • Biomarker

Over the years, markers of cardiac myocyte (CM) injury have contributed to the diagnosis and assessment of myocardial infarction size. Early on, enzymes that are abundant in CM cytoplasm were assayed in blood; more recently, specific and sensitive assays for cardiac contractile proteins have been made available and are now part of international guidelines for the diagnosis of myocardial infarction. It is now almost generally accepted by those in the cardiologic community (eg, American College of Cardiology, European Society of Cardiology, and American Heart Association guidelines)[1] that the widely used, older marker of cardiac injury, creatine kinase isoenzyme (CK-MB), is less specific than troponin (Tn). Moreover, because more troponin is found in the heart per gram of myocardium and a greater quantity is released during injury, troponin is definitely more sensitive than CK-MB for the detection of cardiac damage.[2] Based on these considerations, this article will mainly deal with troponin as a marker of cardiac injury.

Three troponins, C, I, and T, have been identified as part of the contractile system of the cardiac myocyte; however, only TnT and TnI are cardiac-specific, whereas the two isoforms of TnC are indistinguishable between those of cardiac and skeletal muscle, and therefore, TnC is not a specific cardiac marker. Although differences in circulating concentrations and assay characteristics exist between cardiac troponin (cTn) I and T, these differences do not influence substantially their performance in term of markers of cardiac injury; therefore, unless specified, the term "troponin" will be used in the text. In addition to its validated use in the diagnosis of acute coronary events, the use of troponin has been evaluated and tested in other diseases, including heart failure (HF).

MECHANISMS OF RELEASE OF TROPONIN

As shown by the pioneering work of Olivetti, Anversa, and colleagues,[3,4] myocyte cell death occurs at a low but continuous rate during physiologic aging, which is responsible for the onset of myocardial dysfunction in the elderly. It has been shown that cardiac myocytes are continuously lost during the course of chronic HF, leading to the development of dysfunctional, dilated hearts, with different time courses of development, depending of the severity of the disease.[5,6] A continuous release of troponins from the myocardium might reflect ongoing cardiomyocyte death, as seen in animal models of left ventricular dysfunction after myocardial infarction[7] and in patients who have chronic HF.[8,9] This phenomenon is independent of a thrombotic occlusion of a coronary artery, but is attributable to slow, ongoing cardiac myocyte injury or death. The claim that stretching of cardiac myocytes might lead to leakage of the cytosolic pool of troponins because of transient loss of cell membrane integrity is still controversial. No clear proof exists to support the hypothesis that this reversible damage may contribute to the increase of circulating troponin caused by irreversible injury of cardiac myocytes. It is unknown to what extent, if any, apoptosis contributes to TnT elevation in patients who have chronic HF.[10] Clearly, more basic knowledge on the respective roles of these mechanisms is needed.

The authors received grant support and honoraria from Roche Diagnostics, the manufacturer of the high-sensitive troponin assay discussed in this article.

Istituto di Ricerche Farmacologiche "Mario Negri," Milan, Italy

* Corresponding author. Department of Cardiovascular Research, Istituto di Ricerche Farmacologiche "Mario Negri," via Giuseppe La Masa 19, 20156 Milan, Italy

E-mail address: latini@marionegri.it (R. Latini).

Heart Failure Clin 5 (2009) 529–536
doi:10.1016/j.hfc.2009.04.008

Experimental investigations using well-characterized animal models of cardiac damage (eg, myocardial infarction, cardiac overload, diabetes, renal dysfunction, neuroendocrine activation) or cultured, isolated myocytes (eg, hypoxia, hyperglycemia, hormonal stimulation) will probably help in deciphering the biologic complexity behind the apparently naïve measurement of a cardiac contractile protein in the blood of patients who have HF. The expectation is that an understanding of the action of troponins will help in gaining further insight into the pathophysiologic processes believed to be responsible for continuous CM injury and death, such as overactivation of adrenergic or renin-angiotensin-aldosterone systems, endothelins, abnormal calcium handling, inflammatory cytokines, nitric oxide, oxidative stress, and mechanical stretching of cardiac myocytes.

EXPERIMENTAL DATA ON DIFFERENT MODELS OF CARDIAC INJURY

The study of mechanisms and types of injury leading to troponin release has been made possible by the observation that the immunoassay for serum cTnT used in clinical routine could also be used in experimental animals;[11] thanks to this finding, several studies in animals have partially clarified the determinants and mechanisms of troponin release in the bloodstream during ischemic cardiac injury. Though it is still unclear whether apoptotic myocytes can release troponins, it is generally accepted that they can be released from necrotic myocytes.[12,13]

Fishbein and colleagues[12] found that in dogs, pigs, and rats that underwent either permanent coronary ligation or ligation followed by reperfusion, the loss of troponins occurs quickly after ischemic injury and may precede histologic evidence of necrosis, though it does not occur in the myocardium in absence of necrosis. Based on histologic evaluation of the infarcted hearts, the investigators suggested that immunohistochemical staining for cTnI and cTnT may be more sensitive than other stainings, such as hematoxylin & eosin, for identification of areas of myocardial necrosis in experimental animals and in human hearts at autopsy. Zhang and colleagues[13] described two types of cardiac injury caused by isoproterenol use: an early (3–6 hours) transient increase in serum TnT after low doses of isoproterenol, and a marked increase in serum TnT after higher doses, persisting up to 48 hours. The increase in serum concentrations of troponins proportional to the doses of isoproterenol corresponded to a decrease in myocardial immunoreacitvity for TnT, thus supporting the proposed cardiac origin of the circulating protein. However, the troponins appeared to also be released with low doses of isoproterenol, when histologic changes were minimal and mostly reversible.

It appears that myocyte cell death is not required for the release of troponins in the circulation, but some sort of transient reversible stress of the cell can allow leakage of contractile proteins. No experimental studies to date have been done to assess whether, in models of chronic HF, a slow release of troponins can be verified by measuring their presence in serum.

With the development of new drugs, cTnI and cTnT measurement in serum has become an important support to histologic studies of the myocardium for detection of myocardial injury.[14] Recently, several commercially available troponin assays have been tested in different species of experimental animals, including mice, dogs, and monkeys. The performance of the assays varied markedly between species, so the investigators concluded that each troponin assay should be evaluated in individual animal strains or species.[15] As this article is being written, troponin is the preferred translational cardiac safety biomarker and is widely used in the preclinical evaluation of several classes of drugs, such as anthracyclines and other anticancer agents, phosphodiesterase inhibitors, and antiretroviral agents.[14] Indeed, the use of cTn as an early and sensitive marker of cardiac toxicity of anticancer agents is increasing in clinical practice.[16]

NONTHROMBOTIC ELEVATIONS OF CIRCULATING CARDIAC TROPONINS

The detection of cardiac troponins in the plasma of apparently healthy subjects is extremely rare with traditional analytical methods. In general, these elevations can be attributed to spurious findings caused by fibrin interference or cross-reacting antibodies. Transient elevations of troponin have been reported within 24 hours after completion of strenuous exercise, such as that of marathon runners.[17] These elevations have never been found to be associated to increased short-term incidence of adverse cardiac events. In a population-based study, cTnT was elevated (≥ 0.01 ng/mL) in 0.7% of 3557 residents of the Dallas County, and this was statistically associated with a high-risk cardiovascular profile (eg, diabetes mellitus, left ventricular hypertrophy, chronic kidney disease, HF).[18]

Indeed, the high sensitivity of newer troponin assays, which are in the picogram-per-milliliter range, allows detection of minimal cardiac cell injuries, possibly even in the absence of thrombotic occlusion of coronary arteries.[19] With these new assays, the proportion of subjects who have detectable levels of troponin is likely to increase drastically, even in the general population. For instance, circulating cTnI was detectable using a high-sensitive immunoassay in three out of four healthy Caucasian subjects for whom the presence of cardiac or systemic acute or chronic disease was excluded.[20]

A possible alternative cause for elevated circulating cardiac troponin levels, which has not been completely elucidated, is chronic renal insufficiency.[21] The strong association of elevated troponin and cardiac death in patients with end-stage renal failure suggests that cTnT can be used to detect subclinical myocardial injury induced by hemodialyis, thus supporting a cardiac origin for the troponin present in patients who have renal failure. This finding's application for patients who have chronic HF, in whom a high prevalence of mild-to-moderate renal dysfunction is found, is worth studying.

Circulating cardiac troponins are detectable in patients who do not have typical symptoms of acute coronary syndromes. The interpretation for their elevation in this context is challenging to physicians and scientists. In fact, finding measurable concentrations of troponin in unselected patients may lead to unnecessary cardiac evaluation, including invasive testing, which can delay the identification of the true clinical problem. Thus, it is necessary to know the potential causes of troponin elevation independent of coronary thrombosis, which have been reviewed recently.[21]

ELEVATIONS OF TROPONIN IN ACUTE HEART FAILURE

The first evidence that myofibrillar troponin is released into the bloodstream of patients who have HF was published almost simultaneously in 1997 by two independent groups.[22,23] Missov and collaborators[23] studied 35 patients who had severe congestive HF (New York Heart Association [NYHA] class III and IV) with no evidence of myocardial infarction or unstable angina, and provided evidence for ongoing myofibrillar degradation and increased serum levels of cTnI by using a high-sensitive assay (limit of detection 3 pg/mL). Two other markers of myocyte injury were assayed: CK-MB isoenzyme mass and myoglobin concentration. However, both remained within the normal range. La Vecchia and collaborators[22] detected circulating cTnI (limit of detection 0.3 ng/mL) in 6 of 26 patients who had acute HF or severe decompensation of chronic HF. The investigators showed that follow-up measurement of cTnI in these patients was associated with

improvement or deterioration of their clinical status, including death. In fact, two patients, whose levels of TnI were repeatedly abnormal, died 45 and 23 days after admission, whereas in two other patients, whose NYHA class status improved after treatment, TnI levels normalized.

Because of these pioneering studies, knowledge on the clinical utility of measuring circulating troponin is growing steadily. Because low levels of circulating troponin could not be detected by the analytical methods available at that time, most of the clinical investigations that followed those of Missov, La Vecchia, and colleagues were confined to patients who had acute decompensation or severe HF, because a sizeable fraction of these patients had high (ie, measurable) levels of plasma troponin that were positively correlated to the severity of the disease and unfavorable prognoses.[24–27] Repeated measurement of troponin over time is useful for identifying and monitoring high-risk patients[28] and can be effectively combined with measurement of another well-established cardiac marker (ie, natriuretic peptides) to improve risk stratification in patients who have HF.[29,30]

The largest source of data on the prognostic role of cardiac troponins in acute HF comes from a recent report from the Acute Decompensated Heart Failure National Registry (ADHERE).[31] The authors analyzed more than 67,000 patients who were hospitalized for acute decompensated HF and had troponin (either cTnI or cTnT) measured within 24 hours after admission and whose serum creatinine levels were less than 2.0 mg/dL. Overall, 6.2% of the patients were positive for troponin (≥ 1 ng/mL for cTnI or ≥ 0.1 ng/mL for cTnT). On admission, the patients who had elevated troponins had lower systolic blood pressure and lower left ventricular ejection fractions and were less likely to suffer from atrial fibrillation compared with patients who were negative for troponins. Troponin-positive patients had a higher rate of in-hospital mortality (8.0%) than troponin-negative patients (2.7%, $P<.001$), with an adjusted odd ratio of 2.55 (95% CI 2.24–2.89, $P<.001$). The ischemic etiology of HF was not a useful determinant of troponin status and could not be used to predict mortality. A negative troponin test may therefore aid in the identification of patients who have acute HF for whom less intense monitoring and therapy could be appropriate.

ELEVATIONS OF TROPONIN IN CHRONIC HEART FAILURE

In patients who have milder chronic and stable HF, lower levels of troponin should be expected, so that the proportion of patients who have elevated troponin levels should be lower than in those who have acute or severe HF. For instance, only 24% of patients had abnormal cTnT (≥ 0.02 ng/mL) in a recent study[32] that enrolled 136 ambulatory and stable patients who had chronic HF (NYHA class II–IV), a prevalence lower than that observed in less-stable patients (30–83%).[24–27] As already noted, troponin concentration was similar in patients who had acute and chronic HF, including those with or without ischemic etiology, suggesting that troponin release was not related to ischemic events but rather to ongoing myocardial damage or leakage of myofibrillar proteins, reflecting loss of viable cardiac myocytes characteristic of progressive HF.[32] Elevated troponin was an independent predictor of death or readmission for HF at 1 year after enrollment.

The prognostic value of circulating troponin in patients who have stable chronic HF was recently defined in the Valsartan Heart Failure trial (Val-HeFT).[33] The plasma concentration of cTnT and various other biomarkers was measured at study entry in more than 4000 patients who had chronic and symptomatic HF with depressed systolic function.[34] Using a contemporary assay with a limit of detection of 10 pg/mL (0.01 ng/mL), cTnT was measurable in 10.4% of the patients. The median concentration of 27 pg/mL was lower than the diagnostic cutoff for acute myocardial infarction. Patients who had elevated cTnT were more severely ill than those who had undetectable levels of cTnT: they were older, more symptomatic, had more depressed left ventricular function, suffered more frequent comorbidities such as diabetes and atrial fibrillation, had more compromised renal function, and had more pronounced neurohormonal activation (eg, higher levels of natriuretic peptides, norepinephrine, renin, and aldosterone).

With a mean follow-up of 2 years, mortality was almost three times higher in patients who had elevated cTnT (43%) than in those who had undetectable levels (16%). Elevated cTnT was the strongest predictor of death in a multivariable model adjusted for all traditional risk factors.[33]

The threshold for detecting myocyte necrosis has been continuously lowered, and a new generation of high-sensitive troponin assays with improved analytical sensitivity and precision is ready for clinical use.[35] In the Val-HeFT trial, a precommercial version of a high-sensitive cTnT assay (hsTnT) has been evaluated and compared with the traditional assay.[33] The new reagents improved the sensitivity by 5 to 10 fold, lowering the limit of detection to a range of 1 to 2 pg/mL. All the plasma samples from Val-HeFT previously measured using the cTnT reagents were reassayed using the hsTnT method. The fraction of patients who had detectable plasma TnT increased dramatically, from 10% using the traditional assay to 90% using hsTnT reagents. As was already proved using the traditional assay, patients who had elevated hsTnT (more than the median concentration of 12 pg/mL) were more compromised. The circulating concentrations of hsTnT were directly related to left ventricular internal diameter and inversely proportional to the ejection fraction. A similar association between the release of cTnI (measured using a high-sensitive assay) and echocardiographic parameters of increased wall stress (ie, relative left ventricular wall thickness and mitral E/A ratio) was observed in 71 patients who had severe nonischemic HF.[36]

In the Val-HeFT, the risk for adverse clinical events increased steadily with the hsTnT concentration, even at low concentrations in a range that was not previously measurable using the traditional assay.[33] The prognostic accuracy of cardiac troponins was greatly increased, with higher sensitivity observed in those patients who had chronic and stable HF (**Fig. 1**). A striking parallel can be made with brain natriuretic peptides (brain natriuretic peptide [BNP] or N-terminal pro-brain natriuretic peptide [NT-proBNP]) that show good prognostic performance in patients who have cardiovascular diseases, at concentrations much less than their respective diagnostic threshold for the exclusion of HF. Though the high-sensitive cTnT assay is still precommercial, its reliability has been shown in other settings.[37]

Natriuretic peptides are currently the most powerful biomarkers for risk stratification in patients who had HF.[38] Sophisticated statistical analyses were performed in the Val-HeFT trial to compare the prognostic value of B-type natriuretic peptide and hsTnT.[33] It was concluded that the two cardiac markers provided substantially similar prognostic discrimination in these patients who had chronic HF. However, patients who had both cardiac markers elevated (a natriuretic peptide [either BNP or NT-proBNP] and hsTnT) had worse prognoses than those who had a single elevated marker (**Fig. 2**), thus suggesting an additive prognostic value when using hsTnT on top of BNP. In addition, the authors of this article tested whether serial measurement of hsTnT over time could improve its prognostic value and found that the last determination in a sequence of repeated measurement was the best predictor of future adverse events. Similarly, persistently increased cTnT levels were predictive of clinical events (death or hospital readmission for decompensated HF) in a study that enrolled a cohort of 62 patients who had decompensated HF in whom cTnT was

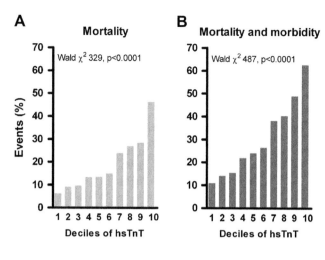

Fig. 1. Relationship between high-sensitive cTnT concentration by deciles and all-cause mortality (*A*) and the combined endpoint of mortality and morbidity (mainly worsening of HF) (*B*) in 4053 patients from the Val-HeFT. The graphs show the association between deciles of baseline plasma high-sensitive TnT (measured using a precommercial assay, Roche Diagnostics, Rotkreuz, Switzerland) and outcome.

measured within 4 days of hospital admission and again 7 days later.[39]

ALTERNATIVE BIOCHEMICAL MARKERS OF MYOCYTE INJURY IN HEART FAILURE

Myocardial cell death can be recognized by the appearance in the blood of proteins released into the circulation from the damaged myocytes. The preferred biomarker for myocardial necrosis is cardiac troponin (I or T) because of its nearly absolute myocardial tissue specificity and high clinical sensitivity.[1] However, other proteins are released by injured myocytes, and their clinical utility has been evaluated in patients who have chronic HF. The circulating concentrations of cardiac proteins

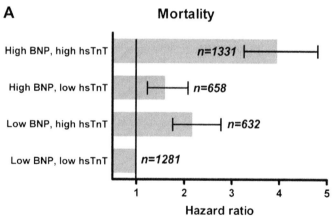

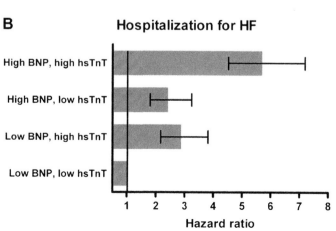

Fig. 2. The additive prognostic value of hsTnT and brain natriuretic peptide in patients from the Val-HeFT who had chronic heart failure. Circulating brain natriuretic peptide (BNP, IRMA Shionogi, Shionogio, Osaka, Japan) and high-sensitive cardiac TnT (hsTnT, precommercial assay, Roche Diagnostics, Rotkreuz, Switzerland) were measured in 3902 patients at randomization in the Val-HeFT. The plots show the hazard ratios and 95% confidence intervals for all-cause mortality (*A*) and for hospitalization for HF (*B*), with a median follow-up time of 24 months. Patients were divided according to their levels of BNP or hsTnT more or less than their median concentration in 4 groups (referent = patients with both BNP and hsTnT less than their respective median). The median concentrations of BNP and hsTnT were 97 pg/mL and 12 pg/mL, respectively.

correlate with the severity of HF.[40] However, some of these proteins present a low cardiac specificity in the presence of skeletal muscle injury or renal insufficiency.

Fatty acid binding proteins are small cytosolic proteins that bind long-chain fatty acids and function as the main transporter of long-chain fatty acids in the cardiomyocyte. Heart-type fatty acid binding protein (H-FABP) is present abundantly in the myocardium and is released into the circulation when the myocardium is injured. Serum levels of H-FABP are elevated in patients who have HF compared with control subjects, and the levels increase with the severity of the disease and may be an independent risk factor in these patients.[25,41] It has been suggested that H-FABP, being cytosolic, may be a more sensitive marker of CM injury in patients who have HF, though its specificity is not as high as that of troponins because H-FABP levels have been found to be elevated in the presence of coexisting skeletal muscle damage or renal failure. Serial measurements and changes in the levels of H-FABP may be associated with corresponding changes in the outcome of HF patients.[42] The prognostic values of cardiac troponins and H-FABP have been compared[43] or combined with that of troponin[44] in single-center studies that enrolled a limited number of patients (≈ 100) who had chronic HF. Larger collaborative studies are required to reach more robust conclusions about the role of H-FABP as a prognostic marker in patients who have HF.

In cases of acute coronary syndromes, when a cardiac troponin assay is not available, the next best alternative as a marker of myocardial necrosis is CK-MB, as measured using a mass assay.[45] Measurement of the circulating levels of CK-MB together with several other myocardial proteins such as myosin light chain-I (MLC-I) can be used to predict acute worsening of HF.[46] In an ancillary study of the Prospective Randomized Flosequinan Longevity Evaluation (PROFILE) trial, a multicenter randomized trial comparing the direct vasodilator flosequinan with placebo in patients who had severe chronic HF (NYHA class III and IV, left ventricular ejection fraction ≤0.35), MLC-1 was measured at baseline and after 1 month in a subgroup of 218 patients.[47] The level of MLC-1 was increased in more than half of the patients, and this increase was associated with increased age, NYHA class IV, and higher serum creatinine levels. At a mean follow-up of 302 days, elevated levels of MLC-1 could be used to predict mortality in the patients randomized to placebo, but not in those in the flosequinan arm. There is unfortunately no clear interpretation for

such interaction between a marker of cardiac integrity and a vasodilator. Overall, elevation of MLC-1 was a weak independent predictor of mortality, significant only if the NYHA class was excluded from the multivariable logistic model.

DO WE NEED A MARKER OF CARDIAC MYOCYTE INJURY IN *CHRONIC* HEART FAILURE?

Given the low circulating concentrations of cTns found in the majority of patients who have chronic heart diseases such as HF, it is likely that the new-generation, high-sensitive assays are the candidates for future studies in this area. However, the recent availability of high-sensitive assays for troponin is generating contrasting reactions in the clinical and scientific communities. The most common criticism from cardiologists is that after having learned how to manage patients who have suspected acute coronary events using well-validated threshold concentrations of troponins assayed using contemporary methods, the use of a new, high-sensitive assay conveys the risk for overdiagnosing acute coronary syndromes and other cardiac diseases. However, the use of serial high-sensitive troponin testing should help in early diagnosis of myocardial disease.[48,49]

High-sensitive assays are likely candidates to provide better understanding of chronic cardiac injury, such as that occurring in chronic HF, stable angina, and cancer chemotherapy. Given that it is unlikely that high-sensitive assays for troponins will find application in the diagnosis of HF, the first question to be answered is whether they will add independent, relevant prognostic information related to the use of the well-accepted natriuretic peptides. From the first large series of the Val-HeFT trial,[33] substantial new prognostic information concerning the use of a high-sensitive troponin assay in patients who have chronic HF seems unlikely, as summarized by Wang in an editorial: "In conclusion, although the data from Latini et al. support a strong association between troponin T and clinical outcomes in chronic HF, hsTnT added only modestly to risk discrimination and did not improve calibration of risk models."[50] In a different sample of elderly male patients, some who had and some who did not have cardiovascular disease, the addition of TnI to a series of other biomarkers substantially improved risk stratification for death from cardiovascular causes.[51]

There is still much experimental and clinical research to be done in this area in the next years, including identification of normal levels of circulating cTns in healthy individuals controlling for age and gender.

SUMMARY

Markers of cardiac myocyte injury have contributed over the years to the diagnosis and to the assessment of size of myocardial infarction. Recent evidence suggests that measurement of the release of cardiac contractile proteins into the bloodstream at lower levels may be useful in the clinical assessment of the patients who have acute or chronic HF. The advent of a new generation of high-sensitive immunoassays for cardiac troponins offers challenges for scientists and clinicians and will likely change the understanding and interpretation of cardiac injury.

REFERENCES

1. Thygesen K, Alpert JS, White HD. Joint ESC/ACCF/AHA/WHF Task Force for the Redefinition of Myocardial Infarction. Universal definition of myocardial infarction. Circulation 2007;116:2634–53.
2. Saenger AK, Jaffe AS. Requiem for a heavyweight: the demise of creatine kinase-MB. Circulation 2008;118:2200–6.
3. Olivetti G, Melissari M, Capasso JM, et al. Cardiomyopathy of the aging human heart. Myocyte loss and reactive cellular hypertrophy. Circ Res 1991;68:1560–8.
4. Olivetti G, Giordano G, Corradi D, et al. Gender differences and aging: effects on the human heart. J Am Coll Cardiol 1995;26:1068–79.
5. Anversa P, Kajstura J, Olivetti G. Myocyte death in heart failure. Curr Opin Cardiol 1996;11:245–51.
6. Mudd JO, Kass DA. Tackling heart failure in the twenty-first century. Nature 2008;451:919–28.
7. Capasso JM, Malhotra A, Li P, et al. Chronic nonocclusive coronary artery constriction impairs ventricular function, myocardial structure, and cardiac contractile protein enzyme activity in rats. Circ Res 1992;70:148–62.
8. Olivetti G, Abbi R, Quaini F, et al. Apoptosis in the failing human heart. N Engl J Med 1997;336:1131–41.
9. Narula J, Pandey P, Arbustini E, et al. Apoptosis in heart failure: release of cytochrome c from mitochondria and activation of caspase-3 in human cardiomyopathy. Proc Natl Acad Sci U S A 1999;96:8144–9.
10. Sobel BE, LeWinter MM. Ingenuous interpretation of elevated blood levels of macromolecular markers of myocardial injury: a recipe for confusion. J Am Coll Cardiol 2000;35:1355–8.
11. Herman EH, Lipshultz SE, Rifai N, et al. Use of cardiac troponin T levels as an indicator of doxorubicin-induced cardiotoxicity. Cancer Res 1998;58:195–7.
12. Fishbein MC, Wang T, Matijasevic M, et al. Myocardial tissue troponins T and I. An immunohistochemical study in experimental models of myocardial ischemia. Cardiovasc Pathol 2003;12:65–71.
13. Zhang J, Knapton A, Lipshultz SE, et al. Isoproterenol-induced cardiotoxicity in Sprague-Dawley rats: correlation of reversible and irreversible myocardial injury with release of cardiac troponin T and roles of iNOS in myocardial injury. Toxicol Pathol 2008;36:277–8.
14. O'Brien PJ. Cardiac troponin is the most effective translational safety biomarker for myocardial injury in cardiotoxicity. Toxicology 2008;245:206–18.
15. Apple FS, Murakami MM, Ler R, et al. for the HESI Technical Committee of Biomarkers Working Group on Cardiac Troponins. Analytical characteristics of commercial cardiac troponin I and T immunoassays in serum from rats, dogs, and monkeys with induced acute myocardial injury. Clin Chem 2008;54:1982–9.
16. Dolci A, Dominici R, Cardinale D, et al. Biochemical markers for prediction of chemotherapy-induced cardiotoxicity: systematic review of the literature and recommendations for use. Am J Clin Pathol 2008;130:688–95.
17. Mingels A, Jacobs L, Michielsen E, et al. Reference population and marathon runner sera assessed by highly sensitive cardiac troponin T and commercial cardiac troponin T and I assays. Clin Chem 2009;55:101–8.
18. Wallace TW, Abdullah SM, Drazner MH, et al. Prevalence and determinants of troponin T elevation in the general population. Circulation 2006;113:1958–65.
19. Wu AH, Fukushima N, Puskas R, et al. Development and preliminary clinical validation of a high sensitivity assay for cardiac troponin using a capillary flow (single molecule) fluorescence detector. Clin Chem 2006;52:2157–9.
20. Clerico A, Fortunato A, Ripoli A, et al. Distribution of plasma cardiac troponin I values in healthy subjects: pathophysiological considerations. Clin Chem Lab Med 2008;46:804–8.
21. Jeremias A, Gibson CM. Narrative review: alternative causes for elevated cardiac troponin levels when acute coronary syndromes are excluded. Ann Intern Med 2005;142:786–91.
22. La Vecchia L, Mezzena G, Ometto R, et al. Detectable serum troponin I in patients with heart failure of nonmyocardial ischemic origin. Am J Cardiol 1997;80:88–90.
23. Missov E, Calzolari C, Pau B. Circulating cardiac troponin I in severe congestive heart failure. Circulation 1997;96:2953–8.
24. Sato Y, Yamada T, Taniguchi R, et al. Persistently increased serum concentrations of cardiac troponin T in patients with idiopathic dilated cardiomyopathy are predictive of adverse outcomes. Circulation 2001;103:369–74.
25. Setsuta K, Seino Y, Ogawa T, et al. Use of cytosolic and myofibril markers in the detection of ongoing myocardial damage in patients with chronic heart failure. Am J Med 2002;113:717–22.

26. Ishii J, Nomura M, Nakamura Y, et al. Risk stratification using a combination of cardiac troponin T and brain natriuretic peptide in patients hospitalized for worsening chronic heart failure. Am J Cardiol 2002;89:691–5.

27. Healey JS, Davies RF, Smith SJ, et al. Prognostic use of cardiac troponin T and troponin I in patients with heart failure. Can J Cardiol 2003;19:383–6.

28. Perna ER, Macin SM, Canella JP, et al. Ongoing myocardial injury in stable severe heart failure: value of cardiac troponin T monitoring for high-risk patient identification. Circulation 2004;110:2376–82.

29. Ishii J, Cui W, Kitagawa F, et al. Prognostic value of combination of cardiac troponin T and B-type natriuretic peptide after initiation of treatment in patients with chronic heart failure. Clin Chem 2003;49: 2020–6.

30. Bertinchant JP, Combes N, Polge A, et al. Prognostic value of cardiac troponin T in patients with both acute and chronic stable congestive heart failure: comparison with atrial natriuretic peptide, brain natriuretic peptide and plasma norepinephrine. Clin Chim Acta 2005;352:143–53.

31. Peacock WF 4th, De Marco T, Fonarow GC, et al. ADHERE Investigators. Cardiac troponin and outcome in acute heart failure. N Engl J Med 2008; 358:2117–26.

32. Hudson MP, O'Connor CM, Gattis WA, et al. Implications of elevated cardiac troponin T in ambulatory patients with heart failure: a prospective analysis. Am Heart J 2004;147:546–52.

33. Latini R, Masson S, Anand IS, et al. Prognostic value of very low plasma concentrations of troponin T in patients with stable chronic heart failure. Circulation 2007;116:1242–9.

34. Cohn JN, Tognoni G. Valsartan heart failure trial investigators. A randomized trial of the angiotensin-receptor blocker valsartan in chronic heart failure. N Engl J Med 2001;345:1667–75.

35. Apple FS, Smith SW, Pearce LA, et al. Use of the Centaur TnI-Ultra assay for detection of myocardial infarction and adverse events in patients presenting with symptoms suggestive of acute coronary syndrome. Clin Chem 2008;54:723–8.

36. Logeart D, Beyne P, Cusson C, et al. Evidence of cardiac myolysis in severe nonischemic heart failure and the potential role of increased wall strain. Am Heart J 2001;141:247–53.

37. Kurz K, Giannitsis E, Zehelein J, et al. Highly sensitive cardiac troponin T values remain constant after brief exercise- or pharmacologic-induced reversible myocardial ischemia. Clin Chem 2008;54:1234–8.

38. Braunwald E. Biomarkers in heart failure. N Engl J Med 2008;358:2148–59.

39. Del Carlo CH, Pereira-Barretto AC, Cassaro-Strunz C, et al. Serial measure of cardiac troponin T levels for prediction of clinical events in decompensated heart failure. J Card Fail 2004;10:43–8.

40. Goto T, Takase H, Toriyama T, et al. Circulating concentrations of cardiac proteins indicate the severity of congestive heart failure. Heart 2003;89:1303–7.

41. Arimoto T, Takeishi Y, Shiga R, et al. Prognostic value of elevated circulating heart-type fatty acid binding protein in patients with congestive heart failure. J Card Fail 2005;11:56–60.

42. Niizeki T, Takeishi Y, Arimoto T, et al. Persistently increased serum concentration of heart-type fatty acid-binding protein predicts adverse clinical outcomes in patients with chronic heart failure. Circ J 2008;72:109–14.

43. Niizeki T, Takeishi Y, Arimoto T, et al. Heart-type fatty acid-binding protein is more sensitive than troponin T to detect the ongoing myocardial damage in chronic heart failure patients. J Card Fail 2007;13:120–7.

44. Setsuta K, Seino Y, Kitahara Y, et al. Elevated levels of both cardiomyocyte membrane and myofibril damage markers predict adverse outcomes in patients with chronic heart failure. Circ J 2008;72: 569–74.

45. Morrow DA, Cannon CP, Jesse RL, et al. National Academy of Clinical Biochemistry. National Academy of Clinical Biochemistry laboratory medicine practice guidelines: clinical characteristics and utilization of biochemical markers in acute coronary syndromes. Circulation 2007;115:e356–75.

46. Sugiura T, Takase H, Toriyama T, et al. Circulating levels of myocardial proteins predict future deterioration of congestive heart failure. J Card Fail 2005; 11:504–9.

47. Hansen MS, Stanton EB, Gawad Y, et al. Canadian PROFILE investigators. Relation of circulating cardiac myosin light chain 1 isoform in stable severe congestive heart failure to survival and treatment with flosequinan. Am J Cardiol 2002;90:969–73.

48. White HD. Will new higher-precision troponins lead to clarity or confusion? Curr Opin Cardiol 2008;23:292–5.

49. Wu AH, Jaffe AS. The clinical need for high-sensitivity cardiac troponin assays for acute coronary syndromes and the role for serial testing. Am Heart J 2008;155(2):208–14.

50. Wang TJ. Significance of circulating troponins in heart failure: if these walls could talk. Circulation 2007;116:1217–20.

51. Zethelius B, Berglund L, Sundström J, et al. Use of multiple biomarkers to improve the prediction of death from cardiovascular causes. N Engl J Med 2008;358:2107–16.

Growth-Differentiation Factor-15 in Heart Failure

Tibor Kempf, MD, Kai C. Wollert, MD*

KEYWORDS

- Biomarker • Growth-differentiation factor-15
- Heart failure • Acute coronary syndrome • Prognosis

Biomarkers reflect distinct disease mechanisms in heart failure (HF), including neurohormonal activation, myocyte stress and injury, inflammation, oxidative stress, and extracellular matrix remodeling.[1] In this regard, changes in biomarker levels in HF are of scientific interest, as they provide insight into the complex pathophysiology of the disease. To be useful clinically, a particular biomarker must provide diagnostic or prognostic information that is not readily available from careful clinical assessment; moreover, measurement of the biomarker level should aid in clinical decision making.[2] These are not trivial requirements. In most patients who have HF, a comprehensive assessment of signs and symptoms in combination with echocardiography will be sufficient to establish the diagnosis.[3] These data, combined with a few routine clinical chemistry values (eg, hemoglobin concentration, serum levels of creatinine, and uric acid), already provide strong prognostic information in chronic HF.[4] Repeat measurements of B-type natriuretic peptide (BNP) or N-terminal proBNP (NT-proBNP) levels have been used to guide treatment decisions in chronic HF. In these studies, HF therapies were intensified to decrease BNP or NT-proBNP levels below a preset cutoff value.[5–7] Although such biomarker-guided, intensified therapy may be associated with improved clinical outcomes, no biomarker has emerged that can guide specific treatment decision in patients who have HF.

The clinical value of many HF biomarkers is limited, because significant parts of the information carried by the particular biomarker are correlated with what is already clinically available or being measured (eg, age, New York Heart Association [NYHA] class, left ventricular ejection fraction [LVEF], renal function). It has been predicted that unrelated biomarkers (ie, biomarkers that carry independent information) will be most valuable in the context of existing clinical markers.[8] Growth-differentiation factor-15 (GDF-15) is emerging as a biomarker that appears to provide insight into a distinct pathophysiological axis in HF and other cardiovascular conditions, and that may provide clinically useful information. GDF-15 is identical to macrophage-inhibitory cytokine-1 (MIC-1), placental bone morphogenetic protein (PLAB), placental-transforming growth factor-β (PTGF-β), prostate-derived factor (PDF), and nonsteroidal anti-inflammatory drug-activated gene-1 (NAG-1).

GROWTH-DIFFERENTIATION FACTOR-15 IS A DISTANT RELATIVE OF TRANSFORMING GROWTH FACTOR-β

The transforming growth factor-β (TGF-β) cytokine superfamily comprises more than 40 members that are thought to be involved in the regulation of development, cell differentiation, and tissue repair. GDF-15 shares the typical seven-cysteine domain but exhibits only 15% to 29% amino acid identity with other TGF-β related cytokines, making it one of the most divergent family members.[9] Like TGF-β, GDF-15 is synthesized

This work was supported by the German Research Foundation (SFB 244) and the German Ministry of Education and Research (BMBF, BioChancePlus).

The authors have applied for a patent, and have a contract with Roche Diagnostics to develop a GDF-15 assay for cardiovascular applications.

Hannover Medical School, Hannover, Germany

* Corresponding author. Klinik für Kardiologie und Angiologie, Medizinische Hochschule Hannover, Carl-Neuberg-Straße 1, 30625 Hannover, Germany.

E-mail address: wollert.kai@mh-hannover.de (K.C. Wollert).

Heart Failure Clin 5 (2009) 537–547

doi:10.1016/j.hfc.2009.04.006

as a precursor protein that undergoes disulfide-linked dimerization. The correctly folded GDF-15 precursor protein then is cleaved proteolytically to release the N-terminal propeptide from the mature C-terminal GDF-15 peptide, which subsequently is secreted as a disulfide-linked approximately 28 kDa dimer.[10]

GDF-15 originally was cloned from an activated macrophage cell line.[9] In the basal state, GDF-15 is expressed weakly in most human tissues, including the heart, lung, kidney, brain, prostate, and colon.[9] Notably, GDF-15 is expressed strongly in the placenta, leading to very high (up to 15,000 ng/L) circulating GDF-15 concentrations in women in the second and third trimester.[11]

As shown in animal models, GDF-15 expression levels may increase sharply in several cell types and tissues in response to pathologic or environmental stress. For example, GDF-15 expression in the liver is induced after carbon tetrachloride (CCl$_4$) poisoning.[12] GDF-15 is induced in the lung after ischemic injury,[13] and in the kidney in response to ischemia or metabolic acidosis.[13,14] Cryoinjury induces GDF-15 expression in neurons and microglia in the brain cortex.[15] It appears, therefore, that GDF-15 is part of a generic gene program that is activated in response to stress. The functional role of GDF-15 in these conditions, however, remains largely unknown. GDF-15 deficient (knock-out, KO) mice, for example, do not show either an enhanced or reduced susceptibility to CCl$_4$ liver poisoning.[12]

GROWTH-DIFFERENTIATION FACTOR-15 IN THE CARDIOVASCULAR SYSTEM

Cultured rat cardiomyocytes strongly express and secrete GDF-15 following simulated ischemia or ischemia/reperfusion injury,[16] and after exposure to mechanical stretch.[17] Up-regulation of GDF-15 following ischemia/reperfusion is mediated, at least in part, by means of induction of nitric oxide (NO) synthase 2, leading to NO and peroxynitrite formation.[16] Similarly, the proinflammatory cytokines interferon-γ and interleukin-1β induce GDF-15 expression in cardiomyocytes by means of a NO-dependent pathway.[16] Expression of GDF-15 in response to mechanical stretch appears to involve an angiotensin 2-dependent signaling cascade.[17]

Consistent with these in vitro observations, GDF-15 expression is increased within the myocardium at risk after coronary artery ligation in mice.[16] Cardiac expression of GDF-15 also is induced following transverse aortic banding, and in genetic mouse models of dilated cardiomyopathy.[18] GDF-15 KO mice develop greater infarct sizes and show more cardiomyocyte apoptosis in the infarct border zone after transient coronary ligation as compared with wild-type littermates.[16] After aortic banding, GDF-15 KO mice develop more hypertrophy associated with worse systolic function, indicating that endogenous GDF-15 suppresses the development of maladaptive hypertrophy.[18] The antiapoptotic and antihypertrophic effects of GDF-15 can be recapitulated using the recombinant protein in isolated cardiomyocytes. These cell culture studies point toward a critical involvement of the PI(3)K-Akt-Bad, ERK1/2, and SMAD2/3 signaling pathways in the cytoprotective effects of GDF-15.[16,18] Together, these observations have identified GDF-15 as a cardioprotective cytokine, and have highlighted, for the first time, a functional role of GDF-15 in vivo.

GDF-15 also is expressed by other cardiovascular cell types, including macrophages, endothelial cells, vascular smooth muscle cells, and adipocytes. Oxidative stress, oxidized low-density lipoprotein (LDL), and proinflammatory cytokines induce GDF-15 expression in macrophages.[9,19] In human endothelial cells, GDF-15 is up-regulated under antiangiogenic stress.[20,21] In human vascular smooth muscle cells, GDF-15 expression levels are increased in response to triglyceride-rich lipoproteins.[22] Moreover, recent studies have shown that human adipocytes express and secrete GDF-15 upon exposure to oxidative stress,[23] and that mouse adipocytes can release paracrine factors that stimulate other cell types to produce GDF-15.[24]

Taken together, these findings indicate that GDF-15 is produced under stressful conditions in many cardiovascular cell types (**Fig. 1**); this prompted the authors to explore the role of GDF-15 as a potential biomarker in patients who have HF and other cardiovascular conditions.

PREANALYTICAL CONSIDERATIONS

Clinical implementation of any new biomarker requires a sensitive and reliable test system.[2] Recently, a GDF-15 immunoradiometric assay (IRMA) using only commercially available antibodies was described.[25] The assay has a theoretical detection limit of 20 ng/L, and is linear over a wide range of GDF-15 concentrations in serum or plasma (200 to 50,000 ng/L). The interassay imprecision of the IRMA is less than or equal to 12.2%. Using this assay, the preanalytical performance of GDF-15 has been assessed; GDF-15 is stable at room temperature in serum, plasma, and whole blood for at least 48 hours. GDF-15 is resistant to at least four freeze-thaw cycles. Neither the choice of the anticoagulant matrix, nor the presence of unrelated biologic substances, such as albumin, bilirubin, or hemoglobin,

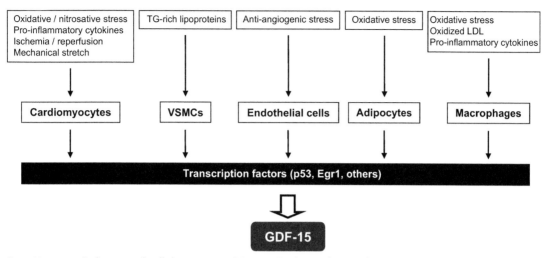

Fig. 1. Upstream inducers and cellular sources of GDF-15 in the cardiovascular system. Data were obtained from neonatal rat cardiomyocytes, otherwise from human cell types. TG, triglycerides; VSMCs, vascular smooth muscle cells.

significantly influences the measured GDF-15 concentrations.[25] Accordingly, the preanalytical characteristics of GDF-15 appear favorable, suggesting that this marker could be measured easily under routine clinical conditions.

The reference range for GDF-15 was determined in a cohort of 429 apparently healthy elderly individuals with a median age of 65 years.[25] Individuals who had an abnormal resting 12-lead ECG, cardiovascular medication, established cardiovascular disease, or other chronic disease or acute illness were excluded from this cohort. GDF-15 plasma concentrations in this cohort

ranged from 184 to 2,241 ng/L. GDF-15 levels were correlated weakly with age, C-reactive protein (CRP), and cystatin C levels, suggesting that individuals who have GDF-15 concentrations at the upper end of the spectrum may have occult (cardiovascular) disease. The rounded 90th percentile in this cohort, 1200 ng/L, therefore was defined as the upper limit of the reference interval in elderly individuals (**Fig. 2**).[25] Recently, GDF-15 serum concentrations have been measured in 200 apparently healthy blood donors of younger age (median age, 40 years); 98% of these individuals had GDF-15 levels below 1200

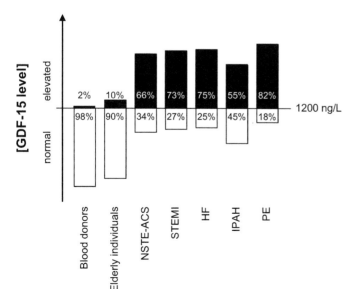

Fig. 2. GDF-15 levels in patients with cardiovascular disease. GDF-15 levels in apparently healthy blood donors (median age, 40 years), apparently healthy elderly individuals (median age, 65 years),[25] in patients with non-ST elevation acute coronary syndrome (NSTE-ACS; data are from the Global Use of Strategies to Open Occluded Arteries [GUSTO] IV trial),[35] ST elevation myocardial infarction (STEMI),[37] chronic heart failure (HF),[26] idiopathic pulmonary arterial hypertension (IPAH),[31] and pulmonary embolism (PE).[34] In each case, the proportion of patients with GDF-15 levels above and below the upper reference limit (1200 ng/L) is shown.

ng/L (Tibor Kempf, Kai C. Wollert, unpublished observation, 2008).

GROWTH-DIFFERENTIATION FACTOR-15 AS A BIOMARKER IN HEART FAILURE AND OTHER CARDIOVASCULAR DISEASE
Heart Failure

The potential role of GDF-15 as a biomarker in HF was assessed in a cohort of 455 patients who had chronic HF with a median LVEF of 32%, most of whom presented with NYHA class 2 and 3 symptoms.[26] Seventy-five percent of these individuals had a GDF-15 level above 1200 ng/L (see **Fig. 2**). GDF-15 levels were elevated in patients who had ischemic or nonischemic HF, and significantly were related to disease severity (**Fig. 3A**). Increased levels of GDF-15 were associated with lower survival rates during 4-year follow-up (see **Fig. 3B**). Survival was especially poor in patients who had GDF-15 levels above the median (approximately 2000 ng/L). GDF-15 added prognostic information to LVEF, NYHA class, and NT-proBNP, and remained independently associated with outcome after multivariate adjustment for age, gender, LVEF, NYHA class, HF etiology, NT-proBNP, creatinine, uric acid, and hemoglobin concentration.[26]

The independent prognostic value of GDF-15 recently was confirmed in 1734 patients who had chronic HF from the Valsartan in Heart Failure (Val-HeFT) trial.[27] GDF-15 levels above 2000 ng/L emerged as an independent predictor of mortality and HF hospitalizations.[27] The prognostic usefulness of repeat GDF-15 measurements is being explored in the Val-HeFT population.

An association of GDF-15 with adverse outcomes also has been observed in 158 patients with severe HF scheduled for cardiac resynchronization therapy (CRT).[28] Notably, combined assessment of GDF-15 and NT-proBNP appeared to identify CRT responders in this small study.[28]

Idiopathic Pulmonary Arterial Hypertension and Right Heart Failure

Idiopathic pulmonary arterial hypertension (IPAH) is a rare disease leading to increased pulmonary vascular resistance and right-sided HF.[29] Functional capacity, hemodynamic variables, and biomarkers (BNP, NT-proBNP, uric acid) have been used for risk stratification in IPAH.[30] Recently, the circulating levels of GDF-15 have been measured in 76 treatment-naïve patients with IPAH, mostly with NYHA class 3 and 4 symptoms, and with a median mean pulmonary artery pressure of 55 mmHg.[31] Fifty-five percent of these individuals had a GDF-15 level above 1200 ng/L (see **Fig. 2**). Elevated GDF-15 levels were associated with an increased risk of death or lung transplantation during 4-year follow-up (**Fig. 4A**). GDF-15 added prognostic information to NT-proBNP and hemodynamic variables, and remained independently associated with a poor outcome after multivariate adjustment.[31] After initiation of medical therapy, changes in GDF-15 levels over time were associated positively with changes in NT-proBNP levels (see **Fig. 4B**), and inversely associated with changes in mixed venous oxygen saturation (see **Fig. 4C**), suggesting that repeat measurements of GDF-15 may be useful to identify IPAH patients who have

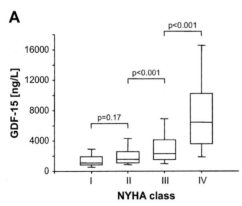

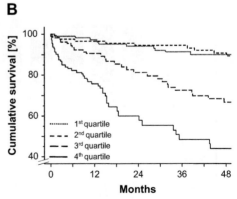

Fig. 3. Growth-differentiation factor-15 (GDF-15) provides prognostic information in heart failure. (*A*) GDF-15 levels in relation to NYHA class (box [25th percentile, median, 75th percentile] and whisker [10th and 90th percentiles] plots). (*B*) Long-term survival in relation to GDF-15 levels at baseline (interquartile boundaries, 1200, 2000, and 3600 ng/L). (*Modified from* Kempf T, von Haehling S, Peter T, et al. Prognostic utility of growth-differentiation factor-15 in patients with chronic heart failure. J Am Coll Cardiol 2007;50:1054; with permission.)

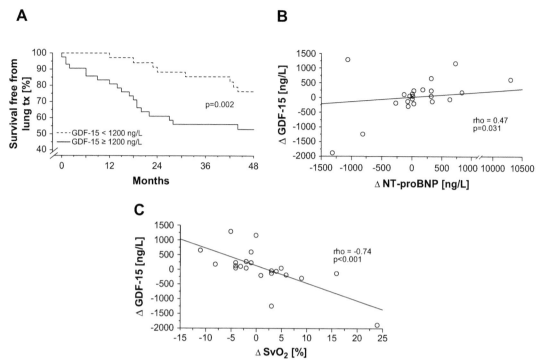

Fig. 4. Growth-differentiation factor-15 (GDF-15) in pulmonary arterial hypertension and right-sided heart failure. (*A*) Long-term risk of death or lung transplantation (tx) according to the GDF-15 levels at baseline in 76 treatment-naïve patients with idiopathic pulmonary arterial hypertension. (*B, C*) In 22 patients, biomarker levels were determined at baseline and 3 to 6 months after the initiation of medical therapy; changes (Δ) in GDF-15 levels were related to changes in NT-proBNP levels (*B*) and inversely related to changes in central venous oxygen saturation (SvO$_2$) (*C*). (*Modified from* Nickel N, Kempf T, Tapken H, et al. Growth-differentiation factor-15 in idiopathic pulmonary arterial hypertension. Am J Respir Crit Care Med 2008;178:534; with permission.)

a favorable response to contemporary treatment regimes.[31]

Pulmonary Embolism

Acute pulmonary embolism (PE) represents a spectrum of syndromes ranging from small peripheral emboli causing no hemodynamic impairment to massive PE resulting in acute right-sided HF and cardiogenic shock.[32] Risk assessment in acute PE is based on hemodynamic parameters (heart rate, blood pressure), imaging of right ventricular (RV) function, and biomarker levels (BNP, NT-proBNP, markers of myocardial necrosis).[33] In a recent study of 123 patients with confirmed acute PE, 82% had a GDF-15 level above 1200 ng/L (see **Fig. 2**).[34] Elevated levels of GDF-15 predicted a complicated 30-day outcome, as defined by PE-related death, cardiopulmonary resuscitation, need for catecholamine administration, or endotracheal intubation (the best GDF-15 cutoff value to discriminate between a favorable and adverse 30-day outcome was 4600 ng/L).[34] GDF-15 remained an independent

predictor of a complicated 30-day outcome after adjustment for clinical parameters, RV function (echocardiography), NT-proBNP, and troponin T.[34] Notably, the prognostic information provided by an echocardiographic assessment of RV function was enhanced by GDF-15 but not by NT-proBNP or troponin T in this study.[34]

Acute Coronary Syndrome

The circulating levels of GDF-15 are increased on admission in patients who have non-ST elevation acute coronary syndrome (NSTE-ACS, ie, unstable angina or non-ST-elevation myocardial infarction). This first was demonstrated in 2081 NSTE-ACS patients from the Global Use of Strategies to Open Occluded Arteries (GUSTO) IV trial who were treated with a conservative strategy.[35] In GUSTO IV, approximately two thirds of the patients presented with GDF-15 levels above 1200 ng/L, and one third presented with levels above 1800 ng/L (see **Fig. 2**). Elevated levels of GDF-15 were associated with an increased risk of death during 1-year follow-up, also after adjustment for clinical risk markers, ECG findings, and clinically available prognostic biomarkers (troponin T, NT-proBNP, creatinine clearance, CRP).[35] Long-term follow-up information on recurrent myocardial infarction was not available in GUSTO IV.

GDF-15 levels were elevated similarly on admission in 2079 NSTE-ACS patients from the Fast Revascularization during InStability in Coronary artery disease (FRISC) II trial.[36] Patients in FRISC II had been randomized to a conservative or an invasive treatment strategy. Elevated levels of GDF-15 independently predicted the 2-year risk of death or recurrent myocardial infarction in the conservative group but not in the invasive group. A significant interaction between GDF-15 levels and treatment strategy was observed. The occurrence of the composite end point was reduced by the invasive strategy by 51% at GDF-15 levels above 1800 ng/L and by 32% at GDF-15 levels between 1200 and 1800 ng/L (**Fig. 5**). Patients who had GDF-15 levels below 1200 ng/L did not benefit significantly from the invasive strategy, even if they presented with ST segment depression or a troponin T level above 0.01 μg/L.[36] These data indicate that GDF-15 may be useful for risk stratification and therapeutic decision making in NSTE-ACS.

The independent predictive value of GDF-15 has been confirmed in patients who have ST elevation myocardial infarction (STEMI)[37] and in patients who have acute chest pain.[38]

BIOLOGIC INFORMATION CARRIED BY GROWTH-DIFFERENTIATION FACTOR-15

Given that GDF-15 is produced by several (cardiovascular) cell types under stressful conditions, it is likely that this biomarker integrates information from different disease pathways (**Fig. 6**).

The significant relation of GDF-15 to NT-proBNP, which has been observed in all cardiovascular disease states, including HF, indicates that GDF-15 reflects, to some extent, cardiac pathologies.[26,31,34–38] Supporting this hypothesis, BNP and GDF-15 are induced similarly by biomechanical stress in isolated rat cardiomyocytes and in the murine heart.[17,18,39] GDF-15 levels in patients who have HF or NSTE-ACS are related inversely to LVEF.[26,36] Moreover, GDF-15 levels are related to HF symptoms, as reflected by NYHA class in chronic HF,[26] Killip class in patients who have STEMI,[37] or the presence of cardiogenic shock in acute PE.[34] As indicated by the inconsistent and weak relation of GDF-15 to troponin levels in patients who have ACS, GDF-15 does not appear to be related directly to myocardial necrosis.[35–37]

GDF-15 levels are related to several cardiovascular risk factors, most consistently to age, smoking, and diabetes.[26,31,34–38] Considering the

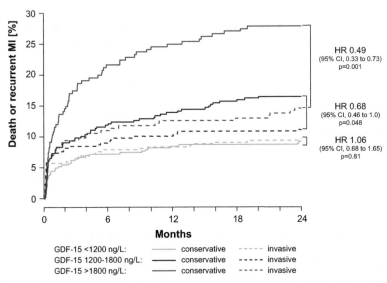

Fig. 5. Interaction of growth-differentiation factor-15 (GDF-15) with treatment strategy in non-ST elevation acute coronary syndrome. The cumulative probability of the composite endpoint of death or recurrent myocardial infarction (MI) during 2 years is shown according to GDF-15 levels on admission (below 1200, between 1200 and 1800, or above 1800 ng/L), and randomization to an invasive or conservative treatment strategy in patients from the FRISC II trial. HR, hazard ratio. (*Modified from* Wollert KC, Kempf T, Lagerqvist B, et al. Growth-differentiation factor-15 for risk stratification and selection of an invasive treatment strategy in non ST elevation acute coronary syndrome. Circulation 2007;116:1540; with permission.)

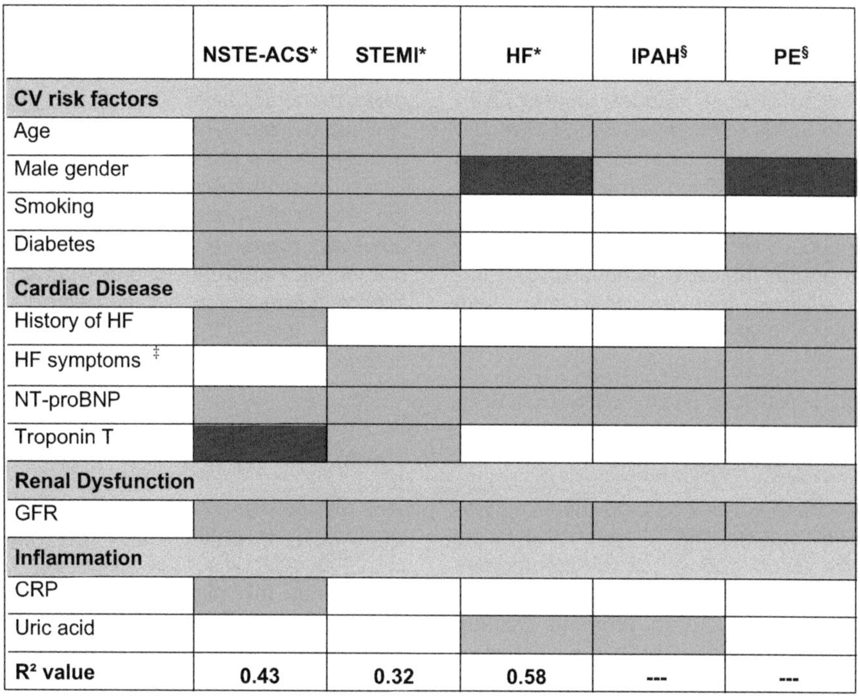

	NSTE-ACS*	STEMI*	HF*	IPAH§	PE§
CV risk factors					
Age					
Male gender					
Smoking					
Diabetes					
Cardiac Disease					
History of HF					
HF symptoms ‡					
NT-proBNP					
Troponin T					
Renal Dysfunction					
GFR					
Inflammation					
CRP					
Uric acid					
R² value	0.43	0.32	0.58	---	---

Fig. 6. Association of growth-differentiation factor-15 (GDF-15) with clinical and biochemical parameters in cardiovascular disease. The relation of GDF-15 to baseline characteristics and other biomarkers was analyzed in patients with non-ST elevation acute coronary syndrome (NSTE-ACS, data are from the Global Use of Strategies to Open Occluded Arteries (GUSTO) IV trial;[35] similar results were obtained in Fast Revascularization during InStability in Coronary artery disease [FRISC] II),[36] ST elevation myocardial infarction (STEMI),[37] chronic heart failure (HF),[26] idiopathic pulmonary arterial hypertension (IPAH),[31] or pulmonary embolism (PE).[34] Significant relations are highlighted in green, absent relations in red (white boxes: parameter not available). Data were derived from *multivariate or §univariate analyses. ‡HF symptoms are represented by New York Heart Association (NYHA) class in HF and IPAH, Killip class in STEMI, and the presence of cardiogenic shock in PE.

relation of GDF-15 to CRP levels in patients who have NSTE-ACS,[35,36] GDF-15 seems to be, in part, a marker of inflammation. Along that line, GDF-15 levels in patients who have HF and IPAH are related to uric acid levels,[26,31] which are thought to reflect inflammation and tissue hypoxia in these conditions.[40] GDF-15 has been identified in macrophages in human carotid endaterectomy specimens, supporting a link between GDF-15 and atherosclerotic disease.[19] Consistent with this idea, GDF-15 levels were associated with the extent of coronary artery disease in the FRISC II NSTE-ACS study population.[36] Together, these data indicate that GDF-15 reflects, to some extent, cardiovascular risk, inflammation, and the extent of atherosclerotic disease.

Finally, higher levels of GDF-15 with decreasing renal function in all investigated cardiovascular disease states suggest that GDF15 is cleared from the circulation through the kidneys or that GDF-15 synthesis is increased in patients who have renal dysfunction.[26,31,34–38]

Notably, these clinical and biochemical indicators of cardiac, vascular, and renal disease explain only part of the variation in the GDF-15 levels in patients who have cardiovascular disease (between 32% and 58%; see R^2 values in Fig. 6), indicating that GDF-15 carries unique additional information. The human GDF-15 promoter contains two p53 and two Egr1 consensus binding sites; both transcription factors are required and sufficient for the induction of GDF-15 in various cell lines.[41–43] p53 and Egr1 are important transcriptional regulators in cardiovascular disease.[44,45] p53 is increased in human atherosclerotic plaques,[46,47] and controls apoptotic cell death in mouse models of atherosclerosis.[48] Notably, p53 colocalizes with GDF-15 in human atherosclerotic plaque macrophages.[19] Increased expression levels of p53 also have been detected in the failing human myocardium,[49] and have been suggested to play a crucial role in the transition from cardiac hypertrophy to HF.[50] Egr1 is induced in human atherosclerotic plaques,[51] and contributes to lesion development in mouse models of atherosclerosis.[52] Egr1 is an essential mediator of pressure overload hypertrophy in mice.[53] Inhibition of Egr1 reduces cardiac GDF-15 expression levels after experimental pressure overload, thus providing a direct link between Egr1 and GDF-15 expression in the heart.[53]

Further characterization of the pathobiology and upstream inducers of GDF-15 in cardiovascular disease may enable the development of new therapies that address the risk associated with elevated GDF-15 levels.

THE FUNCTION OF GROWTH-DIFFERENTIATION FACTOR-15 IN HUMAN CARDIOVASCULAR DISEASE

GDF-15 appears to act as a cardioprotective cytokine in experimental models;[16,18] yet, higher levels of GDF-15 are associated with adverse outcomes in patients. The situation is somewhat reminiscent of BNP, which is thought to promote salutary effects in animal models, while it is indicative of a poor prognosis in patients who have ACS or HF.[39] Elevated levels of GDF-15 in patients may reflect an adaptive response that is overridden by the severity of the underlying disease. Along that line, there might be a state of GDF-15 resistance in patients who have advanced cardiovascular disease, as it has been described for BNP.[39] Identification of the GDF-15 receptor may help settle these questions. It remains possible, however, that elevated levels of GDF-15 promote detrimental effects in the clinical setting. At very high concentrations (above 8500 ng/L), GDF-15 has been shown to act as an appetite suppressant;[54] such an effect may promote cachexia in patients who have advanced HF presenting with very high GDF-15 levels. In line with such a hypothesis, GDF-15 levels are related inversely to body mass index in HF.[26] On the other hand, the very high circulating levels of GDF-15 in pregnant women[11] may argue against an appetite-suppressing effect of GDF-15 in humans.

GROWTH-DIFFERENTIATION FACTOR-15 IN NONCARDIOVASCULAR DISEASE

Increased circulating levels of GDF-15 have been observed in patients who have rheumatoid arthritis, highlighting again, the link to inflammation.[55] Elevated levels of GDF-15 also have been reported in some patients who have malignant disease.[56] Highly elevated levels of GDF-15 are found in β-thalassemia or congenital dyserythropoietic anemia type 1.[57,58] GDF-15 appears to be secreted by erythrocyte precursor cells in these rare conditions that are characterized by an ineffective erythropoiesis.[59]

These observations emphasize that GDF-15 measurements need to be interpreted in the specific clinical context. GDF-15 cannot be used as a diagnostic marker for any particular disease. Like other biomarkers that are not cardiac-specific (eg, renal dysfunction, anemia, hyperuricemia), however, measurement of GDF-15 can provide prognostic information and pathophysiological insight in patients who have been diagnosed, for example, with ACS or HF, by using established criteria. As shown in NSTE-ACS, results from GDF-15 testing may have therapeutic implications.

SUMMARY

The circulating levels of GDF-15 are elevated significantly in patients who have HF and other cardiovascular disorders. GDF-15, however, is not useful for diagnostic purposes, because GDF-15 levels may be elevated in other disease states, and because some patients who have cardiovascular disease present with GDF-15 levels within the normal range (below 1200 ng/L). GDF-15 provides strong and independent prognostic information in HF and all other cardiovascular disease states investigated so far. A GDF-15 value below 1200 ng/L is a strong indicator of a favorable prognosis in HF and other cardiovascular conditions. Like with other HF bio-markers, including BNP, it is currently not known what specific therapies could be used to reduce the risk associated with elevated levels of GDF-15 in HF. Further elucidation of the pathobiology and upstream inducers of this new biomarker may lead to new therapeutic concepts. In NSTE-ACS, GDF-15 levels above 1200 ng/L identify patients who derive the greatest benefit from an invasive treatment strategy. A commercial GDF-15 assay for clinical applications should be available in the near future.

REFERENCES

1. Braunwald E. Biomarkers in heart failure. N Engl J Med 2008;358:2148–59.
2. Morrow DA, de Lemos JA. Benchmarks for the assessment of novel cardiovascular biomarkers. Circulation 2007;115:949–52.
3. Dickstein K, Cohen-Solal A, Filippatos G, et al. ESC Guidelines for the diagnosis and treatment of acute and chronic heart failure 2008: the Task Force for the Diagnosis and Treatment of Acute and Chronic Heart Failure 2008 of the European Society of Cardiology. Developed in collaboration with the Heart Failure Association of the ESC (HFA) and endorsed

by the European Society of Intensive Care Medicine (ESICM). Eur Heart J 2008;29:2388–442.

4. Levy WC, Mozaffarian D, Linker DT, et al. The Seattle Heart Failure Model: prediction of survival in heart failure. Circulation 2006;113:1424–33.

5. Coletta AP, Cullington D, Clark AL, Cleland JG. Clinical trials update from European Society of Cardiology meeting 2008: TIME-CHF, BACH, BEAUTIFUL, GISSI-HF, and HOME-HF. Eur J Heart Fail 2008;10:1264–7.

6. Jourdain P, Jondeau G, Funck F, et al. Plasma brain natriuretic peptide-guided therapy to improve outcome in heart failure: the STARS-BNP Multicenter Study. J Am Coll Cardiol 2007;49:1733–9.

7. Troughton RW, Frampton CM, Yandle TG, Espiner EA, Nicholls MG, Richards AM. Treatment of heart failure guided by plasma aminoterminal brain natriuretic peptide (N-BNP) concentrations. Lancet 2000;355:1126–30.

8. Gerszten RE, Wang TJ. The search for new cardiovascular biomarkers. Nature 2008;451:949–52.

9. Bootcov MR, Bauskin AR, Valenzuela SM, et al. MIC-1, a novel macrophage inhibitory cytokine, is a divergent member of the TGF-beta superfamily. Proc Natl Acad Sci U S A 1997;94:11514–9.

10. Bauskin AR, Zhang HP, Fairlie WD, et al. The propeptide of macrophage inhibitory cytokine (MIC-1), a TGF-beta superfamily member, acts as a quality control determinant for correctly folded MIC-1. Embo J 2000;19:2212–20.

11. Moore AG, Brown DA, Fairlie WD, et al. The transforming growth factor-ss superfamily cytokine macrophage inhibitory cytokine-1 is present in high concentrations in the serum of pregnant women. J Clin Endocrinol Metab 2000;85:4781–8.

12. Hsiao EC, Koniaris LG, Zimmers-Koniaris T, Sebald SM, Huynh TV, Lee SJ. Characterization of growth-differentiation factor 15, a transforming growth factor beta superfamily member induced following liver injury. Mol Cell Biol 2000;20:3742–51.

13. Zimmers TA, Jin X, Hsiao EC, McGrath SA, Esquela AF, Koniaris LG. Growth differentiation factor-15/macrophage inhibitory cytokine-1 induction after kidney and lung injury. Shock 2005;23:543–8.

14. Van Huyen JP, Cheval L, Bloch-Faure M, et al. GDF15 triggers homeostatic proliferation of acid-secreting collecting duct cells. J Am Soc Nephrol 2008;19:1965–74.

15. Schober A, Bottner M, Strelau J, et al. Expression of growth differentiation factor-15/ macrophage inhibitory cytokine-1 (GDF-15/MIC-1) in the perinatal, adult, and injured rat brain. J Comp Neurol 2001;439:32–45.

16. Kempf T, Eden M, Strelau J, et al. The transforming growth factor-beta superfamily member growth-differentiation factor-15 protects the heart from ischemia/reperfusion injury. Circ Res 2006;98:351–60.

17. Frank D, Kuhn C, Brors B, et al. Gene expression pattern in biomechanically stretched cardiomyocytes: evidence for a stretch-specific gene program. Hypertension 2008;51:309–18.

18. Xu J, Kimball TR, Lorenz JN, et al. GDF15/MIC-1 functions as a protective and antihypertrophic factor released from the myocardium in association with SMAD protein activation. Circ Res 2006;98:342–50.

19. Schlittenhardt D, Schober A, Strelau J, et al. Involvement of growth differentiation factor-15/macrophage inhibitory cytokine-1 (GDF-15/MIC-1) in oxLDL-induced apoptosis of human macrophages in vitro and in arteriosclerotic lesions. Cell Tissue Res 2004;318:325–33.

20. Ferrari N, Pfeffer U, Dell'Eva R, Ambrosini C, Noonan DM, Albini A. The transforming growth factor-beta family members bone morphogenetic protein-2 and macrophage inhibitory cytokine-1 as mediators of the antiangiogenic activity of N-(4-hydroxyphenyl)retinamide. Clin Cancer Res 2005;11:4610–9.

21. Secchiero P, Corallini F, Gonelli A, et al. Antiangiogenic activity of the MDM2 antagonist nutlin-3. Circ Res 2007;100:61–9.

22. Bermudez B, Lopez S, Pacheco YM, et al. Influence of postprandial triglyceride-rich lipoproteins on lipid-mediated gene expression in smooth muscle cells of the human coronary artery. Cardiovasc Res 2008;79:294–303.

23. Ding Q, Mracek T, Gonzalez-Muniesa P, et al. Identification of macrophage inhibitory cytokine-1 (MIC-1) in adipose tissue and its secretion as an adipokine by human adipocytes. Endocrinology 2008;150:1688–96.

24. Kim JH, Kim KY, Jeon JH, et al. Adipocyte culture medium stimulates production of macrophage inhibitory cytokine 1 in MDA-MB-231 cells. Cancer Lett 2008;261:253–62.

25. Kempf T, Horn-Wichmann R, Brabant G, et al. Circulating concentrations of growth-differentiation factor 15 in apparently healthy elderly individuals and patients with chronic heart failure as assessed by a new immunoradiometric sandwich assay. Clin Chem 2007;53:284–91.

26. Kempf T, von Haehling S, Peter T, et al. Prognostic utility of growth differentiation factor-15 in patients with chronic heart failure. J Am Coll Cardiol 2007;50:1054–60.

27. Anand IS, Kempf T, Tapken H, et al. Growth-differentiation factor-15 is a strong predictor of adverse outcomes in heart failure: results from Val-HeFT. Circulation 2007;116(Suppl 2):523.

28. Foley P, Chalil S, Ng K, et al. Growth differentiation factor-15 (GDF-15) predicts mortality and morbidity

after cardiac resynchronisation therapy. European Heart Journal 2008;29(Suppl):394.

29. Humbert M, Sitbon O, Simonneau G. Treatment of pulmonary arterial hypertension. N Engl J Med 2004;351:1425–36.

30. Warwick G, Thomas PS, Yates DH. Biomarkers in pulmonary hypertension. Eur Respir J 2008;32:503–12.

31. Nickel N, Kempf T, Tapken H, et al. Growth differentiation factor-15 in idiopathic pulmonary arterial hypertension. Am J Respir Crit Care Med 2008;178:534–41.

32. Piazza G, Goldhaber SZ. Acute pulmonary embolism: part II: treatment and prophylaxis. Circulation 2006;114:e42–7.

33. Torbicki A, Perrier A, Konstantinides S, et al. Guidelines on the diagnosis and management of acute pulmonary embolism: the Task Force for the Diagnosis and Management of Acute Pulmonary Embolism of the European Society of Cardiology (ESC). Eur Heart J 2008;29:2276–315.

34. Lankeit M, Kempf T, Dellas C, et al. Growth differentiation factor-15 for prognostic assessment of patients with acute pulmonary embolism. Am J Respir Crit Care Med 2008;177:1018–25.

35. Wollert KC, Kempf T, Peter T, et al. Prognostic value of growth-differentiation factor-15 in patients with non-ST-elevation acute coronary syndrome. Circulation 2007;115:962–71.

36. Wollert KC, Kempf T, Lagerqvist B, et al. Growth differentiation factor 15 for risk stratification and selection of an invasive treatment strategy in non ST-elevation acute coronary syndrome. Circulation 2007;116:1540–8.

37. Kempf T, Bjorklund E, Olofsson S, et al. Growth-differentiation factor-15 improves risk stratification in ST-segment elevation myocardial infarction. Eur Heart J 2007;28:2858–65.

38. Eggers KM, Kempf T, Allhoff T, Lindahl B, Wallentin L, Wollert KC. Growth-differentiation factor-15 for early risk stratification in patients with acute chest pain. Eur Heart J 2008;29:2327–35.

39. Daniels LB, Maisel AS. Natriuretic peptides. J Am Coll Cardiol 2007;50:2357–68.

40. Anker SD, Doehner W, Rauchhaus M, et al. Uric acid and survival in chronic heart failure: validation and application in metabolic, functional, and hemodynamic staging. Circulation 2003;107:1991–7.

41. Tan M, Wang Y, Guan K, Sun Y. PTGF-beta, a type beta transforming growth factor (TGF-beta) superfamily member, is a p53 target gene that inhibits tumor cell growth via TGF-beta signaling pathway. Proc Natl Acad Sci U S A 2000;97:109–14.

42. Li PX, Wong J, Ayed A, et al. Placental transforming growth factor-beta is a downstream mediator of the growth arrest and apoptotic response of tumor cells to DNA damage and p53 overexpression. J Biol Chem 2000;275:20127–35.

43. Baek SJ, Kim JS, Nixon JB, et al. Expression of NAG-1, a transforming growth factor-beta superfamily member, by troglitazone requires the early growth response gene EGR-1. J Biol Chem 2004;279:6883–92.

44. Mercer J, Bennett M. The role of p53 in atherosclerosis. Cell Cycle 2006;5:1907–9.

45. Khachigian LM. Early growth response-1 in cardiovascular pathobiology. Circ Res 2006;98:186–91.

46. Ihling C, Menzel G, Wellens E, Monting JS, Schaefer HE, Zeiher AM. Topographical association between the cyclin-dependent kinases inhibitor P21, p53 accumulation, and cellular proliferation in human atherosclerotic tissue. Arterioscler Thromb Vasc Biol 1997;17:2218–24.

47. Martinet W, Knaapen MW, De Meyer GR, et al. Elevated levels of oxidative DNA damage and DNA repair enzymes in human atherosclerotic plaques. Circulation 2002;106:927–32.

48. Mercer J, Figg N, Stoneman V, Braganza D, Bennett MR. Endogenous p53 protects vascular smooth muscle cells from apoptosis and reduces atherosclerosis in ApoE knockout mice. Circ Res 2005;96:667–74.

49. Song H, Conte JV Jr, Foster AH, McLaughlin JS, Wei C. Increased p53 protein expression in human failing myocardium. J Heart Lung Transplant 1999;18:744–9.

50. Sano M, Minamino T, Toko H, et al. p53-induced inhibition of Hif-1 causes cardiac dysfunction during pressure overload. Nature 2007;446:444–8.

51. McCaffrey TA, Fu C, Du B, et al. High-level expression of Egr-1 and Egr-1-inducible genes in mouse and human atherosclerosis. J Clin Invest 2000;105:653–62.

52. Harja E, Bucciarelli LG, Lu Y, et al. Early growth response-1 promotes atherogenesis: mice deficient in early growth response-1 and apolipoprotein E display decreased atherosclerosis and vascular inflammation. Circ Res 2004;94:333–9.

53. Buitrago M, Lorenz K, Maass AH, et al. The transcriptional repressor Nab1 is a specific regulator of pathological cardiac hypertrophy. Nat Med 2005;11:837–44.

54. Johnen H, Lin S, Kuffner T, et al. Tumor-induced anorexia and weight loss are mediated by the TGF-beta superfamily cytokine MIC-1. Nat Med 2007;13:1333–40.

55. Brown DA, Moore J, Johnen H, et al. Serum macrophage inhibitory cytokine 1 in rheumatoid arthritis:

a potential marker of erosive joint destruction. Arthritis Rheum 2007;56:753–64.

56. Bauskin AR, Brown DA, Kuffner T, et al. Role of macrophage inhibitory cytokine-1 in tumorigenesis and diagnosis of cancer. Cancer Res 2006;66:4983–6.

57. Tanno T, Bhanu NV, Oneal PA, et al. High levels of GDF15 in thalassemia suppress expression of the iron regulatory protein hepcidin. Nat Med 2007;13: 1096–101.

58. Tamary H, Shalev H, Perez-Avraham G, et al. Elevated growth differentiation factor 15 expression in patients with congenital dyserythropoietic anemia type I. Blood 2008;112:5241–4.

59. Ramirez JM, Schaad O, Durual S, et al. Growth differentiation factor 15 production is necessary for normal erythroid differentiation and is increased in refractory anaemia with ring-sideroblasts. Br J Haematol 2008;144:251–62.

Inflammatory Biomarkers in Heart Failure Revisited: Much More than Innocent Bystanders

Stephan von Haehling, MD[a],*, Joerg C. Schefold, MD[b],
Mitja Lainscak, MD, PhD[c], Wolfram Doehner, MD, PhD[a],
Stefan D. Anker, MD, PhD[a,d]

KEYWORDS

- Heart failure • Immune system
- Biomarker • Inflammation • Cytokine
- Tumor necrosis factor • Acute phase • Adhesion molecule

Chronic heart failure (CHF) is underrecognized and remains underestimated as a public health challenge. This condition is associated with a poor prognosis and has been compared with some types of cancer.[1] Median survival time is 1.7 years in men and 3.2 years in women after the initial diagnosis.[2] The disease affects up to 14 million subjects in the European Union[3,4] and 5 million in the United States,[5] and its treatment consumes a greater percentage of health care costs than HIV infection or cancer.[6,7,8] The etiology of CHF varies from ischemic heart disease to long-standing arterial hypertension and heart valve disease. Literally any heart disease can ultimately result in heart failure (HF). In many cases, however, the causative insult remains unidentified.

Our pathophysiologic understanding of HF has made enormous progress over the last centuries. The discoveries of Frank in 1895 and Starling in 1918 initiated the hemodynamically oriented research into the regulatory mechanisms of heart function and its regulatory proteins.[9] The mechanical model of pump failure has been advanced over the last decades to a much more complex and inclusive concept involving neuroendocrine, immunologic, and metabolic pathways. Meanwhile, groundbreaking research has been undertaken to fine-tune models of HF to establish novel therapeutic avenues that not only increase the affected patients' life expectancy but also improve their quality of life. The latter is a crucial task in the management of patients who have CHF. Indeed, important comorbidities in this regard, such as anemia[10,11,12,13,14] and cardiac cachexia,[15,16,17,18,19] are starting to receive more attention.

Great strides have been made to identify the most important players in HF. In 1958, specific and accurate methods for the measurement of aldosterone secretion became available. In the same year, Gross[20] was the first to suspect a causal relationship between renin and aldosterone secretion, and it soon became clear that the kidney-derived renin is the responsible aldosterone-stimulating hormone.[21] The importance of the renin-angiotensin-aldosterone system in HF

a Charité Medical School, Berlin, Germany
b Charité Medical School, Berlin, Germany
c University Clinic of Respiratory and Allergic Diseases, Golnik, Slovenia
d Centre for Clinical and Basic Research, Rome, Italy
* Corresponding author. Department of Cardiology, Applied Cachexia Research, Charité Medical School, Campus Virchow-Klinikum, Augustenburger Platz 1, D-13353 Berlin, Germany.
E-mail address: stephan.von.haehling@web.de (S. von Haehling).

Heart Failure Clin 5 (2009) 549–560
doi:10.1016/j.hfc.2009.04.001

was clarified in the early 1960s.[21] Captopril, as the first angiotensin-converting enzyme inhibitor, was developed in 1975 and approved for the treatment of hypertension in 1979.[22] The beneficial effects of blocking this system in HF first became clear in 1984.[23] These developments were paralleled by the demonstration of elevated levels of catecholamines in patients who had HF.[24] In 1984, Cohn and colleagues[25] were the first to describe the role of norepinephrine as a prognostic marker that can be readily assessed from the plasma of patients who have CHF. These findings surmounted the paradigm that β-blockers are contraindicated in HF, and the introduction of metoprolol, carvedilol, and bisoprolol into treatment guidelines for patients who had CHF soon followed. It became clear that peripheral tissues were of paramount importance in the HF syndrome. Thus, it is not surprising that CHF is now recognized as a multisystem disorder that affects not only the cardiovascular system but also the musculoskeletal, renal, neuroendocrine, and immune systems. The importance of the immune system in HF was first recognized by Levine and colleagues in 1990.[26] The aim of this review is to provide a broad overview of inflammatory markers in HF and their potential roles in the future.

THE IMPORTANCE OF BIOMARKERS IN HEART FAILURE

Biomarkers have a long history in cardiovascular diseases and in HF.[27] In particular, the troponins have revolutionized clinical decision making in patients presenting with acute chest pain.[28] Some candidate biomarkers have recently emerged that could be useful in patients who have HF. A biomarker in that sense is any objectively quantifiable biologic parameter that is evaluated to determine physiologic or pathologic processes. In HF, an ideal biomarker would be diagnostic and prognostic and would provide a means for guidance of therapy.[29] In addition, it should provide high sensitivity, specificity, and reproducibility and be independent of demographic characteristics. Availability is another important point, because candidate biomarkers should be readily accessible, preferably as a point-of-care device. Finally, the assessment of such a biomarker needs to be cost-effective.

Considering HF alone, the number of potential biomarkers is huge, and it appears that novel candidates are published almost on a weekly basis. It is difficult to keep track of these developments. A big problem is the fact that the number of patients included in biomarker studies remains low in many publications, and it is therefore difficult to estimate the markers' attributes. Convincing data are available for the natriuretic peptides that have recently made their way into HF treatment and management guidelines,[30,31] and these are discussed in other articles found elsewhere in this issue.

THE ORIGIN OF IMMUNE ACTIVATION IN HEART FAILURE

The plasma levels of several proinflammatory cytokines have been found to be elevated in patients who have CHF. The initial description in 1990[26] of elevated levels of tumor necrosis factor α (TNF-α) in patients who had advanced disease sparked substantial research into the origin of this phenomenon. Various hypotheses have been suggested to explain overactivity of the immune system in HF;[31] however, none of these has been proved by direct evidence. The cytokine hypothesis holds that CHF progresses, at least in part, as a consequence of cytokines exacerbating hemodynamic abnormalities or by exerting direct toxic effects on the heart.[32]

Production of proinflammatory cytokines has been attributed mostly to secretion by mononuclear cells such as monocytes and macrophages. It appears that only failing, but not normal, myocardium contributes a significant spillover of cytokines into the blood stream.[33,34] Some data support the view that catecholamine action augments myocardial cytokine production. TNF-α secretion in the peripheral circulation, on the other hand, may be regulated differently when exposed to catecholamines, depending on the duration of exposure.[35] Influences of catecholamines on TNF-α secretion are mainly due to β-receptor desensitization: whereas short-term administration increases β-receptor density,[36] chronic catecholamine exposure, such as seen in CHF, decreases it.[37,38,39] Other concepts have tried to explain the increased production of proinflammatory mediators as a response to myocardial injury[40] or underperfusion of peripheral tissues.[41] Another theory holds that increased edema of the bowel wall causes translocation of bacterial lipopolysaccharide (LPS; also known as endotoxin) from the gut into the bloodstream.[42,43] Indeed, the authors recently demonstrated that the gut wall barrier shows significant differences in terms of wall thickness and permeability in patients who have CHF compared with healthy subjects.[44] LPS is one of the strongest inducers of TNF-α and other proinflammatory substances, and the authors recently demonstrated that very low concentrations of LPS are capable of inducing TNF-α secretion in an ex vivo model in patients who have CHF.[45,46] These very small quantities of LPS were deemed similar to those elevated levels seen in vivo in patients who had CHF during edematous decompensation.[47]

INFLAMMATORY BIOMARKERS IN HEART FAILURE
Proinflammatory Cytokines

Cytokines represent a large family of low molecular weight, pharmacologically active proteins. Different cell types release these mediators for the purpose of altering their own function or that of adjacent cells. Cytokines are redundant in that several different cytokines share some of their major characteristics. In addition, cytokines are pleiotropic in that they alter many different types of cellular functions. One way of differentiating cytokines is to describe whether they primarily promote pro- or anti-inflammatory mechanisms. In HF, cytokines have been implicated in the development and progression of the disease. It has been demonstrated that proinflammatory cytokines are activated earlier in the course of CHF than the classical neurohormones such as angiotensin II or noradrenaline.[48] The most important substances are discussed in the following paragraphs.

Tumor necrosis factor α

TNF-α can be considered the prototypic proinflammatory cytokine in HF. It has been considerably researched since the original description in 1990 of elevated plasma levels in patients who had advanced CHF.[26] The main effects of TNF-α in CHF are summarized in **Box 1**. The cytokine was originally discovered in 1975 by Carswell and colleagues[49] who extracted a substance from the

---

Box 1
Detrimental effects of tumor necrosis factor α in vivo

Left ventricular dysfunction

Left ventricular remodeling

Cardiomyopathy

Myocyte apoptosis

β-receptor uncoupling

Endothelial dysfunction

Pulmonary edema

Cachexia/anorexia

Insulin resistance

Activation of the inducible form of nitric oxide synthase

---

serum of bacille Calmette-Guérin–infected mice treated with endotoxin. This substance was able to mimic the tumor necrotic action of endotoxin itself. It exerts its actions by way of two distinct surface receptors, TNF receptor (TNFR)-1 and TNFR-2. On a cellular level, TNFR-1 is more abundantly expressed and appears to be the main signaling receptor. TNFR-1 mostly mediates deleterious and cytotoxic effects.[50,51] The other TNF-α receptor, TNFR-2, appears to have a more protective role in the heart.[52] Both TNF-α receptors are also shed into the blood stream and become detectable as soluble (s)TNFR-1 and sTNFR-2. In humans, TNF-α is released in response to a large number of inflammatory stimuli such as endotoxin, viruses, and fungal or parasitic antigens.[53] These stimuli increase the transcription and the translation of TNF-α, which is inserted into the cell membrane of the respective cell.[54,55] Membrane-bound TNF-α is then proteolytically cleaved by TNF-α converting enzyme. This step yields its soluble forms, whose biologically active form is a homotrimer.

Plasma levels of TNF-α were found to be associated with poor short-[56] and long-term[57,58] survival in various cohorts of patients who had HF and reduced ejection fraction. Complex regulatory pathways are activated by increased TNF-α levels, such as the sphingomyelin/ceramid pathway, an intracellular and paracrine second messenger signaling cascade that contributes to functional and structural impairment of skeletal muscle tissue in CHF.[59] In addition, TNF-α levels correlate with atrial natriuretic peptide and brain natriuretic peptide (BNP) levels.[60] In one study, sTNFR-1 emerged as the strongest and most accurate prognostic marker among all cytokines, even after adjusting for New York Heart Association (NYHA) class, peak oxygen consumption per unit time, the slope of expired volume per unit time and peak oxygen consumption per unit time (peak VO_2), the slope of minute ventilation divided by carbon dioxide production (VE/VCO_2 slope), left ventricular ejection fraction (LVEF), and the presence of body wasting ($P<.001$).[57] Plasma cytokine parameters were also analyzed in a large substudy of the Vesnarinone Trial.[58] In this study, TNF-α, sTNFR-1, sTNFR-2, interleukin (IL)-6, and soluble IL-6 receptor (IL-6R) were analyzed. When all cytokine parameters were entered into a multivariable model with several clinical variables, only sTNFR-2 remained a significant predictor of mortality ($P = .0001$). Of interest, there was a linear increase in circulating TNF-α values with advancing age, but only in male subjects.[58] Moreover, women 50 years old or younger had relatively low levels of TNF-α, but these were disproportionately higher in women older than 50 years.[58]

A small study comparing patients who had HF with reduced LVEF (systolic HF, n = 17) and those who had preserved LVEF (diastolic HF, n = 17) found that both groups displayed elevated plasma levels of sTNFR-1, sTNFR-2, and IL-6 compared with controls (**Fig. 1**).[61] Levels of TNF-α were elevated only in patients who had reduced LVEF.

Interleukin-6

IL-6 is a proinflammatory cytokine thought to be released in direct response to TNF-α. It is one of the most important inducers of the acute phase reaction. Maintaining this reaction requires an excess of essential amino acids, which yields loss of body proteins.[62,63] IL-6 effects are mediated by way of the IL-6R; however, IL-6 can act on cells lacking the expression of IL-6R because another small transmembrane glycoprotein (gp130, also known as CD130) is responsible for rendering cells susceptible to IL-6 (**Fig. 2**). IL-6R and gp130 are always required for signaling. The soluble form of gp130 inactivates the soluble IL-6/IL-6R complex.

Increased levels of IL-6 have been shown in the circulation of CHF patients.[57,58,59] A point-of-care test is available.[64] IL-6 has been shown to be involved in the development of myocyte hypertrophy, myocardial dysfunction, and muscle wasting. On the other hand, IL-6 seems to block cardiac myocyte apoptosis. Increased levels of IL-6 were found to be associated with a poor prognosis in patients who had CHF,[57,58] whereas increased levels of the soluble IL-6R were not.[58] In sepsis, elimination of IL-6 from the bloodstream has been demonstrated to be a promising therapeutic approach.[65] The prognostic value of gp130 plasma levels was evaluated in a small

study (n = 76) using a composite end point of worsening pump failure and death due to progressive pump failure.[66] Mean soluble gp130 levels were significantly higher in patients who reached an end point (n = 17) compared with stable patients (P<.0001). The rate of freedom from worsening HF was higher in patients who had lower levels of gp130 (P = .03).[66]

Interleukin-1 family of cytokines Along with TNF-α, IL-1 is viewed as a prototypic cytokine. Among the properties of IL-1 is the ability to induce fever, sleep, anorexia, and hypotension.[67] IL-1 is expressed in the myocardium of patients who have HF due to idiopathic dilated cardiomyopathy, and it depresses myocardial contractility in a dose-dependent fashion.[68] This effect is synergistic with that of TNF-α. Additional findings have shown that IL-1 is involved in myocardial apoptosis, hypertrophy, and arrhythmogenesis. Following stimulation with LPS, secretion of the natural IL-1 antagonist (IL-1 receptor antagonist) was higher in patients who had CHF than in normal subjects.[69]

IL-18 was originally termed interferon-γ–inducing factor.[70] It belongs to the IL-1 family of cytokines and has been shown to stimulate specific helper T-cell responses and to induce TNF-α and IL-6 secretion in murine macrophages.[71] Naito and colleagues[72] showed significantly elevated levels of IL-18 in a cohort of 34 patients who had stable CHF. Among 48 patients who had end-stage HF and significantly reduced LVEF, Mallat and colleagues[73] analyzed the expression of IL-18, IL-18 receptor α, and its endogenous inhibitor, IL-18 binding protein. This study found elevated plasma levels of IL-18. Myocardial expression of IL-18 mRNA and

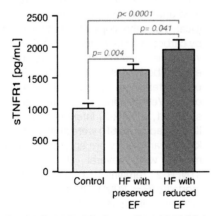
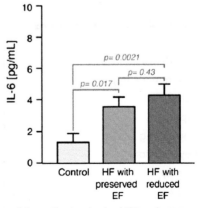

Fig. 1. Serum levels of sTNFR-1 (*left panel*) and IL-6 (*right panel*) in patients who had HF and preserved (n = 17) or reduced (n = 17) left ventricular ejection fraction (EF) compared with control subjects (n = 20). (*From* Niethammer M, Sieber M, von Haehling S, et al. Inflammatory pathways in patients with heart failure and preserved ejection fraction. Int J Cardiol 2008;129:111–7; with permission.)

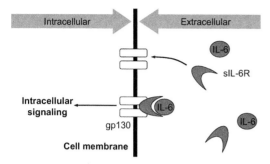

Fig. 2. IL-6 signal transduction by way of IL-6R and gp130. Only the expression of gp130 is required to render cells susceptible to IL-6, because IL-6R can interact with membrane-bound gp130. The activation of the receptor complex leads to the activation of different intracellular transcription factors from the signal transducers and activators of transcriptional family. sIL-6R, soluble IL-6R.

IL-18 receptor α was increased, whereas that of IL-18 binding protein was reduced compared with normal myocardium.[73] Of interest, IL-18 appears to induce myocardial expression of atrial natriuretic peptide mRNA.[74]

Acute Phase Reactants

Inflammation and tissue injury induce a specific reaction of the body known as the acute phase response. Interest in this reaction began in 1930 with the discovery of C-reactive protein (CRP), so named because it reacts with pneumococcal C-polysaccharide.[75] Since then, more than 30 acute phase reactants have been identified, defined as proteins whose plasma concentrations increase (or decrease) by at least 25% during inflammatory processes.[76] The magnitude of the increase varies considerably—from about 50% in the case of ceruloplasmin to as much as 1000-fold for CRP and serum amyloid A.[77]

Acute phase reactants are mainly released by hepatocytes after stimulation by several cytokines such as IL-6, IL-1, TNF-α, interferon-γ, and transforming growth factor β.[77] As mentioned earlier, IL-6 is one of the strongest inducers of the acute phase reaction. Of note, several key players of the acute phase response were found to be elevated in patients who had CHF.

C-reactive protein

CRP has been the most extensively researched among all acute phase reactants. It is produced exclusively in the liver. This protein consists of a single kind of subunit with a molecular weight of 21,500 kD.[78,79] These subunits form cyclic pentamers of 11,000 to 144,000 kD in plasma.[79] Serum levels of CRP increase within 6 hours of an inflammatory stimulus. CRP binds to specific microbial polysaccharides, giving this substance a role in host defense. After binding to these structures, CRP activates the classic complement pathway and opsonizes ligands for phagocytosis.[77]

Leukocyte invasion and inflammatory processes within the arterial wall are key components of atherosclerosis. Because CRP is a marker of inflammatory load, it has been used as a rough proxy for the risk of heart disease. The first study of CRP in patients who had CHF was published in 1990.[80] In this study, 26 (70%) of 37 patients who had varying degrees of HF showed elevated levels of CRP.[80] Another group of researchers measured CRP in 188 patients who had idiopathic dilated cardiomyopathy.[81] All patients had systolic HF with an LVEF of less than 40%. Those patients who died during 5 years of follow-up had significantly higher CRP levels than those who survived (1.05 ± 1.37 mg/dL versus 0.49 ± 1.04 mg/dL, $P<.05$). Caution should be heeded, however, when analyzing CRP data over time. Campbell and colleagues[82] repeatedly analyzed CRP values in 20 apparently healthy individuals. They described considerable intraindividual variation in plasma CRP concentrations over 6 months of follow-up. Therefore, the investigators concluded that the "use of plasma CRP measurement in individual patients is likely to result in many being misclassified in their risk status."[82]

Meanwhile, CRP has been assessed as part of several large-scale studies of patients who had CHF. One study of 4204 patients who had CHF in NYHA classes II through IV found that patients who had baseline high-sensitivity CRP levels above the median of 3.23 mg/L were more likely to have a lower LVEF, to have a higher prevalence of NYHA classes III and IV, to be female, and to receive digoxin and diuretics but were less likely to receive β-blockers, aspirin, or statins.[83] There was a significantly increased risk of death (hazard ratio [HR]: 1.51; 95% confidence interval [CI]: 1.20–1.90; $P<.001$) and of first morbid event (HR: 1.53; 95% CI: 1.28–1.84; $P<.001$) in the highest quartile of baseline CRP after multivariable adjustment.[83]

The value of statins in HF remains a matter of debate, particularly with regard to CRP reduction.[84,85] Recently, the results of the Controlled Rosuvastatin Multinational Trial in Heart Failure (CORONA) were published. CORONA enrolled 5011 patients who had ischemic cardiomyopathy and an impaired LVEF and who were randomized to placebo or the 3-hydroxy-3-methylglutaryl coenzyme A reductase inhibitor rosuvastatin at a dose of 10 mg daily in a double-blind fashion.[86] Median follow-up was 32.8 months. The primary end point was a composite of death from cardiovascular causes, nonfatal myocardial infarction, or nonfatal stroke. When CORONA was terminated, a primary end point had occurred in 692 patients in the rosuvastatin group and in 732 patients in the placebo group (HR: 0.92; 95% CI: 0.83–1.02; $P = .12$). No significant differences were observed between the two groups in terms of the primary outcome. It is interesting to note that rosuvastatin reduced CRP levels significantly during follow-up ($P<.0001$). This reduction, however, failed to translate into beneficial effects in the rosuvastatin-treated patients. It has therefore been questioned whether CRP reduction is an aim worth pursuing in CHF.[87]

Other acute phase reactants

Acute phase proteins include reactants of the complement system (eg, C3, C4, C9), reactants of the coagulation and fibrinolytic system (eg, fibrinogen, plasminogen), antiproteases (eg, α1-antichymotrypsin), transport proteins (eg, ceruloplasmin, haptoglobin, orosomucoid), participants of the inflammatory response (eg, IL-1 receptor antagonist, LPS binding protein [LBP]), and many others. Some of them have been investigated in patients who have CHF.[77]

The role of hepcidin is of particular interest in anemic patients who have CHF. Hepcidin, an acute phase protein, is released from hepatocytes and blocks intestinal iron absorption and iron release from the liver and spleen.[88] It was shown to correlate inversely with hemoglobin levels in patients undergoing hemodialysis.[89] In patients who have CHF, the role of hepcidin is not straightforward,[90] which is partly due to difficulty in its assessment from the plasma. Engström and colleagues[91] analyzed five acute phase reactants from the serum of 6071 men who did not have a history of myocardial infarction or stroke and monitored the incidence of hospitalization for HF for 22 years. Among the 159 subjects who had a primary discharge diagnosis of HF, serum levels of fibrinogen, ceruloplasmin, α1-antitrypsin, and orosomucoid were higher than in subjects not hospitalized for HF (all $P<.001$). This was not the case for haptoglobin ($P = .10$). Subjects in the highest quartile of each of these acute phase reactants displayed the highest risk of developing HF during follow-up.[91]

Adhesion Molecules

Chronic inflammatory processes such as HF involve leukocyte activation and thus adhesion to the vascular endothelium. A large number of adhesion molecules exist. Adhesion molecules represent cell surface receptors that are involved in the binding of leukocytes to each other, to endothelial cells, and to the extracellular matrix. TNF-α is known to induce the expression of different adhesion molecules. Thus, this cytokine may account for mononuclear cell infiltration into the myocardium, which has been reported in CHF. Three main families of adhesion proteins have been identified:[31]

1. The immunoglobulin superfamily includes intracellular adhesion molecule (ICAM)-1, ICAM-2, ICAM-3, vascular-cell adhesion molecule (VCAM)-1, and several others.
2. Integrins form the counterreceptor to members of the immunoglobulin superfamily. They mediate leukocyte adherence to the vascular endothelium and other cell–cell interactions. Examples are lymphocyte function–associated antigen-1 and gpIIb/IIIa.
3. The selectins mediate the adhesion of leukocytes to activated endothelial cells, thus being responsible for the typical "rolling" of leukocytes on the endothelial surface. Such rolling is chiefly mediated by leukocyte selectin and platelet (P)-selectin. Other selectins, such as endothelial selectin, seem to produce a stronger interaction. Such interaction is critically involved in cell extravasation.

Intracellular adhesion molecule-1

Intracellular adhesion molecule (ICAM)-1 is a reliable marker of inflammatory processes because its expression correlates with the degree of inflammation as assessed by light microscopy. Increased ICAM-1 expression therefore suggests endothelial activation due to inflammatory processes. Devaux and colleagues[92] found increased levels of ICAM-1 in cardiac endothelium cells from patients who had CHF compared with control subjects. These data were later confirmed.[93] Tousoulis and colleagues[94] observed elevated levels of soluble (s)ICAM-1 in patients who had HF due to ischemic heart disease or dilated cardiomyopathy compared with healthy control subjects (all $P<.05$). Tsutamoto and colleagues[95] investigated the prognostic value of sICAM-1 plasma values among 102 patients who had CHF. They demonstrated that patients' plasma values increased from the normal level (149 ± 10 ng/mL) to 207 ± 9 in patients who had mild CHF and to 293.18 ng/mL in those who had severe CHF (all $P<.05$). Similar data were obtained in a later study, which showed somewhat higher levels for healthy subjects and patients who had CHF (277 ± 13 versus 383 ± 13 ng/mL, $P<.0001$).[43] In addition, a significant inverse correlation between LVEF and sICAM-1 ($r = -0.36$, $P<.001$) was reported.[41] sICAM-1 levels also predicted impaired survival.

Vascular-cell adhesion molecule-1

Vascular-cell adhesion molecule (VCAM)-1 is a cell surface glycoprotein that is expressed by cytokine-activated endothelial cells. VCAM-1 mediates the adhesion of lymphocytes, monocytes, eosinophils, and basophils to endothelial cells. In addition, it appears to be involved in signal transduction. Wilhemli and colleagues[93] found enhanced VCAM-1 expression in tissue samples from failing myocardium compared with normal myocardium. Devaux and colleagues,[92] on the other hand, failed to demonstrate VCAM-1 expression in failing ventricles obtained at transplantation. Elevated levels of soluble (s)VCAM-1 were observed in 35 patients who had CHF compared with healthy control subjects.[94] Patients in NYHA class IV expressed the highest sVCAM-1 levels in this study. Andreassen and colleagues[96] detected even higher levels of sVCAM-1 among patients awaiting heart transplantation. These patients' plasma levels declined post transplanation; however, they did not normalize during follow-up.

P-selectin

P-selectin is expressed by activated endothelial cells and is essentially involved in leukocyte recruitment to the site of injury during inflammatory processes. Yin and colleagues[97] studied patients who had symptomatic CHF and age-matched control subjects. They reported elevated levels of P-selectin in patients who had CHF that correlated with the levels of sVCAM-1. There was also a trend for a correlation with sICAM-1. Yin and colleagues[97] also found that plasma levels of soluble P-selectin predicted major adverse cardiac events (n = 20), although the overall number of subjects and the number of patients who experienced such an event is too small to allow for any meaningful adjustment. These investigators, however, also detected significant negative correlations between LVEF and sVCAM-1, sICAM-1, and P-selectin (all $P<.01$). Andreassen and colleagues[96] also reported elevated levels of P-selectin in their cohort of patients who had CHF awaiting cardiac transplantation. Of note, the levels of P-selectin were persistently elevated, even 2 years after the procedure. The investigators believed that this finding was due to persistently elevated plasma levels of TNF-α, although they failed to detect a formal correlation between the two.[96]

PROCALCITONIN

Procalcitonin (PCT), a 13-kd propeptide precursor of calcitonin, is mainly produced in the C cells of the thyroid gland and is not released into the systemic circulation under healthy conditions.[98] Thus, PCT plasma concentrations usually remain below 0.1 ng/mL in healthy individuals. Nevertheless, PCT levels are subject to a rapid and profound induction in response to systemic bacterial and fungal infections and in other conditions associated with endotoxinemia.[99] Under such conditions, PCT levels may increase by up to a factor 10,000.[100] Although it is generally accepted that most tissues may produce PCT in conditions of severe systemic inflammation, the exact source of PCT and its biologic function remain to be elucidated. Clinically, PCT is used as an early marker for life-threatening infection (ie, severe sepsis and septic shock). In sepsis, PCT levels correlate with disease severity, are rapidly induced (<1.5 hours), and have a high sensitivity and specificity for diagnosing sepsis (89%–96% and 78%–94%, respectively; cutoff: 1.1–2.0 ng/mL).

Systemic LPS, the most potent inducer of PCT release, may translocate through edematous or ischemic gut walls in patients who have decompensated HF. Little data exist on PCT levels in patients who have stable CHF; however, elevated PCT levels have been observed in patients who have cardiogenic shock.[101] In patients who have uncomplicated acute myocardial infarction, PCT is mainly reported to remain close to normal levels (≤ 0.5 ng/mL).[102] In patients who have acute dyspnea presenting to the emergency room, PCT assessment may be helpful in establishing the differential diagnosis (eg, acute HF versus acute pneumonia).[103,104]

LIPOPOLYSACCHARIDE SIGNALING

LPS may have a significant role in the induction of an immune response in patients who have HF, particularly during edematous decompensation. LPS receptors are shed into the blood stream, and their plasma levels may therefore reflect previous LPS challenges.[43] Indeed, several studies found elevated levels of soluble CD14 in patients who have CHF.[43,57] The measurement of LPS itself is a difficult task, but one study has shown that elevated levels are present in patients who have decompensated HF (**Fig. 3**).[47] These levels normalized with diuretic therapy. The fact that an altered intestinal barrier is present in patients who have CHF buttresses the view that

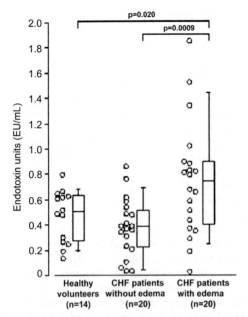

Fig. 3. Plasma endotoxin concentration in healthy volunteers and in HF patients who had and did not have edema. Short horizontal lines represent 10th and 90th percentiles; long horizontal lines represent 25th, 50th, and 75th percentiles. (*From* Niebauer J, Volk HD, Kemp M, et al. Endotoxin and immune activation in chronic heart failure: a prospective cohort study. Lancet 1999;353:1838–42; with permission.)

LPS may enter the circulation through the edematous gut wall.[44,105,106]

The two receptors that render cells responsive to LPS are CD14 and Toll-like receptor 4 (TLR4). LBP is required to initiate binding to CD14.[107] The LBP/CD14 complex then liaises with TLR4.[108] Only the latter is capable of transmitting transmembrane signals and thus able to induce intracellular transcription of, for example, proinflammatory cytokines in response to LPS. Blockade of CD14 can inhibit LPS-stimulated production of TNF-α.[109] The most important intracellular transcription factor in this regard is nuclear factor κB, which is up-regulated in leukocytes from patients who have CHF compared with normal control subjects ($P<.05$).[110] Likewise, TLR4 expression on monocytes isolated from patients who had CHF was recently found to be elevated compared with healthy control subjects ($P<.05$),[111] and TLR4 may represent a potential target for therapeutic interventions.[112] Signal transduction by TLR4 requires complex formation with an additional molecule called MD2.[113] Heat shock protein (Hsp)70 and Hsp90 associate with the TLR4/MD2 complex in response to LPS stimulation.[114,115] Of note, levels of Hsp70 are

significantly higher in patients who have CHF than in healthy control subjects ($P = .004$).[116]

SUMMARY

Biomarkers have the potential to revolutionize the treatment of HF. The first steps in this direction have already been undertaken because BNP and N-terminal-proBNP have recently been added to current management guidelines.[30] These markers, however, do not meet all the requirements of a biomarker outlined earlier. Several investigators have suggested that a multimarker approach may be more promising for several reasons. Such a panel of biomarkers may help in the establishment of the patients' prognosis and diagnosis, may help to identify patients at high risk of decompensation and hospitalization, and therefore, may provide a guide for therapy. Inflammatory biomarkers are interesting candidates in this regard, and it is particularly important to note that inflammatory mediators do not represent a mere epiphenomenon but that they actively take part in the disease process.

A large number of inflammatory markers have been identified to date, and the field is constantly growing. The available evidence best supports proinflammatory cytokines, particularly the receptors sTNFR-1 and sTNFR-2. Many other markers have been assessed only in small studies enrolling less than 100 patients. Thus, future studies need to assess such markers on a larger scale. In many cases, such as the adhesion molecules or most of the acute phase reactants, the pathophysiologic roles of these markers in CHF are not fully understood. Thus, the description of elevated biomarker levels also calls for intensified research to elucidate their roles in the disease process to develop novel therapies for HF.

REFERENCES

1. Stewart S, MacIntyre K, Hole DJ, et al. More 'malignant' than cancer? Five-year survival following a first admission for heart failure. Eur J Heart Fail 2001;3: 315–22.
2. Kannel WB. Vital epidemiologic clues in heart failure. J Clin Epidemiol 2000;53:229–35.
3. Cowie MR, Mosterd A, Wood DA, et al. The epidemiology of heart failure. Eur Heart J 1997;18: 208–25.
4. Davies M, Hobbs F, Davis R, et al. Prevalence of left-ventricular systolic dysfunction and heart failure in the Echocardiographic Heart of England Screening Study: a population based study. Lancet 2001;358:439–44.

5. Hunt SA, Baker DW, Chin MH, et al. American College of Cardiology/American Heart Association. American College of Cardiology/American Heart Association. ACC/AHA guidelines for the evaluation and management of chronic heart failure in the adult: executive summary. A report of the American College of Cardiology/American Heart Association Task Force on Practice Guidelines (Committee to revise the 1995 Guidelines for the Evaluation and Management of Heart Failure). J Am Coll Cardiol 2001;38:2101–13.

6. Meerding WJ, Bonneux L, Polder JJ, et al. Demographic and epidemiological determinants of healthcare costs in Netherlands: cost of illness study. BMJ 1998;317:111–5.

7. O'Connell JB, Bristow MR. Economic impact of heart failure in the United States: time for a different approach. J Heart Lung Transplant 1994;13:S107–12.

8. McMurray JJ, Stewart S. Epidemiology, aetiology, and prognosis of heart failure. Heart 2000;83:596–602.

9. Riegger G. History of heart failure (including hypertension). Z Kardiol 2002;91(Suppl 4):60–3.

10. Silverberg DS, Wexler D, Blum M, et al. The use of subcutaneous erythropoietin and intravenous iron for the treatment of the anemia of severe, resistant congestive heart failure: improves cardiac and renal function and functional cardiac class, and markedly reduces hospitalizations. J Am Coll Cardiol 2000;35:1737–44.

11. Sharma R, Francis DP, Pitt B, et al. Haemoglobin predicts survival in patients with chronic heart failure: a substudy of the ELITE II trial. Eur Heart J 2004;25:1021–8.

12. Szachniewicz J, Petruk-Kowalczyk J, Majda J, et al. Anaemia is an independent predictor of poor outcome in patients with chronic heart failure. Int J Cardiol 2003;90:303–8.

13. Kalra PR, Bolger AP, Francis DP, et al. Effect of anemia on exercise tolerance in chronic heart failure in men. Am J Cardiol 2003;91:888–91.

14. Mozaffarian D, Nye R, Levy WC. Anemia predicts mortality in severe heart failure: the Prospective Randomized Amlodipine Survival Evaluation (PRAISE). J Am Coll Cardiol 2003;41:1933–9.

15. Anker SD, Ponikowski P, Varney S, et al. Wasting as independent risk factor for mortality in chronic heart failure. Lancet 1997;349:1050–3.

16. Evans WJ, Morley JE, Argilés J, et al. Cachexia: a new definition. Clin Nutr 2008;27:793–9.

17. Anker SD, Rauchhaus M. Insights into the pathogenesis of chronic heart failure: immune activation and cachexia. Curr Opin Cardiol 1999;14:211–6.

18. Doehner W, Pflaum CD, Rauchhaus M, et al. Leptin, insulin sensitivity and growth hormone binding protein in chronic heart failure with and without cardiac cachexia. Eur J Endocrinol 2001;145:727–35.

19. von Haehling S, Doehner W, Anker SD. Nutrition, metabolism, and the complex pathophysiology of cachexia in chronic heart failure. Cardiovasc Res 2007;73:298–309.

20. Gross F. Renin und Hypertensin, physiologische oder pathologische Wirkstoffe? [Renin and hypertensin, physiological or pathological substances?] Klin Wochenschr 1958;36:693–706 [in German].

21. Davis JO, Freeman RH. Historical perspectives on the renin-angiotensin-aldosterone system and angiotensin blockade. Am J Cardiol 1982;49:1385–9.

22. von Haehling S, Sandek A, Anker SD. Pleiotropic effects of angiotensin-converting enzyme inhibitors and the future of cachexia therapy. J Am Geriatr Soc 2005;53:2030–1.

23. Riegger GA, Liebau G, Holzschuh M, et al. Role of the renin-angiotensin system in the development of congestive heart failure in the dog as assessed by chronic converting-enzyme blockade. Am J Cardiol 1984;53:614–8.

24. Chidsey CA, Harrison DC, Braunwald E. Augmentation of the plasma norepinephrine response to exercise in patients with congestive heart failure. N Engl J Med 1962;267:650–4.

25. Cohn JN, Levine TB, Olivari MT, et al. Plasma norepinephrine as a guide to prognosis in patients with chronic congestive heart failure. N Engl J Med 1984;311:819–23.

26. Levine B, Kalman J, Mayer L, et al. Elevated circulating levels of tumor necrosis factor in severe chronic heart failure. N Engl J Med 1990;323:236–41.

27. Braunwald E. Biomarkers in heart failure. N Engl J Med 2008;358:2148–59.

28. Lee TH, Goldman L. Evaluation of the patient with acute chest pain. N Engl J Med 2000;342:1187–95.

29. Lainscak M, von Haehling S, Anker SD. Natriuretic peptides and other biomarkers in chronic heart failure: from BNP, NT-proBNP, and MR-proANP to routine biochemical markers. Int J Cardiol 2009;132:303–11.

30. Dickstein K, Cohen-Solal A, Filippatos G, , et alTask Force for Diagnosis and Treatment of Acute and Chronic Heart Failure 2008 of the European Society of Cardiology. ESC Guidelines for the diagnosis and treatment of acute and chronic heart failure 2008: the Task Force for the Diagnosis and Treatment of Acute and Chronic Heart Failure 2008 of the European Society of Cardiology. Developed in collaboration with the Heart Failure Association of the ESC (HFA) and endorsed by the European Society of Intensive Care Medicine (ESICM). Eur Heart J 2008;29:2388–442.

31. Anker SD, von Haehling S. Inflammatory mediators in chronic heart failure: an overview. Heart 2004;90: 464–70.

32. Seta Y, Shan K, Bozkurt B, et al. Basic mechanisms in heart failure: the cytokine hypothesis. J Card Fail 1996;2:243–9.

33. Torre-Amione G, Kapadia S, Lee J, et al. Tumor necrosis factor-alpha and tumor necrosis factor receptors in the failing human heart. Circulation 1996;93:704–11.

34. Torre-Amione G, Stetson SJ, Youker KA, et al. Decreased expression of tumor necrosis factor-alpha in failing human myocardium after mechanical circulatory support: a potential mechanism for cardiac recovery. Circulation 1999;100:1189–93.

35. von Haehling S, Genth-Zotz S, Bolger AP, et al. Effect of noradrenaline and isoproterenol on lipopolysaccharide-induced tumor necrosis factor-alpha production in whole blood from patients with chronic heart failure and the role of beta-adrenergic receptors. Am J Cardiol 2005;95: 885–9.

36. Tohmeh JF, Cryer PE. Biphasic adrenergic modulation of beta-adrenergic receptors in man. Agonist-induced early increment and late decrement in beta-adrenergic receptor number. J Clin Invest 1980;65:836–40.

37. Mancini DM, Frey MJ, Fischberg D, et al. Characterization of lymphocyte beta-adrenergic receptors at rest and during exercise in ambulatory patients with chronic congestive heart failure. Am J Cardiol 1989;63:307–12.

38. Ishida S, Makino N, Masutomo K, et al. Effect of metoprolol on the beta-adrenoceptor density of lymphocytes in patients with dilated cardiomyopathy. Am Heart J 1993;125:1311–5.

39. Wu JR, Chang HR, Huang TY, et al. Reduction in lymphocyte beta-adrenergic receptor density in infants and children with heart failure secondary to congenital heart disease. Am J Cardiol 1996; 77:170–4.

40. Matsumori A, Yamada T, Suzuki H, et al. Increased circulating cytokines in patients with myocarditis and cardiomyopathy. Br Heart J 1994;72:561–6.

41. Tsutamoto T, Hisanaga T, Wada A, et al. Interleukin-6 spillover in the peripheral circulation increases with the severity of heart failure, and the high plasma level of interleukin-6 is an important prognostic predictor in patients with congestive heart failure. J Am Coll Cardiol 1998;31:391–8.

42. Sandek A, Rauchhaus M, Anker SD, et al. The emerging role of the gut in chronic heart failure. Curr Opin Clin Nutr Metab Care 2008;11:632–9.

43. Anker SD, Egerer KR, Volk HD, et al. Elevated soluble CD14 receptors and altered cytokines in chronic heart failure. Am J Cardiol 1997;79: 1426–30.

44. Sandek A, Bauditz J, Swidsinski A, et al. Altered intestinal function in patients with chronic heart failure. J Am Coll Cardiol 2007;50:1561–9.

45. Genth-Zotz S, von Haehling S, Bolger AP, et al. Pathophysiologic quantities of endotoxin-induced tumor necrosis factor-alpha release in whole blood from patients with chronic heart failure. Am J Cardiol 2002;90:1226–30.

46. Sharma R, von Haehling S, Rauchhaus M, et al. Whole blood endotoxin responsiveness in patients with chronic heart failure: the importance of serum lipoproteins. Eur J Heart Fail 2005;7:479–84.

47. Niebauer J, Volk HD, Kemp M, et al. Endotoxin and immune activation in chronic heart failure: a prospective cohort study. Lancet 1999;353:1838–42.

48. Mann DL. Inflammatory mediators and the failing heart: past, present, and the foreseeable future. Circ Res 2002;91:988–98.

49. Carswell EA, Old LJ, Kassel RL, et al. An endotoxin-induced serum factor that causes necrosis of tumors. Proc Natl Acad Sci U S A 1975;72: 3666–70.

50. Beutler B, van Huffel C. Unraveling function in the TNF ligand and receptor families. Science 1994; 264:667–8.

51. von Haehling S, Jankowska EA, Anker SD. Tumour necrosis factor-alpha and the failing heart: pathophysiology and therapeutic implications. Basic Res Cardiol 2004;99:18–28.

52. Heller RA, Song K, Fan N, et al. The p70 tumor necrosis factor receptor mediates cytotoxicity. Cell 1992;70:47–56.

53. Feldman AM, Combes A, Wagner D, et al. The role of tumor necrosis factor in the pathophysiology of heart failure. J Am Coll Cardiol 2000; 35:537–44.

54. Bolger AP, Anker SD. Tumour necrosis factor in chronic heart failure: a peripheral view on pathogenesis, clinical manifestations and therapeutic implications. Drugs 2000;60:1245–57.

55. Kriegler M, Perez C, DeFay K, et al. A novel form of TNF/cachectin is a cell surface cytotoxic transmembrane protein: ramifications for the complex physiology of TNF. Cell 1988;53:45–53.

56. Ferrari R, Bachetti T, Confortini R, et al. Tumor necrosis factor soluble receptors in patients with various degrees of congestive heart failure. Circulation 1995;92:1479–86.

57. Rauchhaus M, Doehner W, Francis DP, et al. Plasma cytokine parameters and mortality in patients with chronic heart failure. Circulation 2000;19:3060–7.

58. Deswal A, Petersen NJ, Feldman AM, et al. Cytokines and cytokine receptors in advanced heart failure: an analysis of the cytokine database from the Vesnarinone Trial (VEST). Circulation 2001; 103:2055–9.

59. Doehner W, Bunck AC, Rauchhaus M, et al. Secretory sphingomyelinase is upregulated in chronic heart failure: a second messenger system of immune activation relates to body composition, muscular functional capacity, and peripheral blood flow. Eur Heart J 2007;28:821–8.

60. Vaz Pérez A, Doehner W, von Haehling S, et al. The relationship between tumor necrosis factor-alpha, brain natriuretic peptide and atrial natriuretic peptide in patients with chronic heart failure. Int J Cardiol 2009.

61. Niethammer M, Sieber M, von Haehling S, et al. Inflammatory pathways in patients with heart failure and preserved ejection fraction. Int J Cardiol 2008; 129:111–7.

62. Kotler DP. Cachexia. Ann Intern Med 2000;133: 622–34.

63. von Haehling S, Lainscak M, Springer J, et al. Cardiac cachexia: a systematic overview. Pharmacol Ther 2009;121:227–52.

64. Schefold JC, Hasper D, von Haehling S, et al. Interleukin-6 serum level assessment using a new qualitative point-of-care test in sepsis: a comparison with ELISA measurements. Clin Biochem 2008;41:893–8.

65. Schefold JC, von Haehling S, Corsepius M, et al. A novel selective extracorporeal intervention in sepsis: immunoadsorption of endotoxin, interleukin 6, and complement-activating product 5a. Shock 2007;28:418–25.

66. Gwechenberger M, Pacher R, Berger R, et al. Comparison of soluble glycoprotein 130 and cardiac natriuretic peptides as long-term predictors of heart failure progression. J Heart Lung Transplant 2005;24:2190–5.

67. Dinarello CA, Wolff SM. The role of interleukin-1 in disease. N Engl J Med 1993;328:106–13.

68. Long CS. The role of interleukin-1 in the failing heart. Heart Fail Rev 2001;6:81–94.

69. Sharma R, Bolger AP, Rauchhaus M, et al. Cellular endotoxin desensitization in patients with severe chronic heart failure. Eur J Heart Fail 2005;7:865–8.

70. Okamura H, Tsutsi H, Komatsu T, et al. Cloning of a new cytokine that induces IFN-gamma production by T cells. Nature 1995;378:88–91.

71. Netea MG, Kullberg BJ, Verschueren I, et al. Interleukin-18 induces production of proinflammatory cytokines in mice: no intermediate role for the cytokines of the tumor necrosis factor family and interleukin-1beta. Eur J Immunol 2000;30:3057–60.

72. Naito Y, Tsujino T, Fujioka Y, et al. Increased circulating interleukin-18 in patients with congestive heart failure. Heart 2002;88:296–7.

73. Mallat Z, Heymes C, Corbaz A, et al. Evidence for altered interleukin 18 (IL)-18 pathway in human heart failure. FASEB J 2004;18:1752–4.

74. Seta Y, Kanda T, Tanaka T, et al. Interleukin-18 in patients with congestive heart failure: induction of atrial natriuretic peptide gene expression. Res Commun Mol Pathol Pharmacol 2000;108:87–95.

75. Tillett WS, Francis T Jr. Serological reactions in pneumonia with nonprotein somatic fraction of pneumococcus. J Exp Med 1930;52:561–71.

76. Morley JJ, Kushner I. Serum C-reactive protein levels in disease. Ann N Y Acad Sci 1982;389:406–18.

77. Gabay C, Kushner I. Acute-phase proteins and other systemic responses to inflammation. N Engl J Med 1999;340:448–54.

78. Oliveira EB, Gotschlich EC, Liu TY. Primary structure of human C-reactive protein. Proc Natl Acad Sci U S A 1977;74:3148–51.

79. Gotschlich EC, Edelman GM. C-reactive protein: a molecule composed of subunits. Proc Natl Acad Sci U S A 1965;54:558–66.

80. Pye M, Rae AP, Cobbe SM. Study of serum C-reactive protein concentration in cardiac failure. Br Heart J 1990;63:228–30.

81. Kaneko K, Kanda T, Yamauchi Y, et al. C-reactive protein in dilated cardiomyopathy. Cardiology 1999;91:215–9.

82. Campbell B, Badrick T, Flatman R, et al. Limited clinical utility of high-sensitivity plasma C-reactive protein assays. Ann Clin Biochem 2002;39:85–8.

83. Anand IS, Latini R, Florea VG, et al. Val-HeFT Investigators. C-reactive protein in heart failure: prognostic value and the effect of valsartan. Circulation 2005;112:1428–34.

84. Farmakis D, Filippatos G, Lainscak M, et al. Anticoagulants, antiplatelets, and statins in heart failure. Cardiol Clin 2008;26:49–58.

85. von Haehling S, Anker SD. Statins for heart failure: at the crossroads between cholesterol reduction and pleiotropism? Heart 2005;91:1–2.

86. Kjekshus J, Apetrei E, Barrios V, et al. The CORONA Group. Rosuvastatin in older patients with systolic heart failure. N Engl J Med 2007;357:2248–61.

87. von Haehling S. Statins for heart failure: still caught in no man's land? Clin Sci 2009;116:37–9.

88. Ganz T. Hepcidin, a key regulator of iron metabolism and mediator of anemia of inflammation. Blood 2003;102:783–8.

89. Malyszko J, Malyszko JS, Hryszko T, et al. Is hepcidin a link between anemia, inflammation and liver function in hemodialized patients? Am J Nephrol 2005;25:586–90.

90. Adlbrecht C, Kommata S, Hülsmann M, et al. Chronic heart failure leads to an expanded plasma volume and pseudoanaemia, but does not lead to a reduction in the body's red cell volume. Eur Heart J 2008;29:2343–50.

91. Engström G, Hedblad B, Tydén P, et al. Inflammation-sensitive plasma proteins are associated with increased incidence of heart failure: a population-based cohort study. Atherosclerosis 2009;202: 617–22.

92. Devaux B, Scholz D, Hirche A, et al. Upregulation of cell adhesion molecules and the presence of low grade inflammation in human chronic heart failure. Eur Heart J 1997;18:470–9.

93. Wilhelmi MH, Leyh RG, Wilhelmi M, et al. Upregulation of endothelial adhesion molecules in hearts with congestive and ischemic cardiomyopathy: immunohistochemical evaluation of inflammatory endothelial cell activation. Eur J Cardiothorac Surg 2005;27:122–7.

94. Tousoulis D, Homaei H, Ahmed N, et al. Increased plasma adhesion molecule levels in patients with heart failure who have ischemic heart disease and dilated cardiomyopathy. Am Heart J 2001;141:277–80.

95. Tsutamoto T, Hisanaga T, Fukai D, et al. Prognostic value of plasma soluble intercellular adhesion molecule-1 and endothelin-1 concentration in patients with chronic congestive heart failure. Am J Cardiol 1995;76:803–8.

96. Andreassen AK, Nordøy I, Simonsen S, et al. Levels of circulating adhesion molecules in congestive heart failure and after heart transplantation. Am J Cardiol 1998;81:604–8.

97. Yin WH, Chen JW, Jen HL, et al. The prognostic value of circulating soluble cell adhesion molecules in patients with chronic congestive heart failure. Eur J Heart Fail 2003;5:507–16.

98. Maruna P, Nedelníková K, Gürlich R. Physiology and genetics of procalcitonin. Physiol Res 2000; 49(Suppl 1):S57–61.

99. Assicot M, Gendrel D, Carsin H, et al. High serum procalcitonin concentrations in patients with sepsis and infection. Lancet 1993;341:515–8.

100. Clec'h C, Fosse JP, Karoubi P, et al. Differential diagnostic value of procalcitonin in surgical and medical patients with septic shock. Crit Care Med 2006;34:102–7.

101. Brunkhorst FM, Clark AL, Forycki ZF, et al. Pyrexia, procalcitonin, immune activation and survival in cardiogenic shock: the potential importance of bacterial translocation. Int J Cardiol 1999;72:3–10.

102. Buratti T, Ricevuti G, Pechlaner C, et al. Plasma levels of procalcitonin and interleukin-6 in acute myocardial infarction. Inflammation 2001;25:97–100.

103. Stolz D, Christ-Crain M, Gencay MM, et al. Diagnostic value of signs, symptoms and laboratory values in lower respiratory tract infection. Swiss Med Wkly 2006;136:434–40.

104. Müller B, Harbarth S, Stolz D, et al. Diagnostic and prognostic accuracy of clinical and laboratory parameters in community-acquired pneumonia. BMC Infect Dis 2007;7:10.

105. Arutyunov GP, Kostyukevich OI, Serov RA, et al. Collagen accumulation and dysfunctional mucosal barrier of the small intestine in patients with chronic heart failure. Int J Cardiol 2008;125:240–5.

106. Sandek A, Anker SD, von Haehling S. The gut and intestinal bacteria in chronic heart failure. Curr Drug Metab 2009;10:22–8.

107. Triantafilou M, Triantafilou K. Lipopolysaccharide recognition: CD14, TLRs and the LPS-activation cluster. Trends Immunol 2002;23:301–4.

108. da Silva Correia J, Soldau K, Christen U, et al. Lipopolysaccharide is in close proximity to each of the proteins in its membrane receptor complex: transfer from CD14 to TLR4 and MD-2. J Biol Chem 2001;276:21129–35.

109. Genth-Zotz S, von Haehling S, Bolger AP, et al. The anti-CD14 antibody IC14 suppresses ex vivo endotoxin stimulated tumor necrosis factor-alpha in patients with chronic heart failure. Eur J Heart Fail 2006;8:366–72.

110. Jankowska EA, von Haehling S, Czarny A, et al. Activation of the NF-kappaB system in peripheral blood leukocytes from patients with chronic heart failure. Eur J Heart Fail 2005;7:984–90.

111. Földes G, von Haehling S, Okonko DO, et al. Fluvastatin reduces increased blood monocyte Toll-like receptor 4 expression in whole blood from patients with chronic heart failure. Int J Cardiol 2008;124:80–5.

112. Földes G, von Haehling S, Anker SD. Toll-like receptor modulation in cardiovascular disease: a target for intervention? Expert Opin Investig Drugs 2006;15:857–71.

113. Shimazu R, Akashi S, Ogata H, et al. MD-2, a molecule that confers lipopolysaccharide responsiveness on Toll-like receptor 4. J Exp Med 1999;189:1777–82.

114. Triantafilou K, Triantafilou M, Dedrick RL. A CD14-independent LPS receptor cluster. Nat Immunol 2001;2:338–45.

115. Triantafilou M, Triantafilou K. Heat-shock protein 70 and heat-shock protein 90 associate with Toll-like receptor 4 in response to bacterial lipopolysaccharide. Biochem Soc Trans 2004;32:636–9.

116. Genth-Zotz S, Bolger AP, Kalra PR, et al. Heat shock protein 70 in patients with chronic heart failure: relation to disease severity and survival. Int J Cardiol 2004;96:397–401.

Biomarkers of Oxidative Stress in Heart Failure

Barry H. Trachtenberg, MD, Joshua M. Hare, MD*

KEYWORDS

- Heart failure • Oxidative stress • Biomarkers
- Myeloperoxidase • Uric acid • Isoprostane
- Malonaldehyde • Oxidized LDL

Production of reactive oxygen species (ROS) occurs as a byproduct of numerous signaling pathways and mitochondrial respiration; ROS, themselves, are signaling molecules. Oxidants play a vital role in processes such as the regulation of cell growth and differentiation, nitric oxide (NO) inactivation, alteration of extracellular matrix activity, and modulation of inflammatory processes.

Oxidative stress may be defined as a state of imbalance, whereby ROS production exceeds endogenous antioxidant mechanisms. ROS include free radicals, such as superoxide anion ($O2 \cdot -$) and hydroxyl ($OH \cdot$), as well as nonradical oxidants such as hydrogen peroxide (H_2O_2). These molecules are generated in most cell and tissue types, including the cardiovascular system.

The potential sources of ROS production in the cardiovascular system are numerous and include: mitochondria, NADPH oxidase, xanthine oxidase (XO), NO synthases, activated neutrophils, cyclo-oxygenases, and auto-oxidation of certain tissue metabolites.[1] Increased amounts of ROS in the myocardium can be caused by: ischemia-reperfusion injury; an increase in inflammatory cytokines; auto-oxidation of catecholamines; and an impairment in antioxidant production.[2] Excess ROS production is implicated in oxidation of lipids, DNA, proteins, and other molecules, which, in turn, can cause impairment in signaling, toxicity, and organ malfunction. Accumulating data suggest that acute and chronic heart failure are

characterized by states of oxidative stress (Reviewed in[2]).

By analogy to oxidative stress, nitrosative stress may be defined by conditions under which the free radical signaling molecule, NO, or other reactive nitrogen species (RNS), are produced in excess relative to their metabolism. There is a growing awareness that RNS interact with ROS, and that optimal physiologic signaling is dependent upon proper nitroso-redox balance.[3,4] Disruptions in this balance have been associated with various pathological conditions including endothelial dysfunction, hypertension, diabetes mellitus, myocardial ischemia, and heart failure (HF).

In a major manifestation of nitroso-redox imbalance, excess superoxide and nitric oxide enhance the production of the highly reactive peroxynitrite, which in turn is implicated in a host of adverse downstream effects associated with several disease states. Peroxynitrite also causes a positive feedback effect on its own formation by inhibiting mitochondrial superoxide dismutase production. It contributes significantly to endothelial dysfunction in various ways, including by decreasing NO availability (and thus causing decreased vasodilation) and triggering lipid peroxidation. Peroxynitrite also activates matrix metalloproteinases and nuclear enzyme poly (ADP-ribose) polymerase-1, causing depletion of cellular ATP stores and activating various inflammatory pathways. The nitrosylation of various proteins also mediates many of the processes leading to organ

Dr. Hare discloses ownership of equity in Duska. Dr. Hare is supported by NIH RO1's HL-65455, AG-025017, HL-HL84275 and U54 HL-81028.

University of Miami, Miami, FL, USA

* Corresponding author. Department of Medicine, Cardiovascular Division, University of Miami Miller School of Medicine, Clinical Research Building, Room 1124, 1120 NW 14th Street C-205, Miami, FL 33136.

E-mail address: jhare@med.miami.edu (J.M. Hare).

Heart Failure Clin 5 (2009) 561–577
doi:10.1016/j.hfc.2009.04.003
1551-7136/09/$ – see front matter © 2009 Published by Elsevier Inc.

malfunction. The nitrosylation of tyrosine, for example, and subsequently prostacyclin synthase, creatine kinase, voltage-gated K channels in the coronary endothelium, and the sarcosplasmic reticulum Ca ATPase (SERCA 2A) lead to impaired cardiac contractility as well as endothelial dysfunction. Other effects of peroxynitrite include apoptosis and damage to DNA. Most importantly, peroxynitrite may disrupt the physiological signaling exerted by protein S-nitrosylation.

Although free radical activity has been measured directly using electron spin resonance spectroscopy,[5] methods such as these are cumbersome and highly sophisticated, rendering them very difficult to apply clinically. Several surrogate urine and serum biomarkers of oxidative stress have been identified including myeloperoxidase, malondialdehyde, oxidized LDL, biopyrrin, isoprostane, and uric acid. A very relevant potential marker of nitric oxide signaling is S-nitrosohemoglobin (SNO-Hb), and nitrotyrosine may offer insights into nitrosative stress. In assessing the utility of biomarkers such as these, it may be helpful to consider key questions such as the ease with which the test can be measured, the additional information provided by the test compared to existing diagnostic tests, and if the tests can aid in clinical decision making.[6] In this article, the authors critically review the literature of a select group of oxidative stress biomarkers in cardiac disease and, in particular, HF.

MYELOPEROXIDASE

Myeloperoxidase (MPO) has emerged as a promising biomarker for predicting prognosis in patients with acute coronary syndrome (ACS), and, to a lesser extent, HF. It is an enzyme abundant in azurophilic granules of neutrophils and monocyte lysosomes. When neutrophils are activated and undergo respiratory burst, MPO is secreted and catalyzes the formation of highly cytotoxic molecules vital to the ability of neutrophils to kill bacteria.

Although MPO is beneficial in host defense, numerous studies have shown its formation of chlorinating, oxidating, and nitrating species can disrupt the biological function of proteins and lipids in a deleterious manner. MPO activity is associated with endothelial dysfunction via its role in the initiation of lipid peroxidation,[7] consumption of NO, and impairment of HDL function.[8]

Animal data suggest that MPO is released by leukocytes within the infarction zone after an acute MI and may contribute to left ventricular (LV) remodeling. MPO knockout mice have significantly decreased LV dilatation and preserved LV function even in the absence of smaller infarct size.[9] Recent clinical evidence in humans supports a role for measuring MPO in patients with chest pain or ACS.

In a study of patients presenting to the emergency room with chest pain of suspected cardiac origin, MPO levels were predictive of major adverse cardiac events in the subsequent 30-day and 6-month periods,[10] even in a cohort of patients with negative troponin T levels (measured serially). The addition of MPO to troponin T levels significantly increased the ability to predict major adverse cardiovascular events (MACE) at 30 days with a modest sensitivity of 66% and specificity of 61%. Furthermore, MPO levels were elevated at baseline (within 2 hours of symptoms) in patients with initially negative troponin T levels, indicating that MPO may serve as a useful tool for risk-stratification, especially in the emergency room or urgent care setting. The fact that MPO portends a worse cardiac prognosis even in patients without evidence of myocardial necrosis offers clinical evidence to support the basic science studies that indicate that MPO levels are correlated with plaque instability.[11] These findings have been reproduced in a study evaluating the ability of MPO and other biomarkers to predict recurrent ischemic events in patients presenting with ACS.[12] Not only was MPO significantly elevated in patients who presented with MI compared to unstable angina, but MPO levels were also predictive of recurrent hospitalization for ACS or MI at 30 days. However, MPO levels may not help guide initial management; there was no difference in 30-day or 6-month outcomes in patients with MPO elevations who were treated with an early invasive versus a conservative strategy. Although in this study the association between MPO elevation and recurrent ischemia was attenuated by 6 months, other data shows that MPO levels above the median can portend up to a two-fold increase in mortality up to 5 years after admission for AMI. This increase in mortality was independent of BNP or LVEF, as well as additive to either LVEF or BNP in predicting mortality.[13]

The potential role for MPO as a biomarker of HF is less clear. There have been data showing MPO elevation in patients with chronic systolic heart failure compared to control patients, and levels are increased with worsening NYHA functional classification.[14] Interestingly, these findings were independent of whether or not the etiology of the HF was due to ischemia. Higher MPO levels in patient with chronic systolic HF are predictive of higher mortality, the need for cardiac transplantation, and HF hospitalization (**Fig. 1**).[15] The correlation between echocardiographic findings in these patients are variable; although there was no association with LVEF or LV end diastolic diameter, increased MPO levels were associated with signs of worsening LV diastolic parameters and right ventricular systolic functioning.

MPO has been studied as a tool, along with C-reactive protein, to provide value additive to BNP in screening for systolic HF in the community. MPO alone detected 27 of 28 patients with

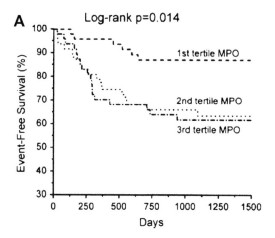

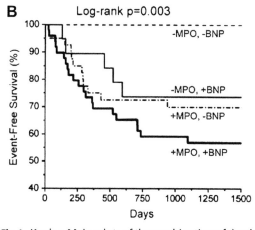

Fig.1. Kaplan-Meier plots of the combination of death, heart transplant, or heart failure hospitalization stratified by myeloperoxidase levels. (*A*) In 140 patients patients with chronic systolic HF and EF<35%, MPO levels stratified in tertiles are predictive of a decreased time from the combination of death, heart transplantation, or HF hospitalization. (*B*) Patients from the two highest tertiles of MPO levels (MPO+) are further stratified by BNP level above the median (65 pg/mL) to predict event-free survival. Thus, prognostic information provided by MPO is independent of BNP levels. (*From* Tang WH, Tong W, Troughton RW, et al. Prognostic value and echocardiographic determinants of plasma myeloperoxidase levels in chronic heart failure. J Am Coll Cardiol 2007;49:2368; with permission.)

undiagnosed systolic dysfunction out of 1360 patients screened. Both MPO and CRP have diagnostic value additive to BNP alone, and surprisingly, the specificity of MPO was higher than plasma BNP (74% versus 41%, respectively; **Fig. 2**).[16]

Although MPO may prove useful in chronic HF, MPO levels are not significantly different in patients presenting with dyspnea who were determined to have acute decompensated HF versus those who had other causes of dyspnea. MPO levels increased in both groups, suggesting that many causes of dyspnea other than HF can cause MPO elevations.[17] Nor was MPO predictive of mortality. This discordance in data among studies of MPO in HF may be explained by the variability of cutoff values used in the clinical studies, which is a key limitation in the role of MPO as a biomarker.

On the positive side, serum MPO measurement is commercially available and inexpensive. Correlation among different assays is high. In patients presenting with chest pain or ACS, the information provided by MPO is additive to currently used biomarkers and has been reproduced. Further trials may lead to an enhanced role of MPO in these patients. It would be particularly valuable to determine if the risk heralded by an elevated MPO can be modified by a specific therapy. Statins may decrease MPO levels via down-regulation of MPO gene expression,[18] but currently there is no therapy specific for MPO. In HF, the data are more discordant and more studies are warranted to evaluate if it can aid in clinical decision-making.

BIOPYRRINS

Heme-oxygenase, the rate-limiting enzyme of bilirubin synthesis, is induced during oxidative stress. Bilirubin has been shown to scavenge ROS in vivo as well as protect low density lipoprotein from oxidation via the interaction of bilirubin with alpha-tocopherol.[19] In fact, studies have shown an inverse relationship between serum bilirubin and coronary artery disease, suggesting that bilirubin may have a cardiovascular protective effect.[20,21]

Using an antibilirubin monoclonal antibody, oxidative metabolites of bilirubin excreted in urine (called biopyrrins) have been identified. Ischemia-reperfusion injuries are classic models of tissue damage caused by the production of excess ROS, which overwhelms natural antioxidant defense mechanisms. In a rat model of myocardial ischemia-reperfusion injury, biopyrrin levels were shown to increase in a biphasic manner at 8 hours and 24 hours. Rats injected with an NO synthase

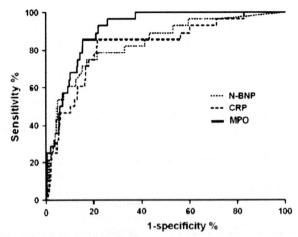

Fig. 2. Receiver operating characteristic curves for N-BNP, CRP, and MPO in screening for left ventricular systolic dysfunction (LVSD). 1360 patients in the community were screened by echocardiogram and 28 patients were found to have LVSD. Using a cutoff of 33.9 ng/mL, 27/28 patients with LVSD were detected. Area under the curve for N-BNP, MPO, and CRP respectively is 0.84, 0.91, and 0.82. MPO had the highest specificity and positive predictive value as an individual marker. Specificity was best using all three markers. (*From* Ng LL, Pathik B, Loke IW, et al. Myeloperoxidase and C-reactive protein augment the specificity of B-type natriuretic peptide in community screening for systolic heart failure. Am Heart J 2006;152:98; with permission.)

inhibitor had not only decreased MI size and improved hemodynamics, but they also had decreased urinary biopyrrin excretion and decreased histological evidence of biopyrrin formation in both the heart and lungs.

Although the number of human studies evaluating the role of biopyrrins as biomarker is limited, they have yielded interesting results. Urinary levels of biopyrrin (corrected for serum creatinine) are elevated in patients with MI, and they are significantly higher in patients with AMI compared those with stable angina. Reperfusion of coronary arteries leads to an increased urinary biopyrrin/creatinine level, peaking at 4 hours and trending towards normal from 24 hours to 7 days.[22]

In one study, levels of biopyrrin were significantly higher in patients with HF compared to controls, and correlated with NYHA functional classification[23] (**Fig. 3**). Log biopyrrin/creatinine levels had a significant positive correlation with

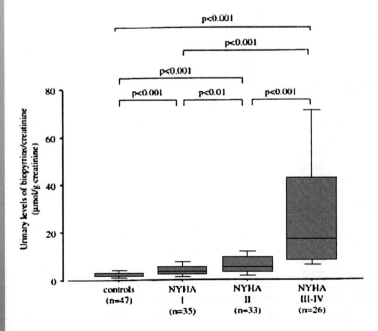

Fig. 3. Box plot of urinary levels of biopyrrins (corrected for creatinine) associated with New York Heart Association (NYHA) functional classes. The biopyrrin/creatinine level is not only significantly higher in patients who have heart failure versus controls, but the level is also significantly increased in association with higher NYHA classification. NYHA III/IV patients are combined. The *horizontal line* in the box represents the median value; the *boxed area* is the interquartile range; and the *whiskers* represent the 10% to 90% range. (*From* Hokamaki J, Kawano H, Yoshimura M, et al. Urinary biopyrrins levels are elevated in relation to severity of heart failure. J Am Coll Cardiol 2004;43:1882; with permission.)

pulmonary artery wedge pressure, pulmonary artery pressure, and log BNP, while having a significant negative correlation with cardiac index and LVEF. Standard medical therapy of HF was shown to reduce both biopyrrin levels and NYHA functional classification in parallel. In addition, a study of cardiac transplanted rats revealed a significant increase in biopyrrins in rats with allograft vasculopathy versus those treated with immunosuppressive therapy. The detection of elevated urinary biopyrrin preceded the detection of myocardial necrosis, which was represented by troponin elevation.[24]

Biopyrrin is a relatively new biomarker of oxidative stress. Compared to other biomarkers, there is a scarcity of data evaluating its potential role in heart disease. Thus, its clinical utility in adding to diagnostic precision or prognosis is currently limited. Although some studies have shown promise, more data, particularly in humans, are needed.

ISOPROSTANE

Isoprostanes (iPs), structural isomers of prostaglandins, are products of peroxidation of unsaturated fatty acid residues in lipids. Although some iPs exist in plasma, most are formed in the phospholipid layer of cell membranes and excreted in urine.

A major limitation of using isoprostanes as biomarkers is the discrepancy in the method and type of measurement. Isoprostanes have traditionally been measured in urine or plasma via gas chromatomography–mass spectrometry though some researchers have detected iP levels by enzyme linked immunosorbent assay, which is a less costly method but with less reliability and precision.[25,26] The vast majority of isoprostane studies have focused on F2-isoprostanes, products of the arachidonic acid peroxidation. In this group alone, there are as many as 64 compounds in four structural classes that can be formed. The selection of which class of iP is measured can lead to starkly different conclusions, particularly in CHF. Although isomers from all four classes of $PGF_2\alpha$ (F2-iPs) are significantly elevated in certain diseases (ie, homozygous familial hypercholesteremia or HFH), only selected F2-iPs are elevated in HF.[27]

Numerous studies have been performed using isoprostanes as markers of oxidative stress in general and, more specifically, of lipid peroxidation. iPs are commonly regarded as promising biomarkers because they: represent a nonenzymatic process of lipid peroxidation; are rapidly excreted (thus varying in temporal proximity to changes in oxidative stress); and can be measured noninvasively in the urine. In fact, a study from the National Institute of Environmental Health Sciences (NIEHS) that used acute CCl4 poisoning as a rodent model of oxidative stress determined that serum and urine iPs, along with serum malondialdehyde, represented the most reliable biomarkers of oxidative stress out of ten potential markers,[28] although this group did not include biomarkers such as oxidized LDL, uric acid, or MPO.

Urinary excretion of $iPF_2\alpha$-III is elevated in patients with coronary heart disease, and its levels increase in tandem with the number of traditional coronary heart disease risk factors (**Fig. 4**).[29] Large cohort studies have shown significant correlations between iPs and smoking, diabetes mellitus, and obesity, although the data have been disparate with regards to dyslipidemia.[30–32] These conflicting data may be accounted for by the use of different measurement techniques.

Several studies have investigated iPs in patients who have HF. Urinary, plasma, and even pericardial levels of iPs have been correlated with CHF and have been found to increase significantly with higher NYHA functional class.[33–35] One study found levels of certain antioxidants (vitamins C, A, E, lutein, and lycopene) to decrease with higher NYHA classification.[33] Vitamin E can lower iP levels in apo-E deficient mice in accord with decreased atherosclerotic lesions.[36] Evidence for a similar effect from vitamin E in humans is conflicting.[37,38] Thus, although there are substantial amounts of data using isoprostane levels as a marker of oxidant stress, its potential as a biomarker is limited by the variety of iP isomers and the lack of uniformity in method of measurement.

MALONDIALDEHYDE/THIOBARBITURIC ACID REACTIVE SUBSTANCES

Malondialdehyde (MDA) and thiobarbituric acid reactivity (TBAR) are measurements of lipid peroxidation and peroxidative tissue injury. Whereas MDA is an aldehyde produced from the peroxidation of lipids, thiobarbituric acid reactive substances (TBARS) are products of lipid oxidation that estimate MDA measurement. TBA assays are limited as they also measure nonlipid-related materials and fatty peroxide-derived decomposition products, in addition to MDA.[39] MDA has cardiovascular toxicity, particularly in atherogenesis by converting LDL to its atherogenic form, and by promoting collagen cross-linkage in the extracellular matrix.[40]

MDA and TBARS levels vary widely among normal controls and between laboratories because of variations in measurement techniques. More reliable, newer techniques are more time-consuming and expensive, which limits their

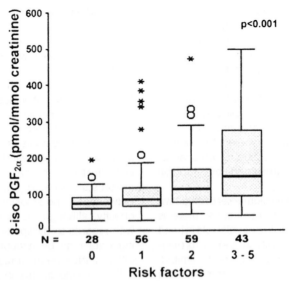

Fig. 4. Box plot of urinary excretion of 8-iso-PGF$_{2\alpha}$ (corrected for creatinine) versus the number of risk factors for coronary heart disease (CHD). This study involved 93 patients with known CHD and 93 controls frequency-matched by age and sex. Urinary levels of 8-iso-PGF$_{2\alpha}$ were measured in all patients and were found to increase with the number of CHD risk factors. Risk factors are obesity, diabetes mellitus, hyperlipidemia, hypertension, and cigarette smoking. The *horizontal line* in the box represents the median; the *box* is the interquartile range; the *open circles* represent outliers; and *asterisks* are extreme values. (*From* Schwedhelm E, Bartling A, Lenzen H, et al. Urinary 8-iso-prostaglandin F2alpha as a risk marker in patients with coronary heart disease: a matched case-control study. Circulation 2004;109:847; with permission.)

adoption.[41] These limitations on reproducibility and general availability restrict the advancement of MDA/TBARS as a useful biomarker.

MDA and TBARs are elevated dose-dependently in: tobacco smokers,[41] patients with diabetes mellitus, those with impaired glucose tolerance,[40,42] and those with coronary artery disease (CAD).[43] In patients on hemodialysis, elevated MDA may be associated with the acceleration of CAD.[44] MDA may be alternatively elevated or reduced following post-MI reperfusion,[45,46] limiting its application in this setting.

Several studies with small sample sizes have shown that MDA levels are elevated in patients who have HF and that MDA levels are inversely correlated with ejection fraction.[47–49] Metoprolol and carvedilol therapy have been shown to lead to a decline in TBARs in patients who have idiopathic and ischemic HF.[50] However, other trials have failed to show that MDA is significantly elevated in HF patients with recent MI or in stable ischemic and nonischemic HF patients.[51] Larger trials with ischemic and nonischemic cardiomyopathy patients are needed.

As mentioned previously, a recent study by the NIEHS determined that isoprostanes and serum MDA (detected by gas chromatography and mass spectrometry) have excellent potential as general markers of oxidative stress because of their

sensitivity and specificity. However, MDA levels are limited by several factors, first and foremost by the challenges of a reproducible and uniform measurement. At present, it has not been demonstrated that MDA levels enhance clinical decision-making or provide additional information to existing data. Further insights into the use of MDA/TBARS as a biomarker of oxidative stress in HF or CAD will depend on additional studies.

OXIDIZED LDL

While many oxidative stress biomarkers represent an indirect measurement of lipid oxidation, several methods of measuring oxidized (Ox) LDL in a more direct manner have been developed. Original methods measured auto-antibodies as indirect indices of Ox-LDL, but a series of new tests using ELISA have been developed to measure Ox-LDL directly. Three different procedures have been developed to measure anti–Ox-LDL mAbs (DLH3 Ab, E06 Ab, and the 4E6 Ab). The methodology, expense, and sensitivity/specifity of these tests vary.

LDL contains one apoB molecule plus many triacylglycerol, free cholesterol, cholesteryl ester, and phospholipid molecules. Upon oxidation of LDL, many oxidized lipids are produced and some of these lipids modify apoB. OxLDL contains fragmented and aggregate forms of apoB, and monoclonal Abs of OxLDL recognize only the fragments.[52] It is presumed that these assays measure only minimally oxidized LDL, because LDL that is more oxidized should be recognized and cleared rapidly. The proportion of LDL that is oxidized has been reported to range from 0.001% to 0.65% in healthy subjects[53,54] to significantly higher levels in patients who have cardiovascular disease (up to 5% in patients with ACS).[55] Small, dense LDL is most susceptible to oxidation because it contains smaller amounts of antioxidants.

OxLDL has been studied extensively in association with coronary and carotid artery disease. Not only is OxLDL elevated in patients who have coronary and cerebral artery disease,[56] but the level of OxLDL within carotid artery plaque is also greater than in plasma by approximately 70-fold. Patients who have carotid artery disease and elevated plaque OxLDL are more likely to have greater macrophage infiltration of plaque, which is associated with thin fibrous caps, large lipid cores, and a greater propensity for plaque rupture. Levels of OxLDL are also elevated in patients with acute cerebral ischemia and may be predictive of enlargement of the size of infarction.[57,58]

In one of the more promising studies of the role of OxLDL as a biomarker for CAD, plasma OxLDL had a sensitivity of 76% and a specificity of 90% for CAD.[59] OxLDL has been shown to be increased in patients with AMI versus patients with stable angina,[60] and other studies have shown that OxLDL levels are predictive of future adverse cardiac events in patients with known CAD.[61] One of the largest cohort studies investigating the ability of OxLDL to predict coronary events found a positive association, but it should be noted that this was not independent of the cheaper and more readily available levels of apo B or total cholesterol/HDL ratio.[62] This study, using the widely-used 4E6 mAb, conflicts with smaller studies using other available mAbs which found that OxLDL can predict coronary events independent of apoB.[63,64] Underlying the association with cardiovascular events may be the fact that OxLDL contributes to endothelial dysfunction by enhancing the degradation and inhibiting the synthesis of NO. Using intracoronary bradykinin to assess endothelial function in patients without CAD, OxLDL was correlated with a more resistant vasomotor response.[65]

Plasma levels of OxLDL are also elevated in patients with chronic HF of ischemic and nonischemic etiology and are positively correlated with NYHA classification, inversely correlated with ejection fraction, and may serve as an independent predictor of mortality (**Fig. 5**).[66] A recent study of more than 2500 healthy controls found that OxLDL may be associated with early ventricular remodeling using sensitive tissue doppler echocardiographic variables,[54] suggesting a potential for screening in the community. However, the effect size was small, implying that any potential utility would be only as an additive test to other screening tests or biomarkers. The source of elevation of plasma OxLDL was evaluated in a small Japanese study. Measurements of OxLDL were taken from the coronary sinus, aortic root, and femoral vein in patients with idiopathic dilated cardiomyopathy. In control subjects, there was no difference between measurements regardless of the source, although in DCM patients there was a significant increase in oxLDL sampled from the coronary sinus versus the aorta or periphery, suggesting a myocardial source of OxLDL in the failing heart.

A recent study showed not only a significantly elevated baseline OxLDL in patients with newly diagnosed peripartum cardiomyopathy, but also that levels decreased significantly in patients who had clinical improvement after 6 months versus those without improvement.[67] The sample size was small, but if these initial findings are investigated further, they may lead to novel insights into the mechanism and treatment of peripartum cardiomyopathy. Holvoet and colleagues[68] also found that OxLDL was increased significantly in heart transplant patients with allograft vasculopathy, independent of time after transplantation, age, and serum levels of LDL and high density lipoprotein cholesterol.

Ox-LDL is associated with diabetes mellitus[69] and is positively correlated with blood glucose levels.[70] Recent investigations have supported an association of Ox-LDL with the metabolic syndrome.[71,72] However, other studies do not support an association;[73] this discrepancy may be dependent on which of the three major antibodies is used to measure OxLDL.

OxLDL measurements have some advantages over some of the other biomarkers, especially the fact that it measures lipid peroxidation in a direct manner. It is also commercially available (4e6) and is potentially modifiable with therapies such as statins. It has a good sensitivity and specificity for diagnosing coronary artery disease and initial studies suggest a potential role in HF detection and prognosis. Its utility is limited by disparity between methods, expense, and the finding that at least one of the methods is not additive to existing tests (ie, 4E6 mAb and apo B, total cholesterol/HDL level).

URIC ACID

Xanthine oxidoreductase (XOR), the enzyme that catalyzes the conversion of hypothanthine to uric

A

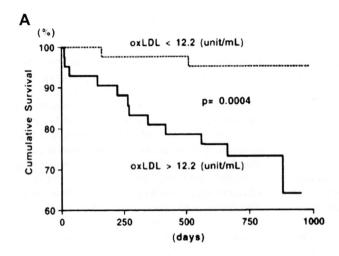

B

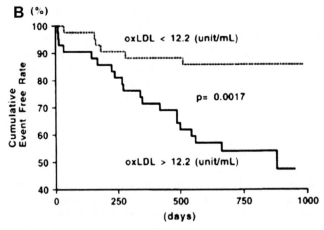

Fig. 5. The Kaplan-Meier survival (A) and cumulative cardiac event-free rate (B) plots for congestive heart failure patients subdivided into two groups according to the median level of oxidized low-density lipoprotein (OxLDL) (12.2 U/mL). 84 patients with chronic CHF were followed for a mean of 780 days after OxLDL was measured. Cardiac events include cardiac death or hospitalization for worsening HF, MI, or fatal arrhythmia. Using the median level of OxLDL 12.2 U/mL as a stratifier, patients with levels below the median were 1.9 times more likely to survive and 2.5 times more likely to be free of cardiac events. (From Tsutsui T, Tsutamoto T, Wada A, et al. Plasma oxidized low-density lipoprotein as a prognostic predictor in patients with chronic congestive heart failure. J Am Coll Cardiol 2002;39:962; with permission.)

acid in the final steps of purine degradation, also produces ROS as part of this process.[3] Xanthine oxidase (XO) and XOR activity are upregulated in myocardial ischemia/referfusion injury and in HF.[3] Because the enzyme produces uric acid in proportion to ROS generation, uric acid may be a very valuable and easily accessible biomarker of oxidative stress in the cardiovascular system.

The association of increased XO activity and increased levels of uric acid (UA) may be of clinical relevance in a broad array of cardiovascular disorders, including HF and several diseases that are risk factors for HF, including hypertension, the metabolic syndrome, vascular disease, dyslipidemia, diabetes mellitus, obesity and obstructive sleep apnea. Elevated uric acid levels predict the onset of hypertension, a phenomenon more pronounced in younger patients. In one study of patients with a mean age of 13 years who were referred for new onset of HTN, UA was elevated in 89% of patients with essential HTN and 30% with secondary HTN.[74] Adult studies have shown varying degrees of uric acid elevation but generally

have been much more modest. Because uric acid directly results from XO activity, there are important therapeutic implications, such as a recent study showing blood pressure lowering effects of XO inhibition in young patients with HTN and elevated serum uric acid.[75]

There are numerous biomarker evaluations of serum uric acid. Hyperuricemia independently predicts: mortality in patients with type II diabetes mellitus;[76] the presence of ischemic heart disease and cardiovascular mortality in the general population;[77] and mortality and the need for cardiac transplantation in patients with chronic HF[78] (Fig. 6). In chronic HF patients, receiver operating curve analysis identified a cutoff of 565 μmol/L (9.5 mg/dL) as the best mortality predictor, and every 1 mg/dL increase in SUA increases the risk of death in these patients by 31.7%. Perhaps the most remarkable finding from this study was that UA predicted prognosis better than established indicators such as age, renal function, sodium, and exercise capacity.[78] Hyperuricemia is also unique in that it is the only marker of oxidative stress

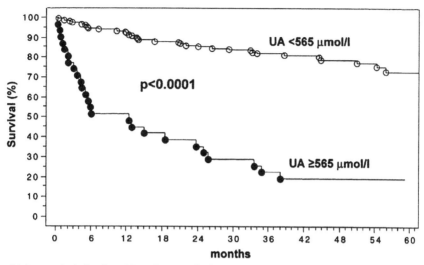

Fig. 6. Kaplan-Meier survival plot for 182 patients with chronic HF using serum uric acid (SUA) levels. In a separate study, it was determined using receiver operating curve analyses that a using a cutoff SUA level of 565 μmol/L (9.5 mg/dL) yielded the best prediction of mortality. This level was used to predict survival (mean follow-up time = 41 months) for 182 patients with chronic heart failure of ischemic and nonischemic etiology, P<0.001. (*From* Anker SD, Doehner W, Rauchhaus M, et al. Uric acid and survival in chronic heart failure: validation and application in metabolic, functional, and hemodynamic staging. Circulation 2003;107:1994; with permission.)

used in a clinically validated model to predict survival in HF, displaying independent predictive power in the Seattle Heart Failure Model.[79]

Hyperuricemia is also associated with hemodynamic compromise. In a study of patients with HF undergoing right heart catheterization, hyperuricemia was positively associated with pulmonary artery pressures and inversely associated with cardiac index. Importantly, these findings were independent of BNP levels.[80] In patients who have chronic HF, elevated uric acid levels are associated with elevated inflammatory markers such as IL-6, TNFα, AND ICAM-1,[81] and are inversely correlated with anaerobic threshold on metabolic testing.[82]

Another unique advantage of serum uric acid as a biomarker is the availability of targeted therapy to reduce UA levels. Allopurinol and its active metabolite oxypurinol are both XO inhibitors, widely used for gout, which have been used in various studies exploring the effects of XO inhibition on HF. A number of animal studies have shown significant efficacy for XO inhibitors in HF. In murine models of induced MI, XO inhibition lead to improved survival,[83] improved LV function,[84] and reversal of ventricular remodeling.[85] Allopurinol in dogs with pacing-induced HF attenuates the increase in afterload and the decrease in myocardial contractility versus controls.[86]

The studies of XO inhibition in human trials of HF have shown promise; however, they have not shown enough benefit to justify its widespread

use in this patient population. A small study of patients with ischemic cardiomyopathy given a single dose of IV oxypurinol with cardiac MR imaging before and after showed a significant improvement in ejection fraction and a decreased end-systolic volume.[87] Studies have also shown an improvement in endothelial function with XO inhibition in patients with CAD[88] as well as an improvement in myocardial efficiency.[89]

A prospective trial of 60 patients with an LVEF<40% showed a significant improvement in LVEF after 4 weeks of oxypurinol, although these results were only significant after a post-hoc elimination of 13 patients who were screened despite having an EF>40%. In a larger double-blinded, randomized control trial of oxypurinol in greater than 400 patients with Class II–IV NYHA HF on maximally tolerated medical therapy (OPT-CHF study), oxypurinol was found to have no benefit in the composite end-point that measured mortality, morbidity, and quality of life. In a subgroup analysis of patients with a UA>9.5 mg/dL, there was a nonsignificant trend towards clinical improvement; the degree to which SUA was lowered by oxypurinol correlated with patient outcome in a number of important clinical domains (**Fig. 7**).[90] This key finding strongly supports the notion that serum uric acid may be a biomarker that can be used to target XO inhibitor therapy.

A recent study suggests that most clinical trials, such as the OPT-CHF, may not have used sufficient dosing of XO inhibitors.[91] This study

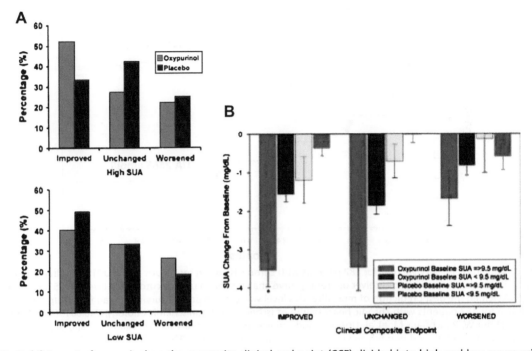

Fig. 7. (*A*) Impact of oxypurinol on the composite clinical end point (CCE) divided into high and low serum uric acid levels. 405 patients with symptomatic HF (NYHA III or IV) on maximum medical therapy were randomized to oxypurinol therapy or placebo. Overall, there was no difference in the composite clinical end point. However, a subgroup analysis using a SUA level of 9.5 mg/dL as a cutoff, showed a trend toward improvement in the group with high SUA levels ($P = 0.02$ for interaction between high and low SUA groups). (*B*) Degree of SUA reduction in patients with low and high SUA in relation to change in CCE. The *y*-axis is represented by the change in SUA and the *x*-axis is grouped according to an improved, unchanged, or worsened CCE. In the cohort of patients treated with oxypurinol, there was a significant association between improvement in CCE and reduction in SUA. For example, patients in the oxypurinol/high SUA category who improved had an average SUA decrease of 3.5 mg/dL compared with 1.7 mg/dL in the patients who had a worsened CCE. (*From* Hare JM, Mangal B, Brown J, et al. Impact of oxypurinol in patients with symptomatic heart failure. Results of the OPT-CHF study. J Am Coll Cardiol 2008;51:2305; with permission.)

demonstrated that high-dose allopurinol can lead to improvement in endothelial function, independent of its ability to lower uric acid levels.

Recently, allantoin has been proposed as a novel marker of oxidative stress. Most mammals use the enzyme uricase to convert uric acid into allantoin. Humans have a mutation resulting in the absence of this enzyme, though oxidation of UA may lead to production of allantoin. Allantoin is elevated in HF and is reduced with allopurinol;[92] thus, allantoin also has potential both as a marker and a therapeutic target.

MARKERS OF NITRO-REDOX IMBALANCE: S-NITROSOHEMOGLOBIN

As previously mentioned, nitric oxide plays a central regulatory role largely via post-translational modification of effector molecules, a process termed "S-nitrosylation". This ubiquitous signaling process is disrupted by oxidative stress (**Fig. 8**). Accordingly, biomarkers of S-nitrosylation could

play a pivotal role in assessing a patient's nitroso-redox balance. This data, in turn, could give much greater insights into a patient's status than assessing the degree of oxidative stress alone.

Over the past decades, it has become clear that circulating hemoglobin is a crucial molecule influenced by nitroso-redox balance. In this regard, Hb is the largest reservoir of both O2 and NO in the body. O2 is carried at hemes, and NO at both hemes and cysteine thiols to form S-nitroso-hemoglobin(SNO-Hb).[93] SNO-Hb forms preferentially in the oxygenated form of Hb, whereas conditions of low oxygen content cause release of NO from Hb, thus causing vasodilation and enhanced oxygen delivery to tissues. SNO-Hb is regenerated with the rebinding of O2 to Hb in the lungs. Hemoglobin is also a source of superoxide, and this production of ROS by Hb is increased in states of persistent hypoxia, such as chronic HF.[4] This increased production of ROS impairs S-nitrosylation. These important considerations

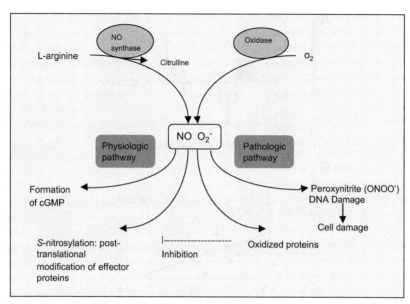

Fig. 8. The interaction between NO and superoxide production (termed the nitroso-redox balance). The nitroso-redox balance is critical to cellular and organ functioning. In patients who have heart failure, the production of superoxide is increased, inhibiting the post-translational modification of effector molecules by NO. (*From* Hare JM. Nitroso-redox balance in the cardiovascular system. New Engl J Med 2004;351:2113; with permission. Copyright © 2004, Massachusetts Medical Society.)

provide the basis for measurements of Hb and its level of S-NO having the potential to be a valuable biomarker, particularly in HF and other cardiovascular diseases.

SNO-Hb stores NO in a stable form and transports it in an endocrine fashion. Datta and colleagues[94] showed that, in vitro, the ability of red blood cells (RBCs) to vasodilate correlated directly with SNO-Hb content. In a clinical study by the same group, patients with CHF demonstrated an impaired ability to deliver SNO-Hb versus controls (**Fig. 9**). Thus, the impaired delivery of NO to the vasculature would be implicated in the vasoconstriction and poor oxygen delivery that are characteristic of heart failure. Perhaps future studies can investigate peripheral SNO-Hb levels as markers of HF severity.

Evidence also supports a role for the anion nitrite in delivery of NO to the vasculature. Nitrite is reduced to NO by deoxygenated hemoglobin. Recent studies have shown that nitrite predominantly causes vasodilation of capacitance vessels during periods of normoxia, but, under hypoxic conditions, nitrite causes profound arterial vasodilation without an incremental increase in venous vasodilation.[95] This finding suggests a potential role for nitrite therapy in the setting of a myocardial infarction, which in canine models has been shown to reduce infarct size.[96]

In addition to SNO-Hb as a potential biomarker to examine the health of the SNO system, other biomarkers may give insight into nitrosative stress, the state in which NO production is excessive and deleterious (a condition often associated with inflammation). Nitrotyrosine has been examined in this capacity and shown to correlate with MPO and TNFα, in a manner that increased with worsening heart failure.[97]

THERAPEUTICS

Despite substantial enthusiasm for the OS hypothesis of disease, the vast majority of large clinical outcome trials of antioxidant vitamins have been largely disappointing. A recent long-term study of greater than 14,000 male physicians, for example, showed no cardiovascular benefit from the use of vitamin E or C supplementation.[98] Trials of dietary modification such as the DASH diet have shown, however, to decrease markers of oxidative stress.[99] Interestingly, many of the cardioprotective benefits linked to red wine consumption are caused by decreased lipid peroxidation and increased bioavailability of nitric oxide.[100]

FP15 is a peroxynitrite decomposition catalyst molecule that has been studied in animal models that tested the effect of directly antagonizing the effects of oxidative and nitrosative stress. This novel agent has been shown to decrease myocardial necrosis, improve attenuate diabetic cardiomyopathy, and improve survival in a doxorubicin-induced cardiomyopathy model.[2]

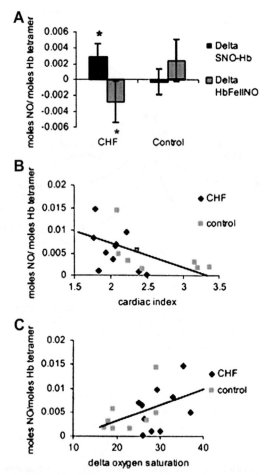

Fig. 9. (*A*) Change in Hb-bound nitric oxide (NO) as measured from pulmonary artery to left ventricle in patients with CHF and control patients. HbFeNO represents iron-nitrosylhemoglobin, which is produced when NO binds deoxygenated Hb. During pulmonary oxygenation, SNO-Hb is formed when some NO bind to a cysteine residue of Hb. Shown here is the change in Hb-bound NO from PA to LV in CHF patients (n = 10) and control subjects (n = 8). In CHF patients, SNO-Hb was found to increase with pulmonary oxygenation while HbFeNO decreases with oxygenation. *Significant change in metabolite flux ($P<0.05$). (*B*) Change in total NO metabolite flux across pulmonary circulation versus cardiac index. The change in NO metabolite flux correlates inversely with cardiac index for CHF patients and control subjects ($P<0.05$). (*C*) Change in total NO metabolite flux across pulmonary circulation versus delta Hb oxygen saturation ($dSaO_2$). The change in NO metabolite flux correlates positively with $dSaO_2$ for CHF patients and control subjects.($P<0.05$). These findings suggest that there are transpulmonary gradients of Hb-bound NO in CHF and that they are more pronounced with worsening hemodynamics (*B*) and with the increased peripheral oxygen extraction (*C*) characteristic of heart failure. Hemoglobin may transport these NO metabolites and release NO or its metabolites peripherally to hypoxic areas. (*From* Datta B, Tufnell-Barrett T, Bleasdale RA, et al. Red blood cell nitric oxide as an endocrine vasoregulator: a potential role in congestive heart failure. Circulation 2004;109:1341; with permission.)

A full review of medications with potential or proven antioxidant properties is beyond the scope of this review. It should be noted, however, that some of the benefits from HF medications. such as statins, carvedilol, hydralazine, angiotensin receptor blockers, and angiotensin converting enzyme inhibitors, are attributed to their antioxidant capabilities, while nitrates directly stimulate nitric oxide.

SUMMARY

The past few decades have seen a wealth of studies advancing insights into the role of oxidative and nitrosative stress in cardiovascular disease. Perhaps the greatest insight in this regard is that ROS and RNS exhibit numerous important physiological and pathophysiological interactions. As knowledge of pathophysiology has advanced,

Table 1
Comparison of biomarkers of oxidative stress

	Aids in Diagnosis?	Aids in Prognosis or Risk-Stratification?	Modifiable with Specific Targeted Therapy?
MPO	++	++	−
Biopyrrin	−	+	−
Isoprostane	+	+	−
MDA/TBARS	±	±	−
OxLDL	++	++	+++
Uric acid	++	++++	++++

−: Not enough data, ±: Evidence neither supports nor conflicts, +: Minimal evidence to support, ++: Some evidence to support, +++: Good evidence to support, ++++: Very good evidence to support.
Abbreviations: MDA/TBARS, malondialdehyde/thiobarbituric acid reactive substances; MPO, myeloperoxidase.

so have attempts to assess OS and NS with biomarkers. Several novel serum and urine biomarkers have been used to reflect these pathways, which are critical in the pathophysiology of HF. Some have shown promise as targets of therapy, but none, except perhaps uric acid, has emerged in a uniform manner to currently enhance care for the average clinician (**Table 1**). Although measuring UA clearly adds to existing prognostic indicators, it is still unclear if XO inhibition should be recommended for patients with HF and elevated serum uric acid. Investigations into the use of a profile combining multiple biomarkers, including oxidative stress, neurohormonal, and inflammatory markers, rather than any single biomarker may ultimately provide the most utility. One of the main limitations of many of the individual oxidative stress biomarkers is the lack of uniformity and standardization among many of the specific tests. Also, more large clinical trials using biomarkers, particularly interventional studies, need to be performed. Finally, it would be of particular value to conduct a large-scale population-based study that measures all known oxidative stress biomarkers so as to determine the relative value and additive information provided by their measurement (see **Fig 1**).

REFERENCES

1. Cave AC, Brewer AC, Narayanapanicker A, et al. NADPH oxidases in cardiovascular health and disease. Antioxid Redox Signal 2006;8(5–6): 691–728.
2. Ungvari Z, Gupte SA, Recchia FA, et al. Role of oxidative-nitrosative stress and downstream pathways in various forms of cardiomyopathy and heart failure. Curr Vasc Pharmacol 2005;3(3):221–9.
3. Zimmet JM, Hare JM. Nitroso-redox interactions in the cardiovascular system. Circulation 2006; 114(14):1531–44.
4. Hare JM, Stamler JS. NO/redox disequilibrium in the failing heart and cardiovascular system. J Clin Invest 2005;115(3):509–17.
5. Spiekermann S, Landmesser U, Dikalov S, et al. Electron spin resonance characterization of vascular xanthine and NAD(P)H oxidase activity in patients with coronary artery disease: relation to endothelium-dependent vasodilation. Circulation 2003;107(10):1383–9.
6. Morrow DA, de Lemos JA. Benchmarks for the assessment of novel cardiovascular biomarkers. Circulation 2007;115(8):949–52.
7. Zhang R, Brennan ML, Fu X, et al. Association between myeloperoxidase levels and risk of coronary artery disease. JAMA 2001;286(17): 2136–42.
8. Nicholls SJ, Zheng L, Hazen SL. Formation of dysfunctional high-density lipoprotein by myeloperoxidase. Trends Cardiovasc Med 2005;15(6): 212–9.
9. Vasilyev N, Williams T, Brennan ML, et al. Myeloperoxidase-generated oxidants modulate left ventricular remodeling but not infarct size after myocardial infarction. Circulation 2005;112(18):2812–20.
10. Brennan ML, Penn MS, Van LF, et al. Prognostic value of myeloperoxidase in patients with chest pain. N Engl J Med 2003;349(17):1595–604.
11. Fu X, Kassim SY, Parks WC, et al. Hypochlorous acid oxygenates the cysteine switch domain of pro-matrilysin (MMP-7). A mechanism for matrix metalloproteinase activation and atherosclerotic plaque rupture by myeloperoxidase. J Biol Chem 2001;276(44):41279–87.
12. Morrow DA, Sabatine MS, Brennan ML, et al. Concurrent evaluation of novel cardiac biomarkers

in acute coronary syndrome: myeloperoxidase and soluble CD40 ligand and the risk of recurrent ischaemic events in TACTICS-TIMI 18. Eur Heart J 2008;29(9):1096–102.

13. Mocatta TJ, Pilbrow AP, Cameron VA, et al. Plasma concentrations of myeloperoxidase predict mortality after myocardial infarction. J Am Coll Cardiol 2007;49(20):1993–2000.

14. Tang WH, Brennan ML, Philip K, et al. Plasma myeloperoxidase levels in patients with chronic heart failure. Am J Cardiol 2006;98(6):796–9.

15. Tang WH, Tong W, Troughton RW, et al. Prognostic value and echocardiographic determinants of plasma myeloperoxidase levels in chronic heart failure. J Am Coll Cardiol 2007;49(24):2364–70.

16. Ng LL, Pathik B, Loke IW, et al. Myeloperoxidase and C-reactive protein augment the specificity of B-type natriuretic peptide in community screening for systolic heart failure. Am Heart J 2006;152(1):94–101.

17. Shah KB, Kop WJ, Christenson RH, et al. Lack of diagnostic and prognostic utility of circulating plasma myeloperoxidase concentrations in patients presenting with dyspnea. Clin Chem 2009;55(1):59–67.

18. Kumar AP, Reynolds WF. Statins downregulate myeloperoxidase gene expression in macrophages. Biochem Biophys Res Commun 2005;331(2):442–51.

19. Neuzil J, Stocker R. Free and albumin-bound bilirubin are efficient co-antioxidants for alpha-tocopherol, inhibiting plasma and low density lipoprotein lipid peroxidation. J Biol Chem 1994;269(24):16712–9.

20. Schwertner HA, Jackson WG, Tolan G. Association of low serum concentration of bilirubin with increased risk of coronary artery disease. Clin Chem 1994;40(1):18–23.

21. Hopkins PN, Wu LL, Hunt SC, et al. Higher serum bilirubin is associated with decreased risk for early familial coronary artery disease. Arterioscler Thromb Vasc Biol 1996;16(2):250–5.

22. Shimomura H, Ogawa H, Takazoe K, et al. Comparison of urinary biopyrrin levels in acute myocardial infarction (after reperfusion therapy) versus stable angina pectoris and their usefulness in predicting subsequent cardiac events. Am J Cardiol 2002;90(2):108–11.

23. Hokamaki J, Kawano H, Yoshimura M, et al. Urinary biopyrrins levels are elevated in relation to severity of heart failure. J Am Coll Cardiol 2004;43(10):1880–5.

24. Yamamoto M, Maeda H, Hirose N, et al. Bilirubin oxidation provoked by nitric oxide radicals predicts the progression of acute cardiac allograft rejection. Am J Transplant 2007;7(8):1897–906.

25. Bessard J, Cracowski JL, Stanke-Labesque F, et al. Determination of isoprostaglandin F2alpha type III in human urine by gas chromatography-electronic impact mass spectrometry. Comparison with enzyme immunoassay. J Chromatogr B Biomed Sci Appl 2001;754(2):333–43.

26. Proudfoot J, Barden A, Mori TA, et al. Measurement of urinary F(2)-isoprostanes as markers of in vivo lipid peroxidation-A comparison of enzyme immunoassay with gas chromatography/mass spectrometry. Anal Biochem 1999;272(2):209–15.

27. Li H, Lawson JA, Reilly M, et al. Quantitative high performance liquid chromatography/tandem mass spectrometric analysis of the four classes of F(2)-isoprostanes in human urine. Proc Natl Acad Sci U S A 1999;96(23):13381–6.

28. Kadiiska MB, Gladen BC, Baird DD, et al. Biomarkers of oxidative stress study II: are oxidation products of lipids, proteins, and DNA markers of CCl4 poisoning? Free Radic Biol Med 2005;38(6):698–710.

29. Schwedhelm E, Bartling A, Lenzen H, et al. Urinary 8-iso-prostaglandin F2alpha as a risk marker in patients with coronary heart disease: a matched case-control study. Circulation 2004;109(7):843–8.

30. Keaney JF Jr, Larson MG, Vasan RS, et al. Obesity and systemic oxidative stress: clinical correlates of oxidative stress in the Framingham Study. Arterioscler Thromb Vasc Biol 2003;23(3):434–9.

31. Reilly MP, Pratico D, Delanty N, et al. Increased formation of distinct F2 isoprostanes in hypercholesterolemia. Circulation 1998;98(25):2822–8.

32. Gross M, Steffes M, Jacobs DR Jr, et al. Plasma F2-isoprostanes and coronary artery calcification: the CARDIA Study. Clin Chem 2005;51(1):125–31.

33. Polidori MC, Pratico D, Savino K, et al. Increased F2 isoprostane plasma levels in patients with congestive heart failure are correlated with antioxidant status and disease severity. J Card Fail 2004;10(4):334–8.

34. Cracowski JL, Tremel F, Marpeau C, et al. Increased formation of F(2)-isoprostanes in patients with severe heart failure. Heart 2000;84(4):439–40.

35. Mallat Z, Philip I, Lebret M, et al. Elevated levels of 8-iso-prostaglandin F2alpha in pericardial fluid of patients with heart failure: a potential role for in vivo oxidant stress in ventricular dilatation and progression to heart failure. Circulation 1998;97(16):1536–9.

36. Pratico D, Tangirala RK, Rader DJ, et al. Vitamin E suppresses isoprostane generation in vivo and reduces atherosclerosis in ApoE-deficient mice. Nat Med 1998;4(10):1189–92.

37. De CR, Cipollone F, Filardo FP, et al. Low-density lipoprotein level reduction by the 3-hydroxy-3-

methylglutaryl coenzyme-A inhibitor simvastatin is accompanied by a related reduction of F2-isoprostane formation in hypercholesterolemic subjects: no further effect of vitamin E. Circulation 2002; 106(20):2543–9.

38. Desideri G, Croce G, Tucci M, et al. Effects of bezafibrate and simvastatin on endothelial activation and lipid peroxidation in hypercholesterolemia: evidence of different vascular protection by different lipid-lowering treatments. J Clin Endocrinol Metab 2003;88(11):5341–7.

39. Janero DR. Malondialdehyde and thiobarbituric acid-reactivity as diagnostic indices of lipid peroxidation and peroxidative tissue injury. Free Radic Biol Med 1990;9(6):515–40.

40. Slatter DA, Bolton CH, Bailey AJ. The importance of lipid-derived malondialdehyde in diabetes mellitus. Diabetologia 2000;43(5):550–7.

41. Lykkesfeldt J. Malondialdehyde as biomarker of oxidative damage to lipids caused by smoking. Clin Chim Acta 2007;380(1–2):50–8.

42. Niskanen LK, Salonen JT, Nyyssonen K, et al. Plasma lipid peroxidation and hyperglycaemia: a connection through hyperinsulinaemia? Diabet Med 1995;12(9):802–8.

43. Tamer L, Sucu N, Polat G, et al. Decreased serum total antioxidant status and erythrocyte-reduced glutathione levels are associated with increased serum malondialdehyde in atherosclerotic patients. Arch Med Res 2002;33(3):257–60.

44. Boaz M, Matas Z, Biro A, et al. Comparison of hemostatic factors and serum malondialdehyde as predictive factors for cardiovascular disease in hemodialysis patients. Am J Kidney Dis 1999; 34(3):438–44.

45. Pucheu S, Coudray C, Vanzetto G, et al. Assessment of radical activity during the acute phase of myocardial infarction following fibrinolysis: utility of assaying plasma malondialdehyde. Free Radic Biol Med 1995;19(6):873–81.

46. Olsson KA, Harnek J, Ohlin AK, et al. No increase of plasma malondialdehyde after primary coronary angioplasty for acute myocardial infarction. Scand Cardiovasc J 2002;36(4):237–40.

47. Diaz-Velez CR, Garcia-Castineiras S, Mendoza-Ramos E, et al. Increased malondialdehyde in peripheral blood of patients with congestive heart failure. Am Heart J 1996;131(1):146–52.

48. Polidori MC, Savino K, Alunni G, et al. Plasma lipophilic antioxidants and malondialdehyde in congestive heart failure patients: relationship to disease severity. Free Radic Biol Med 2002;32(2): 148–52.

49. Keith M, Geranmayegan A, Sole MJ, et al. Increased oxidative stress in patients with congestive heart failure. J Am Coll Cardiol 1998;31(6): 1352–6.

50. Kukin ML, Kalman J, Charney RH, et al. Prospective, randomized comparison of effect of long-term treatment with metoprolol or carvedilol on symptoms, exercise, ejection fraction, and oxidative stress in heart failure. Circulation 1999;99(20): 2645–51.

51. Tingberg E, Ohlin AK, Gottsater A, et al. Lipid peroxidation is not increased in heart failure patients on modern pharmacological therapy. Int J Cardiol 2006;112(3):275–81.

52. Itabe H, Ueda M. Measurement of plasma oxidized low-density lipoprotein and its clinical implications. J Atheroscler Thromb 2007;14(1):1–11.

53. Shoji T, Nishizawa Y, Fukumoto M, et al. Inverse relationship between circulating oxidized low density lipoprotein (oxLDL) and anti-oxLDL antibody levels in healthy subjects. Atherosclerosis 2000;148(1):171–7.

54. Rietzschel ER, Langlois M, De Buyzere ML, et al. Oxidized low-density lipoprotein cholesterol is associated with decreases in cardiac function independent of vascular alterations. Hypertension 2008;52(3):535–41.

55. Holvoet P, Vanhaecke J, Janssens S, et al. Oxidized LDL and malondialdehyde-modified LDL in patients with acute coronary syndromes and stable coronary artery disease. Circulation 1998; 98(15):1487–94.

56. Nishi K, Itabe H, Uno M, et al. Oxidized LDL in carotid plaques and plasma associates with plaque instability. Arterioscler Thromb Vasc Biol 2002;22(10):1649–54.

57. Uno M, Kitazato KT, Suzue A, et al. Inhibition of brain damage by edaravone, a free radical scavenger, can be monitored by plasma biomarkers that detect oxidative and astrocyte damage in patients with acute cerebral infarction. Free Radic Biol Med 2005;39(8):1109–16.

58. Uno M, Harada M, Takimoto O, et al. Elevation of plasma oxidized LDL in acute stroke patients is associated with ischemic lesions depicted by DWI and predictive of infarct enlargement. Neurol Res 2005;27(1):94–102.

59. Holvoet P, Mertens A, Verhamme P, et al. Circulating oxidized LDL is a useful marker for identifying patients with coronary artery disease. Arterioscler Thromb Vasc Biol 2001;21(5):844–8.

60. Ehara S, Naruko T, Shirai N, et al. Small coronary calcium deposits and elevated plasma levels of oxidized low density lipoprotein are characteristic of acute myocardial infarction. J Atheroscler Thromb 2008;15(2):75–81.

61. Shimada K, Mokuno H, Matsunaga E, et al. Circulating oxidized low-density lipoprotein is an independent predictor for cardiac event in patients with coronary artery disease. Atherosclerosis 2004;174(2):343–7.

62. Wu T, Willett WC, Rifai N, et al. Is plasma oxidized low-density lipoprotein, measured with the widely used antibody 4E6, an independent predictor of coronary heart disease among U.S. men and women? J Am Coll Cardiol 2006;48(5):973–9.

63. Tsimikas S, Brilakis ES, Miller ER, et al. Oxidized phospholipids, Lp(a) lipoprotein, and coronary artery disease. N Engl J Med 2005;353(1):46–57.

64. Toshima S, Hasegawa A, Kurabayashi M, et al. Circulating oxidized low density lipoprotein levels. A biochemical risk marker for coronary heart disease. Arterioscler Thromb Vasc Biol 2000; 20(10):2243–7.

65. Matsumoto T, Takashima H, Ohira N, et al. Plasma level of oxidized low-density lipoprotein is an independent determinant of coronary macrovasomotor and microvasomotor responses induced by bradykinin. J Am Coll Cardiol 2004;44(2):451–7.

66. Tsutsui T, Tsutamoto T, Wada A, et al. Plasma oxidized low-density lipoprotein as a prognostic predictor in patients with chronic congestive heart failure. J Am Coll Cardiol 2002;39(6):957–62.

67. Forster O, Hilfiker-Kleiner D, Ansari AA, et al. Reversal of IFN-gamma, oxLDL and prolactin serum levels correlate with clinical improvement in patients with peripartum cardiomyopathy. Eur J Heart Fail 2008;10(9):861–8.

68. Holvoet P, Van CJ, Collen D, et al. Oxidized low density lipoprotein is a prognostic marker of transplant-associated coronary artery disease. Arterioscler Thromb Vasc Biol 2000;20(3):698–702.

69. Ehara S, Ueda M, Naruko T, et al. Pathophysiological role of oxidized low-density lipoprotein in plaque instability in coronary artery diseases. J Diabetes Complicat 2002;16(1):60–4.

70. Chen NG, Azhar S, Abbasi F, et al. The relationship between plasma glucose and insulin responses to oral glucose, LDL oxidation, and soluble intercellular adhesion molecule-1 in healthy volunteers. Atherosclerosis 2000;152(1):203–8.

71. Holvoet P, Lee DH, Steffes M, et al. Association between circulating oxidized low-density lipoprotein and incidence of the metabolic syndrome. JAMA 2008;299(19):2287–93.

72. Ueba T, Nomura S, Nishikawa T, et al. Circulating oxidized LDL, measured with FOH1a/DLH3 antibody, is associated with metabolic syndrome and the coronary heart disease risk score in healthy Japanese. Atherosclerosis 2009;203(1):243–8.

73. Sjogren P, Basu S, Rosell M, et al. Measures of oxidized low-density lipoprotein and oxidative stress are not related and not elevated in otherwise healthy men with the metabolic syndrome. Arteriocler Thromb Vasc Biol 2005;25(12):2580–6.

74. Feig DI, Johnson RJ. Hyperuricemia in childhood primary hypertension. Hypertension 2003;42(3): 247–52.

75. Feig DI, Soletsky B, Johnson RJ. Effect of allopurinol on blood pressure of adolescents with newly diagnosed essential hypertension: a randomized trial. JAMA 2008;300(8):924–32.

76. Ioachimescu AG, Brennan DM, Hoar BM, et al. Serum uric acid, mortality and glucose control in patients with Type 2 diabetes mellitus: a PreCIS database study. Diabet Med 2007;24(12):1369–74.

77. Fang J, Alderman MH. Serum uric acid and cardiovascular mortality the NHANES I epidemiologic follow-up study, 1971–1992. National Health and Nutrition Examination Survey. JAMA 2000;283(18): 2404–10.

78. Anker SD, Doehner W, Rauchhaus M, et al. Uric acid and survival in chronic heart failure: validation and application in metabolic, functional, and hemodynamic staging. Circulation 2003;107(15): 1991–7.

79. Levy WC, Mozaffarian D, Linker DT, et al. The Seattle Heart Failure Model: prediction of survival in heart failure. Circulation 2006;113(11):1424–33.

80. Kittleson MM, St John ME, Bead V, et al. Increased levels of uric acid predict haemodynamic compromise in patients with heart failure independently of B-type natriuretic peptide levels. Heart 2007;93(3): 365–7.

81. Leyva F, Anker SD, Godsland IF, et al. Uric acid in chronic heart failure: a marker of chronic inflammation. Eur Heart J 1998;19(12):1814–22.

82. Leyva F, Chua TP, Anker SD, et al. Uric acid in chronic heart failure: a measure of the anaerobic threshold. Metabolism 1998;47(9):1156–9.

83. Stull LB, Leppo MK, Szweda L, et al. Chronic treatment with allopurinol boosts survival and cardiac contractility in murine postischemic cardiomyopathy. Circ Res 2004;95(10):1005–11.

84. Naumova AV, Chacko VP, Ouwerkerk R, et al. Xanthine oxidase inhibitors improve energetics and function after infarction in failing mouse hearts. Am J Physiol Heart Circ Physiol 2006;290(2): H837–43.

85. Minhas KM, Saraiva RM, Schuleri KH, et al. Xanthine oxidoreductase inhibition causes reverse remodeling in rats with dilated cardiomyopathy. Circ Res 2006;98(2):271–9.

86. Amado LC, Saliaris AP, Raju SV, et al. Xanthine oxidase inhibition ameliorates cardiovascular dysfunction in dogs with pacing-induced heart failure. J Mol Cell Cardiol 2005;39(3):531–6.

87. Baldus S, Mullerleile K, Chumley P, et al. Inhibition of xanthine oxidase improves myocardial contractility in patients with ischemic cardiomyopathy. Free Radic Biol Med 2006;41(8):1282–8.

88. Baldus S, Koster R, Chumley P, et al. Oxypurinol improves coronary and peripheral endothelial function in patients with coronary artery disease. Free Radic Biol Med 2005;39(9):1184–90.

89. Cappola TP, Kass DA, Nelson GS, et al. Allopurinol improves myocardial efficiency in patients with idiopathic dilated cardiomyopathy. Circulation 2001;104(20):2407–11.

90. Hare JM, Mangal B, Brown J, et al. Impact of oxypurinol in patients with symptomatic heart failure. Results of the OPT-CHF study. J Am Coll Cardiol 2008;51(24):2301–9.

91. George J, Carr E, Davies J, et al. High-dose allopurinol improves endothelial function by profoundly reducing vascular oxidative stress and not by lowering uric acid. Circulation 2006;114(23):2508–16.

92. Doehner W, Schoene N, Rauchhaus M, et al. Effects of xanthine oxidase inhibition with allopurinol on endothelial function and peripheral blood flow in hyperuricemic patients with chronic heart failure: results from 2 placebo-controlled studies. Circulation 2002;105(22):2619–24.

93. Hare JM. Nitroso-redox balance in the cardiovascular system. N Engl J Med 2004;351(20):2112–4.

94. Datta B, Tufnell-Barrett T, Bleasdale RA, et al. Red blood cell nitric oxide as an endocrine vasoregulator: a potential role in congestive heart failure. Circulation 2004;109(11):1339–42.

95. Maher AR, Milsom AB, Gunaruwan P, et al. Hypoxic modulation of exogenous nitrite-induced vasodilation in humans. Circulation 2008;117(5):670–7.

96. Gonzalez FM, Shiva S, Vincent PS, et al. Nitrite anion provides potent cytoprotective and antiapoptotic effects as adjunctive therapy to reperfusion for acute myocardial infarction. Circulation 2008;117(23):2986–94.

97. Eleuteri E, Di SA, Ricciardolo FL, et al. Increased nitrotyrosine plasma levels in relation to systemic markers of inflammation and myeloperoxidase in chronic heart failure. Int J Cardiol, in press.

98. Sesso HD, Buring JE, Christen WG, et al. Vitamins E and C in the prevention of cardiovascular disease in men: the Physicians' Health Study II randomized controlled trial. JAMA 2008;300(18):2123–33.

99. Miller ER III, Erlinger TP, Sacks FM, et al. A dietary pattern that lowers oxidative stress increases antibodies to oxidized LDL: results from a randomized controlled feeding study. Atherosclerosis 2005;183(1):175–82.

100. Opie LH, Lecour S. The red wine hypothesis: from concepts to protective signalling molecules. Eur Heart J 2007;28(14):1683–93.

Newer Biomarkers in Heart Failure

Sachin Gupta, MD, Mark H. Drazner, MD, MSc,
James A. de Lemos, MD*

KEYWORDS

- Biomarkers • Heart failure • Osteoprotegerin
- Galectins • Cystatins • Chromogranin A • Adipokines

The pathophysiology of heart failure is complex, and the list of biomarkers representing distinct pathophysiologic pathways is growing rapidly. Other articles in this issue of the *Heart Failure Clinics* have reviewed the role of existing biomarkers in heart failure diagnosis and risk assessment. This article focuses on some promising newer biomarkers (**Box 1**) for which less data are currently available.

OSTEOPROTEGERIN

Osteoprotegerin (OPG), a member of the tumor necrosis factor (TNF) receptor superfamily, is a secreted glycoprotein with pleiotrophic functions including the regulation of bone resorption.[1] OPG also plays a regulatory role in inflammatory pathways, acting as a decoy for the receptor activator of nuclear factor B ligand (RANKL), competitively inhibiting interactions between RANKL and RANK.[1,2] Because RANKL and RANK are difficult to measure in vivo, OPG has gained attention as a measurable indicator of activity of the RANKL/RANK pathway. This pathway is involved in the pathogenesis of heart failure, mediating autocrine, paracrine, and endocrine interactions between cells expressing RANKL and cardiomyocytes expressing RANK.[3] The binding of RANKL to RANK promotes the activity of matrix metalloproteinase, leading to degradation of extracellular matrix and increased apoptosis.[3]

In rats, expression of OPG, RANKL, and RANK is persistently increased after myocardial infarction in ischemic cardiomyocytes, whereas only OPG expression is up-regulated in the nonischemic region.[3] Moreover, these mediators localize to the cardiomyocytes within the infarcted ventricle, suggesting that the OPG/RANK/RANKL system is activated within the myocardium in ischemic heart failure.

Recent studies have evaluated circulating OPG levels in patients who have heart failure. Elevated serum levels of OPG are present in humans who have ischemic and nonischemic heart failure[4] and correlate positively with progressively increasing severity of heart failure, including higher New York Heart Association (NYHA) functional class, amino-terminal pro–brain natriuretic peptide (NTproBNP) level, and lower cardiac index (**Fig. 1**).[3] In a substudy of 234 subjects who had ischemic heart failure enrolled in the Optimal Trial in Myocardial Infarction with Angiotensin II Antagonist Losartan, baseline fasting plasma OPG levels were obtained within 3 days of myocardial infarction, and again after 1 month and 2 years.[4] For comparison, plasma OPG levels were also measured in 15 age- and sex-matched healthy control subjects. The plasma OPG levels were significantly elevated in patients who had heart failure compared with control subjects at all the time points. Patients who had OPG levels in the fourth quartile (ie, ≥ 4.1 ng/mL) had a significantly higher mortality rate than those who had lower OPG levels (**Fig. 2**). In multivariate analysis, OPG was independently associated with all-cause mortality and cardiovascular death. Increasing quartiles of OPG were also associated with increasing risk of angina, nonfatal myocardial infarction, and cardiac and all-cause mortality during the median 2.7-year follow-up period.

OPG levels may also rise in advance of clinical heart failure due to the development of subclinical cardiac structural abnormalities. In apparently healthy subjects from the community enrolled in

The University of Texas Southwestern Medical Center, Dallas, TX, USA
* Corresponding author. Division of Cardiology, Department of Internal Medicine, The University of Texas Southwestern Medical Center, 5909 Harry Hines Boulevard, HA 9.133, Dallas, TX 75390.
E-mail address: james.delemos@utsouthwestern.edu (J.A. de Lemos).

Heart Failure Clin 5 (2009) 579–588
doi:10.1016/j.hfc.2009.04.004

the Dallas Heart Study, higher OPG levels were associated with greater left ventricular mass and lower left ventricular ejection fraction,[5] findings that would be expected to lead to increased heart failure development over time.

GALECTIN-3

Galectin-3, a protein produced by activated macrophages, is a member of a family of β-galactoside-binding lectins and promotes cardiac fibroblast proliferation and collagen synthesis.[6] Increased myocardial expression of galectin-3 is seen at an early stage in the progression of heart failure and may help to identify patients who have preclinical risk factors who are more likely to develop overt heart failure.[6]

In the Pro-BNP Investigation of Dyspnea in the Emergency Department study, higher levels of galectin-3 were observed in patients who had acute heart failure compared with those who had dyspnea from other causes (9.2 pg/mL versus 6.9 pg/mL, $P<.001$).[7] The galectin-3 concentration, however, did not correlate with NYHA functional classification. Significantly higher concentrations of galectin-3 were observed in patients who died during the 60 days of follow-up compared with those who survived (median 12.9 ng/mL versus 9.0 ng/mL, $P<.001$). In multivariate analysis adjusting for NTproBNP, log-transformed galectin-3 levels remained independently associated with death within 60 days (odds ratio [OR]: 10.3 per log change, 95% confidence interval [CI]: 1.6–174.1;

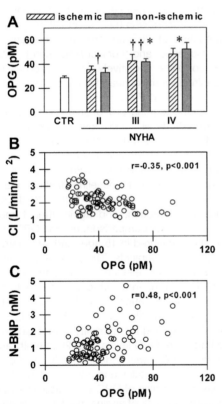

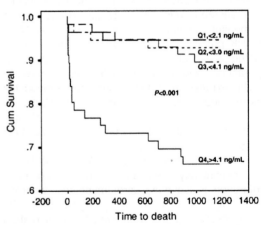

Fig. 1. (A) Serum levels of OPG in patients who have congestive heart failure according to NYHA functional class II through IV and etiology compared with healthy controls (CTR). (B) Relationship between serum OPG and cardiac index (CI). (C) Relationship between serum OPG and serum levels of NTproBNP (N-BNP) in patients who have congestive heart failure. Values are expressed as mean ± SEM, and statistical comparisons are based on entire heart failure group regardless of etiology. *$P<.05$ versus control subjects; †$P<.05$; ††$P<.01$ versus NYHA class IV. (From Ueland T, Yndestad A, Oie E, et al. Dysregulated osteoprotegerin/RANK ligand/RANK axis in clinical and experimental heart failure. Circulation 2005;111:2465; with permission).

Fig. 2. Kaplan-Meier curves showing the cumulative (Cum) incidence of death during the entire study (median follow-up 27 months) according to the quartiles (Q) of plasma OPG at enrollment. (From Ueland T, Jemtland R, Godang K, et al. Prognostic value of osteoprotegerin in heart failure after acute myocardial infarction. J Am Coll Cardiol 2004;44:1973; with permission).

$P<.01$). The combination of galectin-3 and NTpro BNP provided incremental prognostic information for short-term death (**Fig. 3**). Although individuals who had elevation of NTproBNP but not galectin-3 did not demonstrate increased risk of death and heart failure in this study, this finding is likely explained by the small size of this subgroup ($n = 36$) (see **Fig. 3**).

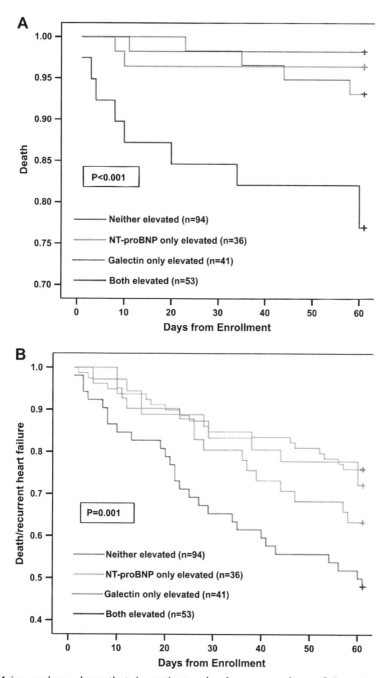

Fig. 3. Kaplan-Meier analyses show that in patients who have acute heart failure at presentation, the combination of galectin-3 in excess of 9.42 ng/mL and NTproBNP above the optimal cut point (5562 pg/mL) was associated with higher rates of death (*A*) and of mortality/recurrent heart failure (*B*) than with either of the two markers alone. (*From* van Kimmenade RR, Januzzi JL Jr, Ellinor PT, et al. Utility of amino-terminal pro-brain natriuretic peptide, galectin-3, and apelin for the evaluation of patients with acute heart failure. J Am Coll Cardiol 2006;48:1222; with permission).

CYSTATIN C

Cystatin C, a 13-kd cysteine protease inhibitor, is expressed in most human tissues and is believed to play a role in tissue remodeling.[8] Cystatin C has recently gained attention as a novel marker of renal function. Compared to creatinine or creatinine-based equations that estimate the glomerular filtration rate, cystatin C is more sensitive for detecting mild to moderate renal dysfunction and is not influenced by age, sex, or muscle mass.[9,10] Similarly to other markers of renal dysfunction,[11,12] elevated levels of cystatin C are associated with cardiac structural abnormalities[13,14] and incident heart failure.[10,15,16]

In a subgroup analysis from the Heart and Soul Study, serum cystatin C was measured in participants who had coronary artery disease but not a reported history of heart failure.[13] Left ventricular hypertrophy was present in 68% of participants in quartile 4 (cystatin C ≥1.28 mg/L) compared with 44% of those in quartile 1 (cystatin C ≤0.91 mg/L) (adjusted OR: 2.17, 95% CI: 1.34–3.52; P = .002). Diastolic dysfunction was present in 52% of participants in quartile 4 compared with 24% of

those in quartile 1 (OR: 1.79, 95% CI: 1.04–3.11; P = .04). In the same population, compared with patients in the lowest quartile of serum cystatin C, those in the highest quartile were found to be at an increased risk of incident heart failure, cardiovascular events, and all-cause mortality after multivariable adjustment.[10]

Among elderly subjects who had prevalent heart failure enrolled in the Cardiovascular Health Study, higher concentrations of cystatin C predicted an adverse prognosis independent of creatinine-based measures of renal function (**Fig. 4**).[17] Moreover, a change of one standard deviation in cystatin C was associated with a greater mortality risk (hazard ratio [HR]: 1.31, 95% CI: 1.17–1.47) compared with a similar change in creatinine (HR: 1.17, 95% CI: 1.01–1.36).[17]

Similar findings were observed in a study of 480 patients hospitalized for acutely decompensated heart failure.[18] In this study, 39% of the patients who had cystatin C levels above the median value (1.30 mg/L) died compared with 12% of those who had cystatin C levels below the median ($P<$.0001). Increasing tertiles of cystatin C were associated with a progressive increase in mortality (**Fig. 5**).

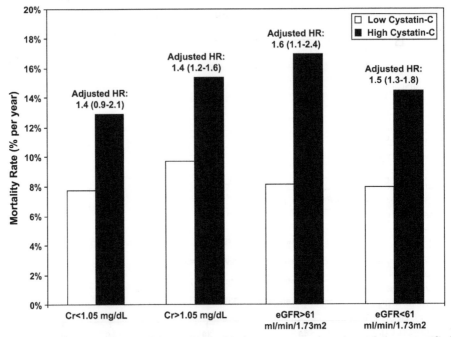

Fig. 4. Association of cystatin C levels with mortality in elderly persons who have heart failure, stratified by creatinine (Cr) and estimated glomerular filtration rate (eGFR) levels. The figure shows annual mortality risk for participants who have cystatin C levels above ("high"; *black columns*) or below ("low"; *white columns*) the median of 1.26 mg/L. The adjusted hazard ratios (HR) compare high versus low cystatin C levels among subgroups of participants who have high creatinine (above the median value of 1.05 mg/dL) or low creatinine (<1.05 mg/dL), and who have high eGFR (>61 mL/min/1.73 m^2) or low eGFR (<61 mL/min/1.73 m^2). (*From* Shlipak MG, Katz R, Fried LF, et al. Cystatin-C and mortality in elderly persons with heart failure. J Am Coll Cardiol 2005;45:270; with permission).

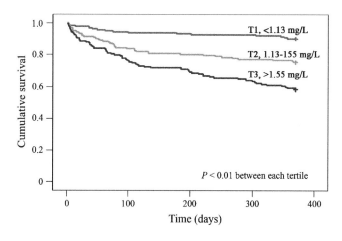

Fig. 5. One-year survival by tertiles (T) of cystatin C. All-cause mortality at 12 months: 9.9% for first tertile (cystatin C <1.13 mg/L), 24.8% for second tertile (cystatin C 1.13–1.55 mg/L), and 41.8% for third tertile (cystatin C >1.55 mg/L). *P* (log rank) for difference between tertiles: T1 versus T2, *P*<.001; T2 versus T3, *P*<.01; T1 versus T3, *P*<.0001. (*From* Lassus J, Harjola VP, Sund R, et al. Prognostic value of cystatin C in acute heart failure in relation to other markers of renal function and NT-proBNP. Eur Heart J 2007;28:1845; with permission.)

Moreover, cystatin C in combination with NTproBNP provided better risk stratification than either biomarker alone.

In summary, higher levels of cystatin C identify apparently healthy individuals in the population who are more likely to have subclinical cardiac structural abnormalities and to develop heart failure in the future. Among individuals who have existing heart failure, higher cystatin C levels appear to predict subsequent mortality. Future studies are needed to determine whether cystatin C elevation is exclusively due to renal disease or whether it also reflects primary cardiovascular pathology.

CHROMOGRANIN A

Chromogranin A (CgA), a 49-kd acidic, soluble protein, is present in secretory granules throughout the neuroendocrine and nervous systems.[19] Although predominantly found in the chromaffin granules in the adrenal medulla, CgA is also present in the secretory granules of other peptidergic cells, peripheral sympathetic neurons, cholinergic nerve terminals in skeletal muscle, and the central nervous system.[20] The coexistence of CgA with other peptide hormones and sympathetic amines in the secretory vesicles suggests that blood levels of CgA may be an important marker of sympathetic nervous system activity. CgA is a prohormone and undergoes several tissue-specific posttranslational modifications, resulting in the production of several biologically active peptides. One such group of peptides (vasostatin I and II) inhibits vasoconstriction mediated by adrenergic agonists.[19] Another such compound, catestatin, inhibits the release of catecholamines; reduced catestatin levels have been associated with hypertension.[21] In addition to inhibiting vasoconstriction, exogenous infusion of

vasostatin produces significant dose-dependent negative inotropic and lusitropic actions in animal models.[22]

Recent reports have shown increased myocardial expression of CgA in patients who have dilated and hypertrophic cardiomyopathy compared with control subjects.[22] A significant decrease in expression of CgA protein occurs after unloading of the left ventricle with a ventricular assist device.[23] Furthermore, significantly higher CgA levels are seen in patients who have chronic heart failure from ischemic and nonischemic cardiomyopathy compared with healthy subjects.[22,24] CgA levels increase progressively with increasing severity of heart failure and correlate positively with left ventricular end-diastolic pressure and BNP levels.[22] Moreover, increased CgA levels have been shown to independently predict increased mortality in patients who have myocardial infarction (HR: 1.17 per 10-ng/mL increase, 95% CI: 1.06–1.28)[25] and in those who have chronic heart failure (**Fig. 6**) (risk ratio: 1.22 between the first and third quartiles, 95% CI: 1.06–1.41) (*P* = .005).[24]

Enhanced expression of CgA in the failing myocardium and its antiadrenergic actions suggest that CgA functions in an autocrine or paracrine manner, with protective effects similar to β-blockers. At the same time, its negative lusitropic effects may be due to activation of fibroblasts and endothelial cells, thereby contributing to cardiac remodeling and diastolic dysfunction.

ADIPOKINES

Heart failure, although often considered primarily a disease of heart muscle, is a systemic disorder with secondary effects in various organ systems. Along with the progression of cardiac dysfunction and the decrease in cardiac output, an increase in

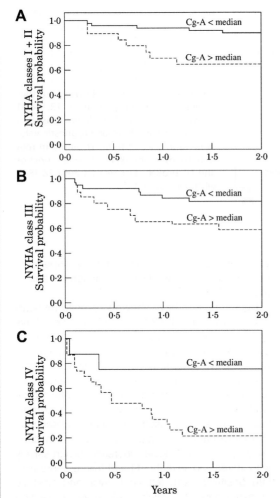

Fig. 6. Kaplan-Meier survival curves represented by NYHA class and the categorized CgA variable. The median CgA levels were 109.7 ng/mL for NYHA class I (*A*), 146.9 ng/mL for NYHA class II (*A*), 279 ng/mL for NYHA class III (*B*), and 545 ng/mL for NYHA class IV (*C*). (*From* Ceconi C, Ferrari R, Bachetti T, et al. Chromogranin A in heart failure: a novel neurohumoral factor and a predictor for mortality. Eur Heart J 2002;23:971; with permission).

systemic inflammation occurs, as reflected by elevated levels of proinflammatory cytokines such as TNF-α, interleukin-1, C-reactive protein, and OPG.[26] The inflammatory state, along with visceral congestion, may result in decreased appetite. Moreover, heart failure increases catabolism, leading to a decrease in lean muscle mass, skeletal muscle atrophy, exercise intolerance, and weight loss. Cardiac cachexia has been shown to be an independent predictor of increased mortality.[27]

The metabolic abnormalities in chronic heart failure are accompanied by alterations in several biomarkers produced by adipose tissue (called

adipokines), including adiponectin, leptin, and resistin. These adipokines exert local autocrine/paracrine effects on the myocardium in addition to systemic endocrine effects.[28] All of these adipokines are linked to cardiovascular diseases through their roles in regulation of energy balance, insulin sensitivity, angiogenesis, blood pressure, and lipid metabolism.

Adiponectin

Adiponectin, a cytokine produced by the adipose tissue, is involved in the pathophysiology of disorders linked with obesity, such as insulin resistance, type 2 diabetes mellitus, and diastolic cardiac dysfunction. Lower levels of adiponectin are seen in obese subjects compared with healthy controls, and adiponectin is negatively correlated with body mass index (BMI) and type 2 diabetes mellitus. Recently, adiponectin has received much attention as a biomarker of cardiovascular diseases in obese individuals.

Although studies have shown that low levels of adiponectin are associated with hypertension, hyperlipidemia, and coronary artery disease,[29,30] the association between adiponectin and cardiovascular disease is not consistent.[26,27] For example, patients who have heart failure have higher levels of adiponectin. Moreover, higher adiponectin levels are associated with an adverse prognosis in heart failure.[31–33]

In a study of 4046 elderly British men, high adiponectin levels were associated with increased all-cause and cardiovascular mortality independent of renal function, even in subjects who did not have known cardiovascular disease or heart failure (**Fig. 7**).[33] The interaction of adiponectin and obesity in chronic heart failure is complex and poorly understood. Obese people are more likely to develop heart failure,[34] but at the same time, high BMI is associated with a more favorable prognosis in chronic heart failure.[35] Further, there is an inverse relationship between BMI and adiponectin such that obese people have lower adiponectin levels[32,36] and patients who have heart failure and cachexia have a higher concentration of adiponectin compared with patients who have heart failure without cachexia.[37] The mechanisms behind this paradoxic relationship are unclear. Exogenous administration of adipocyte complement–related protein to mice results in profound and sustained weight loss,[38] suggesting that adiponectin, similar to TNF-α, promotes wasting, and therefore, low adiponectin concentration favors survival in heart failure. Identification of the mechanisms causing adiponectin levels to rise in heart failure requires further research.

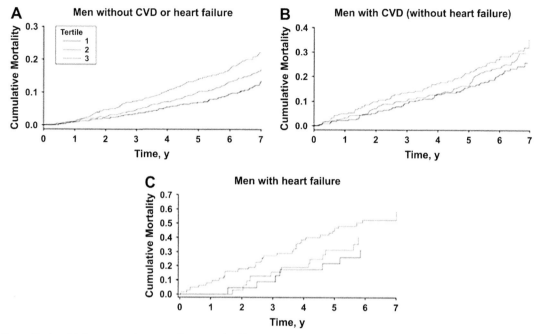

Fig. 7. Kaplan-Meier curves for mortality stratified by tertiles (T) of adiponectin levels in men who had no physician-diagnosed prevalent cardiovascular disease (CVD) or heart failure (A), in men who had CVD but no heart failure (B), and in men who had physician-diagnosed heart failure (C). (*From* Wannamethee SG, Whincup PH, Lennon L, et al. Circulating adiponectin levels and mortality in elderly men with and without cardiovascular disease and heart failure. Arch Intern Med 2007;167:1514; with permission.)

Leptin

Leptin, a 16-kd peptide predominantly secreted by adipocytes and to a small extent by other tissues including cardiomyoctyes, is integral in the regulation of body weight by inducing satiety and by increasing energy expenditure.[28] Although leptin induces satiety and promotes weight loss, a paradoxic increase in leptin levels is present in obesity due to leptin resistance in the peripheral tissues.[39] The secretion of leptin is regulated by insulin, inflammatory cytokines, catecholamines, and glucocorticoids. Of interest, elevated levels of leptin are present in patients who have heart failure and correlate with higher levels of insulin, catecholamines, TNF-α, and other inflammatory cytokines.[40–42]

Leptin has potent effects on several central and peripheral tissues including hypothalamus, sympathetic nervous system, skeletal muscle, liver, myocardium, and vascular tissue. In the central tissues, leptin mediates its action through the long-signal transducing form of its receptor, the OB-Rb receptor, leading to a decrease in appetite and an increase in sympathetic activity and energy expenditure. In skeletal muscle, leptin inhibits insulin signaling, resulting in reduced glucose uptake and increased fatty acid oxidation, thereby promoting a reduction in fat mass and

weight loss. The effects of leptin on central tissues and myocardium may remain preserved even in the presence of peripheral leptin resistance.[43]

Higher leptin levels may contribute to the unexplained weight loss and reduction in fat mass

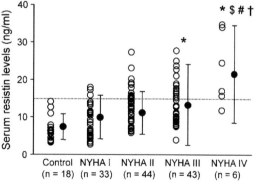

Fig. 8. Serum resistin levels in control subjects and in patients who have chronic heart failure. *P<.01 versus control; $P<.01 versus NYHA class I; #P<.01 versus NYHA class II; †P<.05 versus NYHA class III. Dashed line indicates normal upper limit of resistin, determined as mean plus 2 SD value of control subjects (14.1 ng/mL). (*From* Takeishi Y, Niizeki T, Arimoto T, et al. Serum resistin is associated with high risk in patients with congestive heart failure—a novel link between metabolic signals and heart failure. Circ J 2007;71:462; with permission.)

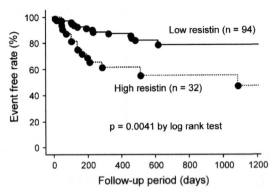

Fig. 9. Kaplan-Meier survival curves between patients who have high and low resistin levels. The follow-up end points were cardiac death and rehospitalization caused by worsening of heart failure. (*From* Takeishi Y, Niizeki T, Arimoto T, et al. Serum resistin is associated with high risk in patients with congestive heart failure—a novel link between metabolic signals and heart failure. Circ J 2007;71:462; with permission.)

commonly seen in advanced heart failure.[40] Moreover, increased leptin levels may contribute to sympathetic activation seen in heart failure.[44] In vitro, leptin promotes cardiomyocyte hypertrophy[45] (although the evidence is inconsistent),[46] oxygen free radical production, increased cardiac oxygen consumption, and decreased cardiac efficiency after cardiac injury, thereby contributing to myocardial remodeling and progression of heart failure.[28,45] In addition, the catabolic effects of leptin on skeletal muscle may contribute to the respiratory and functional limitation often seen in heart failure.[47]

Despite intriguing data linking leptin to a number of pathophysiologic pathways in heart failure, the value of leptin as a clinical biomarker has not been established. Given the close correlation between fat mass and leptin levels, interpretation of circulating leptin levels may prove to be challenging. For example, in analyses unadjusted for fat mass, leptin levels are higher in noncachectic versus cachectic patients who have heart failure; moreover, in cachectic patients, leptin levels may be similar to or lower than in healthy individuals.[48] In contrast, after adjustment for the total fat mass, a similar increase in leptin levels may be seen in cachectic and noncachectic patients, although the evidence is conflicting.[40,48] These findings highlight the need to identify appropriate indexing methods for leptin so that associations of leptin with cardiovascular phenotypes that are independent of fat mass can be characterized.

Resistin

Resistin, a 12.5-kd cysteine-rich polypeptide, has recently been identified as a unique signaling molecule associated with insulin resistance that links obesity to diabetes.[49] Increased levels of resistin are seen in mice that have diet-induced obesity and in genetic models of obesity and insulin resistance. Moreover, neutralization of resistin with antiserum enhances insulin-stimulated glucose uptake, and recombinant resistin has been shown to blunt the action of insulin.[49] In humans, inflammatory cells, not adipocytes, are the major source of circulating resistin,[50] and obese individuals have been noted to have elevated resistin levels.[51] Plasma resistin levels correlate with levels of several inflammatory markers such as soluble TNF-α receptor 2, interleukin-6, and lipoprotein-associated phospholipase A_2 and are predictive of coronary atherosclerosis in asymptomatic individuals.[52]

Serum resistin levels have been found to be higher in patients who have heart failure compared with healthy subjects, and a positive correlation is seen between increasing resistin levels and NHYA functional class (**Fig. 8**).[53] In this study that included 126 subjects who had heart failure, higher resistin levels were associated with an increased rate of hospitalization and cardiac death (**Fig. 9**).[53] In addition, resistin was a significant independent predictor of future cardiac events in multivariable models also adjusting for BNP levels, age, and BMI.

SUMMARY

Several novel biomarkers have been identified that contribute to a better understanding of pathophysiologic mechanisms involved in heart failure. For example, OPG may reflect the role of RANK/RANKL activity, and CgA may reflect the response to sympathetic activation among individuals who have heart failure. Cystatin C, a promising marker of heart failure risk in the population, may provide information beyond renal function. Several members of the adipokine family, including adiponectin, leptin, and resistin, likely play important roles in the complex and often paradoxic associations between obesity, heart failure, and outcomes.

A note of caution is warranted, however. Despite the intriguing early information from these newer markers, none is ready for clinical use. The biomarker field is becoming ever more crowded with candidate markers, and the pathway from early development to clinical application is appropriately steep. Much additional study is needed to determine how these biomarkers will fit into diagnostic and treatment algorithms for patients who have heart failure.

REFERENCES

1. Simonet WS, Lacey DL, Dunstan CR, et al. Osteoprotegerin: a novel secreted protein involved in the regulation of bone density. Cell 1997;89:309–19.
2. Yun TJ, Chaudhary PM, Shu GL, et al. OPG/FDCR-1, a TNF receptor family member, is expressed in lymphoid cells and is up-regulated by ligating CD40. J Immunol 1998;161:6113–21.
3. Ueland T, Yndestad A, Oie E, et al. Dysregulated osteoprotegerin/RANK ligand/RANK axis in clinical and experimental heart failure. Circulation 2005;111:2461–8.
4. Ueland T, Jemtland R, Godang K, et al. Prognostic value of osteoprotegerin in heart failure after acute myocardial infarction. J Am Coll Cardiol 2004;44:1970–6.
5. Omland T, Drazner MH, Ueland T, et al. Plasma osteoprotegerin levels in the general population: relation to indices of left ventricular structure and function. Hypertension 2007;49:1392–8.
6. Sharma UC, Pokharel S, van Brakel TJ, et al. Galectin-3 marks activated macrophages in failure-prone hypertrophied hearts and contributes to cardiac dysfunction. Circulation 2004;110:3121–8.
7. van Kimmenade RR, Januzzi JL Jr, Ellinor PT, et al. Utility of amino-terminal pro-brain natriuretic peptide, galectin-3, and apelin for the evaluation of patients with acute heart failure. J Am Coll Cardiol 2006;48:1217–24.
8. Abrahamson M, Olafsson I, Palsdottir A, et al. Structure and expression of the human cystatin C gene. Biochem J 1990;268:287–94.
9. Fliser D, Ritz E. Serum cystatin C concentration as a marker of renal dysfunction in the elderly. Am J Kidney Dis 2001;37:79–83.
10. Ix JH, Shlipak MG, Chertow GM, et al. Association of cystatin C with mortality, cardiovascular events, and incident heart failure among persons with coronary heart disease: data from the Heart and Soul Study. Circulation 2007;115:173–9.
11. Go AS, Chertow GM, Fan D, et al. Chronic kidney disease and the risks of death, cardiovascular events, and hospitalization. N Engl J Med 2004;351:1296–305.
12. Dries DL, Exner DV, Domanski MJ, et al. The prognostic implications of renal insufficiency in asymptomatic and symptomatic patients with left ventricular systolic dysfunction. J Am Coll Cardiol 2000;35:681–9.
13. Ix JH, Shlipak MG, Chertow GM, et al. Cystatin C left ventricular hypertrophy, and diastolic dysfunction: data from the Heart and Soul Study. J Card Fail 2006;12:601–7.
14. Patel PC, Ayers CR, Murphy SA, et al. Association of ystatin C with left ventricular structure and function: the Dallas Heart Study. Circ Heart Fail 2009;2:98–104.
15. Djousse L, Kurth T, Gaziano JM. Cystatin C and risk of heart failure in the Physicians' Health Study (PHS). Am Heart J 2008;155:82–6.
16. Watanabe S, Okura T, Liu J, et al. Serum cystatin C level is a marker of end-organ damage in patients with essential hypertension. Hypertens Res 2003;26:895–9.
17. Shlipak MG, Katz R, Fried LF, et al. Cystatin-C and mortality in elderly persons with heart failure. J Am Coll Cardiol 2005;45:268–71.
18. Lassus J, Harjola VP, Sund R, et al. Prognostic value of cystatin C in acute heart failure in relation to other markers of renal function and NT-proBNP. Eur Heart J 2007;28:1841–7.
19. Taupenot L, Harper KL, O'Connor DT. The chromogranin-secretogranin family. N Engl J Med 2003;348:1134–49.
20. Munoz DG, Kobylinski L, Henry DD, et al. Chromogranin A-like immunoreactivity in the human brain: distribution in bulbar medulla and cerebral cortex. Neuroscience 1990;34:533–43.
21. O'Connor DT, Kailasam MT, Kennedy BP, et al. Early decline in the catecholamine release-inhibitory peptide catestatin in humans at genetic risk of hypertension. J Hypertens 2002;20:1335–45.
22. Pieroni M, Corti A, Tota B, et al. Myocardial production of chromogranin A in human heart: a new regulatory peptide of cardiac function. Eur Heart J 2007;28:1117–27.
23. Wohlschlaeger J, von Winterfeld M, Milting H, et al. Decreased myocardial chromogranin a expression and colocalization with brain natriuretic peptide during reverse cardiac remodeling after ventricular unloading. J Heart Lung Transplant 2008;27:442–9.
24. Ceconi C, Ferrari R, Bachetti T, et al. Chromogranin A in heart failure: a novel neurohumoral factor and a predictor for mortality. Eur Heart J 2002;23:967–74.
25. Omland T, Dickstein K, Syversen U. Association between plasma chromogranin A concentration

and long-term mortality after myocardial infarction. Am J Med 2003;114:25–30.

26. Braunwald E. Biomarkers in heart failure. N Engl J Med 2008;358:2148–59.

27. Anker SD, Ponikowski P, Varney S, et al. Wasting as independent risk factor for mortality in chronic heart failure. Lancet 1997;349:1050–3.

28. Schulze PC, Kratzsch J. Leptin as a new diagnostic tool in chronic heart failure. Clin Chim Acta 2005; 362:1–11.

29. Hopkins TA, Ouchi N, Shibata R, et al. Adiponectin actions in the cardiovascular system. Cardiovasc Res 2007;74:11–8.

30. Lawlor DA, Davey Smith G, Ebrahim S, et al. Plasma adiponectin levels are associated with insulin resistance, but do not predict future risk of coronary heart disease in women. J Clin Endocrinol Metab 2005;90: 5677–83.

31. Kistorp C, Faber J, Galatius S, et al. Plasma adiponectin, body mass index, and mortality in patients with chronic heart failure. Circulation 2005;112: 1756–62.

32. Tamura T, Furukawa Y, Taniguchi R, et al. Serum adiponectin level as an independent predictor of mortality in patients with congestive heart failure. Circ J 2007;71:623–30.

33. Wannamethee SG, Whincup PH, Lennon L, et al. Circulating adiponectin levels and mortality in elderly men with and without cardiovascular disease and heart failure. Arch Intern Med 2007;167:1510–7.

34. Kenchaiah S, Evans JC, Levy D, et al. Obesity and the risk of heart failure. N Engl J Med 2002;347:305–13.

35. Lavie CJ, Osman AF, Milani RV, et al. Body composition and prognosis in chronic systolic heart failure: the obesity paradox. Am J Cardiol 2003;91:891–4.

36. Cnop M, Havel PJ, Utzschneider KM, et al. Relationship of adiponectin to body fat distribution, insulin sensitivity and plasma lipoproteins: evidence for independent roles of age and sex. Diabetologia 2003;46:459–69.

37. McEntegart MB, Awede B, Petrie MC, et al. Increase in serum adiponectin concentration in patients with heart failure and cachexia: relationship with leptin, other cytokines, and B-type natriuretic peptide. Eur Heart J 2007;28:829–35.

38. Fruebis J, Tsao TS, Javorschi S, et al. Proteolytic cleavage product of 30-kDa adipocyte complement-related protein increases fatty acid oxidation in muscle and causes weight loss in mice. Proc Natl Acad Sci U S A 2001;98:2005–10.

39. Ahima RS, Flier JS. Leptin. Annu Rev Physiol 2000; 62:413–37.

40. Doehner W, Pflaum CD, Rauchhaus M, et al. Leptin, insulin sensitivity and growth hormone binding protein in chronic heart failure with and without cardiac cachexia. Eur J Endocrinol 2001;145:727–35.

41. Doehner W, Rauchhaus M, Godsland IF, et al. Insulin resistance in moderate chronic heart failure is related to hyperleptinaemia, but not to norepinephrine or TNF-alpha. Int J Cardiol 2002;83:73–81.

42. Leyva F, Anker SD, Egerer K, et al. Hyperleptinaemia in chronic heart failure. Relationships with insulin. Eur Heart J 1998;19:1547–51.

43. Hintz KK, Aberle NS, Ren J. Insulin resistance induces hyperleptinemia, cardiac contractile dysfunction but not cardiac leptin resistance in ventricular myocytes. Int J Obes Relat Metab Disord 2003;27:1196–203.

44. Haynes WG, Morgan DA, Walsh SA, et al. Receptor-mediated regional sympathetic nerve activation by leptin. J Clin Invest 1997;100:270–8.

45. Abe Y, Ono K, Kawamura T, et al. Leptin induces elongation of cardiac myocytes and causes eccentric left ventricular dilatation with compensation. Am J Physiol Heart Circ Physiol 2007;292: H2387–96.

46. Barouch LA, Berkowitz DE, Harrison RW, et al. Disruption of leptin signaling contributes to cardiac hypertrophy independently of body weight in mice. Circulation 2003;108:754–9.

47. Wolk R, Johnson BD, Somers VK. Leptin and the ventilatory response to exercise in heart failure. J Am Coll Cardiol 2003;42:1644–9.

48. Murdoch DR, Rooney E, Dargie HJ, et al. Inappropriately low plasma leptin concentration in the cachexia associated with chronic heart failure. Heart 1999;82:352–6.

49. Steppan CM, Bailey ST, Bhat S, et al. The hormone resistin links obesity to diabetes. Nature 2001;409: 307–12.

50. Patel L, Buckels AC, Kinghorn IJ, et al. Resistin is expressed in human macrophages and directly regulated by PPAR gamma activators. Biochem Biophys Res Commun 2003;300:472–6.

51. Azuma K, Katsukawa F, Oguchi S, et al. Correlation between serum resistin level and adiposity in obese individuals. Obes Res 2003;11:997–1001.

52. Reilly MP, Lehrke M, Wolfe ML, et al. Resistin is an inflammatory marker of atherosclerosis in humans. Circulation 2005;111:932–9.

53. Takeishi Y, Niizeki T, Arimoto T, et al. Serum resistin is associated with high risk in patients with congestive heart failure—a novel link between metabolic signals and heart failure. Circ J 2007;71:460–4.

Biomarkers of Extracellular Matrix Turnover

Faiez Zannad, MD, PhD[a,b,c], Bertram Pitt, MD[d,*]

KEYWORDS

- Heart failure • Extracellular matrix • Fibrosis
- Collagen • Biomarkers • Metalloproteinases

The extracellular cardiac matrix (ECCM) plays an important role in the support of myocytes and fibroblasts. Collagen is the principal structural protein, and collagen types 1 and 3 are the most abundant in the myocardium. Collagen type 1 has a poor specificity but represents most cardiac collagen (85%) and confers tensile strength and resistance to stretch and deformation. Type 3 is less abundant but more specific to the heart and confers resilience.[1–3] Fibrillar collagens within the myocardium are substrates for matrix metalloproteinases (MMPs). Among the MMPs, MMP-1 has the highest affinity for fibrillar collagen and preferentially degrades collagen 1 and 3.[3] The net level of MMP-1 activity depends on the relative concentrations of active enzyme and of a family of tissue inhibitors of metalloproteinases (TIMP). MMP-1 and TIMP-1 are coexpressed in cardiac fibroblasts and are regulated to maintain the architecture of the ECCM.[4] Type I C-terminal telopeptide (CITP) is a pyridinoline cross-linked telopeptide produced as a result of the hydrolysis of collagen type 1 fibrils by MMP-1; additionally, it is a marker of collagen type 1 degradation.[5]

The disruption of the equilibrium between the synthesis and degradation of the ECCM results in an excessive accumulation of collagen type 1 and 3 fibers within the myocardium. ECCM remodeling is an essential process in cardiac remodeling, hypertensive cardiac hypertrophy, dilated cardiomyopathy, and postinfarction healing.[5] ECCM turnover is influenced by ischemia, stretch, inflammation, and neurohormonal mediators. Myocardial fibrosis is therefore the consequence of several pathologic processes mediated by mechanical, neurohormonal, and cytokine factors. Cardiac fibrosis, a major determinant of diastolic dysfunction and pumping capacity, results in tissue heterogeneity and anisotropy and provides the structural substrate for dys-synchrony and arrhythmogenicity, thus potentially contributing to the progression of congestive heart failure (HF) and sudden cardiac death. ECCM turnover may be the target of therapeutic agents aimed at preventing or limiting the progression of adverse cardiac remodeling in HF and therefore hospitalization for HF and death due to progressive HF and sudden cardiac death.

NONINVASIVE ASSESSMENT OF EXTRACELLULAR CARDIAC MATRIX

Given the importance of fibrous tissue in the pathophysiology of myocardial dysfunction and failure, the noninvasive assessment of fibrosis could prove to be a clinically useful tool, particularly given the potential for cardioprotective and cardioreparative pharmacologic strategies.[6] The

Faiez Zannad is a consultant for Servier, Boehringer, Otsuka, and Boston Scientific. Bertram Pitt is a consultant for Pfizer, Merck, Novartis, Takeda, and Astra Zeneca.
a Hôpital Jeanne d'Arc, Dommartin-les-Toul, France
b Centre Hospitalier Universitaire de Nancy, France
c Nancy-Université, Vandoeuvre-les-Nancy, France
d University of Michigan, Ann Arbor, MI, USA
* Corresponding author. Department of Medicine, University of Michigan School of Medicine, Cardiovascular Center, 1500 East Medical Center Drive, Ann Arbor, MI 48109.
E-mail address: bpitt@umich.edu (B. Pitt).

Heart Failure Clin 5 (2009) 589–599
doi:10.1016/j.hfc.2009.04.010

measurement of various serum peptides arising from the metabolism of collagen types 1 and 3 may provide information on the extent of myocardial fibrosis[7] and thus prognosis and clues to appropriate strategies to improve prognosis. Because procollagen type I C-terminal propeptide (PICP), aminoterminal propeptides of type-I procollagen (PINP), and N terminal type III collagen peptide (PIIINP) are released with collagen type 1 or 3 molecules in a stoichiometric manner during collagen biosynthesis, they are important markers of this process (**Fig. 1**).[6,8,9]

Although these markers are not specific to the myocardium, Querejeta and colleagues have shown a correlation between myocardial collagen content and the serum concentration of PICP in patients have hypertension[10] and have demonstrated that serum PICP is secreted by the heart by means of the coronary sinus in patients who have hypertensive heart disease (**Fig. 2**).[11] The procollagen type I N-terminal propeptide (PIP)/CITP ratio, an index of coupling between the synthesis and degradation of collagen type 1, was found to be higher in hypertensive patients who had increased collagen accumulation in myocardial tissue than in those who had normal collagen accumulation.[12] In patients who had dilated cardiomyopathy, Izawa and colleagues showed that both collagen volume fraction and the abundance of collagen type 1 and 3 mRNAs in the left ventricular (LV) myocardium were higher in patients who had an increased serum PICP/CITP ratio than in those who had a lower PIP/CITP ratio. Changes in blood procollagen PIIINP correlate with changes in LV end diastolic volume

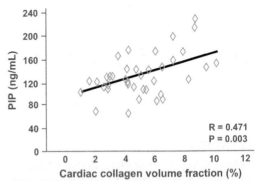

Fig. 2. Correlation between myocardial collagen content and the serum concentration of procollagen I C-terminal peptide (PICP) in patients with hypertension. It has been demonstrated that serum PICP is secreted by the heart by means of the coronary sinus in patients with hypertensive heart disease. (*Adapted from* Querejeta R, Varo N, Lopez B, et al. Serum carboxy-terminal propeptide of procollagen type I is a marker of myocardial fibrosis in hypertensive heart disease. Circulation 2000;101:1729–35; with permission.)

index in patients from baseline to 1 month after acute myocardial infarction (MI) (**Fig. 3**).[13]

This evidence linking serum ECCM markers to the heart's ECCM content provides a rationale for their use as biomarkers of ECCM remodeling in cardiac disease.[14] MMP-1 and TIMP-1 levels in coronary sinus blood were higher than in

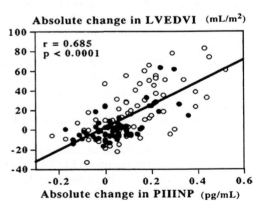

Fig. 3. Changes in blood procollagen type III N-terminal peptide (PIIINP) correlate to changes in left ventricular end diastolic volume index (LVEDVI) in patients from baseline to 1 month after acute myocardial infarction. (*From* Hayashi M, Tsutamoto T, Wada A, et al. Immediate administration of mineralocorticoid receptor antagonist spironolactone prevents postinfarct left ventricular remodeling associated with suppression of a marker of myocardial collagen synthesis in patients with first anterior acute myocardial infarction. Circulation 2003;107:2559–65; with permission.)

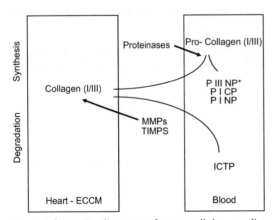

Fig. 1. Schematic diagram of extracellular cardiac matrix (ECCM) turnover. ICTP, type I pyridinoline cross-linked C-terminal telopeptide; MMPs, metalloproteinases; PIIINP*, procollagen III N-terminal peptide; P ICP, procollagen I C-terminal peptide; PINP, procollagen I N-terminal peptide; TIMPs, tissue inhibitors of metalloproteinases.

peripheral venous blood in hypertensive patients, but not in normotensive subjects, although there was no association between blood levels and myocardial expression of MMP-1 and TIMP-1 or the amount and distribution of fibrillar collagen.[15]

Several studies have shown that changes in plasma MMP/TIMP levels may be indicative of a myocardial source. For example, Lalu and colleagues[16] measured right atrial and plasma MMP-2 and MMP-9 levels in patients undergoing cardiac surgery. In that study, equivalent directional changes in myocardial and plasma MMP-2 and MMP-9 levels were reported. Inokubo and colleagues[17] reported that the changes in plasma MMP levels that occurred in patients who had an acute coronary syndrome were directly reflective of myocardial production based upon aorto–coronary sinus gradients.

EXTRACELLULAR CARDIAC MATRIX IN HYPERTENSION, DIABETES, OBESITY, LEFT VENTRICULAR HYPERTROPHY, AND DIASTOLIC HEART FAILURE

In experimental models of HF, an increase in mechanical load increases collagen synthesis by fibroblasts, as indicated by an increase in procollagen type 3 mRNA[18,19] Nakahara and colleagues showed that serum PIIINP concentration was correlated significantly with relative wall thickness in hypertensive patients who had LV hypertrophy (LVH). Interestingly, despite the fact that the eccentric and concentric LVH subgroups showed no differences in LV mass index or brain-type natriuretic peptide (BNP) concentration, the serum PIIINP concentration was significantly higher in the concentric hypertrophy group than in the essential hypertension group. They suggested that plasma aldosterone levels are associated with PIIINP concentration and may be the cause of eccentric hypertrophy by promoting cardiac fibrosis.[20] Experimental and clinical data have demonstrated serologic and morphometric evidence of increased myocardial fibrosis in hypertensive patients who have diastolic HF. An association between elevated levels of TIMP-1,[21] PICP, PIIINP,[22] ICTP, MMP-2, MMP-9, and diastolic dysfunction have been reported and suggest that greater collagen turnover is seen in more severe phases of diastolic dysfunction.

In other reports, TIMP-1 correlated with markers of diastolic filling, namely the E:A ratio and E Dec. A plasma TIMP-1 level of greater than 500 ng/mL has a specificity of 97% and a positive predictive value of 96% in predicting diastolic dysfunction.[23] PICP levels are related to blood pressure and LV filling parameters, but not to LV mass (LVM).

Therefore, it appears that myocardial fibrotic markers are increased in hypertension before LVH develops and are associated with diastolic dysfunction.[24] Poulsen and colleagues[25] reported a significant association between serum PIINP and reduced LV longitudinal contractility as assessed by the mean strain, measured by tissue Doppler echocardiography.

In selected patients who had uncomplicated type 2 diabetes, parameters of cardiac function were positively correlated with serum PICP.[26] Patients who have both arterial hypertension and diabetes mellitus have a high risk of heart failure. In a recent report, serum levels of PIIINP levels were significantly higher in hypertensive diabetic patients than in controls, although lower than in patients who had HF and systolic LV dysfunction. Collagen type 1 markers (PICP and PINP) were not influenced by HF but were lower in hypertensive diabetic patients than in controls.[27] Myocardial fibrosis and collagen deposition are the primary structural changes observed in diabetic cardiomyopathy. Collagen interacts with glucose, forming Schiff bases, which transform into glycated collagen to form advanced glycation end products (AGEs). The advanced glycation end products are a stable form of cross-linked collagen and are thought to contribute to arterial and myocardial stiffness, endothelial dysfunction, and atherosclerotic plaque formation. Correlations between advanced glycation end product serum levels and isovolumetric relaxation time and LV diameter during diastole have been reported.[28] Therefore, the impaired cardiac diastolic and systolic function observed in patients who have diabetes mellitus can be the result of fibrosis and altered collagen structure, specifically because of increased collagen cross-linking or formations of advanced glycation end products. In obese subjects without cardiovascular disease, hypertension, cardiac hypertrophy, or diabetes mellitus serum levels of markers of cardiac collagen synthesis were associated significantly with insulin resistance but not related to LVM.[29] Therefore, changes in collagen turnover may occur early in the disease process in high-risk patients before HF is clinically detectable.

Alterations of collagen and elastin fibers also are involved in the arterial stiffening that is associated with aging and disease states such as hypertension, diabetes mellitus, atherosclerosis, and chronic renal failure[30] and may contribute to the progression to diastolic HF. In older hypertensive patients who had LVH, brachial-ankle pulse wave velocity (baPWV), a measure of arterial stiffness, was reported to be correlated with the plasma level of PICP and ICTP and independently correlated to the total TIMP-1/MMP-1 ratio and negatively correlated with the E/A ratio of LV inflow, but not with LVM index (LVMI).[31]

Few studies have explored the prognostic potential of ECCM circulating levels in patients who have HF and a preserved EF. A small study from Japan suggested that CITP is an independent predictor of cardiac events in patients who had preserved LV systolic function, but not in those who had systolic dysfunction.[32] These results, however, were inconsistent with other studies in patients who had systolic dysfunction.

EXTRACELLULAR CARDIAC MATRIX IN MYOCARDIAL ISCHEMIA AND INFARCTION

Collagen 1 generally is involved in thick collagen fibers showing numerous cross-links and is associated with high tensile strength, whereas collagen 3 is observed mainly in much thinner and elastic fibers.[33] Collagen 1 is therefore more efficient for structural support and is much more abundant in the healthy heart and in mature infarct scar.[33,34] In contrast, collagen 3 seems to be the main component of reactive ischemic-related fibrosis within viable myocardium, outside of infarcted areas, and it can be synthesized in a more rapid and reactive way leading to the development of new areas of myocardial fibrosis.[33] In patients who had chronic coronary artery disease, exercise single positon emission computed tomography ischemia was associated with increased collagen 3 turnover, independent of concomitant medications, even when LV ejection fraction was normal.[35] This suggests that active ischemia may promote cardiac fibrosis, which may relate to chronic adverse cardiac remodeling in patients who have ischemic cardiomyopathy. In the postmyocardial infarct heart, there is time-dependent damage to myocytes and ECCM in the infarct zone, followed by gradual reparation with fibrosis. The noninfarct zone exhibits reactive hypertrophy, interstitial fibrosis, and increased collagen, leading to cardiac dysfunction and progressive dilation.[33]

The synthesis of collagen 3 has been shown to be enhanced in the days following an acute MI,[36,37] especially when revascularization is unsuccessful.[36] New collagen is mostly thin type 3, whereas subsequent collagen maturation involves a conversion to thick type 1 that provides an increased resistance to distension. On the degradation side, early after MI (first 24 hours), collagen degradation clearly exceeds synthesis as shown by increased MMP-1 levels.[34] In the later stages after MI (2 weeks to 1 year or more), healing and scarring processes to actively repair the damaged site[33,38] exceed ECCM degradation, as shown by decreased MMP and increased TIMP or a decreased MMP/TIMP ratio.[34,38] In a substudy of Eplerenone Post-Acute Myocardial Infarction Heart Failure Efficacy and Survival Study (EPHESUS), which evaluated the effects of the selective aldosterone receptor antagonist eplerenone versus placebo in patients who had HF and LVSD after MI, serum levels of collagen biomarkers were measured in 476 patients. Baseline collagen biomarkers were correlated with serum BNP and hs-CRP levels. Important changes in these collagen biomarkers levels occurred within the first month after acute MI. PINP levels increased significantly from baseline to month 1 and declined modestly thereafter. The overall profile was similar for PIIINP, but remained above baseline through month 9. At baseline, CITP levels were significantly higher than reference levels. There was a sustained and statistically significant fall in CITP levels from baseline to month 1 and subsequent stabilization at levels slightly lower than the upper reference value through month 9.[39] In other recent studies, CITP levels were reported to increase in the 10 days following acute MI,[40] and high baseline levels of CITP in post-MI patients were associated with LV remodeling.[41] Serum CITP levels were associated strongly with long-term outcome independent from BNP levels. Risks for all-cause death and cardiovascular death increased by 17% and 21% respectively with each increment of 2 ng/mL in baseline CITP levels.

Although increased levels of specific MMP types have been reported early following myocardial ischemia, plasma TIMP levels do not follow the same pattern.[42] Troponin levels, indicative of the extent of myocardial injury, appear to be related only weakly to plasma levels of MMPs. This suggests that the degree of matrix remodeling that occurs in the post-MI period is independent of the extent of myocyte loss and myocardial injury. Indeed, changes in plasma levels of MMPs in the post-MI period are emerging as an independent predictor of the degree of adverse LV remodeling and progression to HF. An early increase in MMP-9 levels is associated with an increased risk for the subsequent development of HF.[42] Thus, plasma profiling of MMPs and TIMPs in patients after MI is likely to be of prognostic and diagnostic importance. Whether and to what degree modifying these changes in plasma MMP/TIMP profiles in the post-MI period may alter the course of LV remodeling and the risk of HF beneficially remain to be established, however.

EXTRACELLULAR CARDIAC MATRIX IN HEART FAILURE WITH SYSTOLIC DYSFUNCTION

Synthesis of collagen 3 has been shown to be enhanced in severe or uncompensated cardiomyopathy of various origins.[43,44] In a sample of patients from the Randomized Aldactone Evaluation Study (RALES), baseline PIIINP was associated with an increased risk of death (relative risk [RR] 2.36, 95% CI 1.34 to 4.18) and of death plus hospitalization (RR 1.83, 95% CI 1.18 to 2.83) (**Fig. 4**).[45] In 1009 patients with HF enrolled in the Research into Etanercept CytOkine Antagonism in VentriculaR dysfunction (RECOVER) trial, multivariable analysis adjusted for clinical correlates (age, sex, New York Heart Association class, heart rate, beta-blocker use, ischemic etiology) revealed that PIIINP and MMP-1 had a negative association with exercise capacity assessed by the 6-minutes walk test, accounting for 28% of variance in the model. PIIINP also independently predicted survival and event-free survival.[46] Importantly, a positive correlation was detected between ECCM and inflammatory markers (PIIINP to interleukin [IL]-18, MMP-1 and TIMP-1 to C-reactive protein [CRP], TIMP-1 to IL-18, MMP-1 to IL-10). PIIINP was the only biomarker independently associated with death and HF hospitalization, which is consistent with results from a previous study.[45] Also, in the adjusted multivariable model including all biomarkers, PIIINP and MMP-1 were independent predictors of the 6-minute walk test, a measure of functional capacity and disease severity. The independent association of ECCM functional capacity and PIIINP with HF morbidity and mortality suggests that excessive ECCM turnover may be associated with functional capacity deterioration and poor outcome.

In other studies, other more classical prognostic factors (Troponin, BNP) have outweighed ECCM markers as an independent significant predictor of outcome.[47] In patients who had dilated cardiomyopathy and LV systolic dysfunction, the degree of diastolic dysfunction was associated with PIIINP concentrations independent of LV volume and ejection fraction. Patients who had the extreme diastolic dysfunction characterized by irreversible RF with unloading had the highest PIIINP concentrations and the worst prognosis.[48] Large artery fibrosis is associated with aortic stiffening, which imposes an additional systolic load and impairs exercise tolerance in patients who have HF. High serum PIIINP levels were found to be independently associated with aortic stiffening in patients who had a dilated cardiomyopathy (DCM), suggesting that abnormalities in the extracellular cardiac matrix turnover might involve the proximal elastic vasculature and could explain partially the progressive large artery stiffening process characterizing HF.[49]

EXTRACELLULAR CARDIAC MATRIX, ARRHYTHMIAS, AND SUDDEN DEATH

Structural alterations and fibrosis have been implicated in the generation and perpetuation of atrial fibrillation (AF) and ventricular arrhythmias.

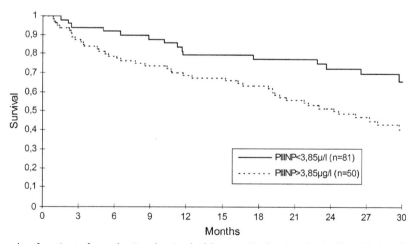

Fig. 4. In a sample of patients from the Randomized Aldactone Evaluation Study (RALES), baseline procollagen type III N-terminal peptide (PIIINP) was associated with an increased risk of death (relative risk [RR] 2.36, 95% CI 1.34 to 4.18) and of death and hospitalization (RR 1.83, 95% CI 1.18 to 2.83). (*From* Zannad F, Alla F, Dousset B, et al. Limitation of excessive extracellular matrix turnover may contribute to survival benefit of spironolactone therapy in patients with congestive heart failure: insights from the Randomized Aldactone Evaluation Study (RALES). RALES Investigators. Circulation 2000;102:2700–6; with permission.)

AF is associated commonly with HF. Atrial interstitial fibrosis has been observed in patients who have HF and in animal models of pacing-induced HF. Atrial fibrosis results in conduction abnormalities and an increase in AF vulnerability. The precise signaling processes involved in the development of atrial fibrosis are unknown. Angiotensin 2 appears to play a role, as inhibition of the angiotensin-converting enzyme (or angiotensin-receptor blockade) blunts atrial fibrosis in animal models of HF and decreases the incidence of AF in patients who have HF. Transforming growth factor-beta (TGF-beta) also appears to play an important role.[50] Qualitative and quantitative analyses of intraoperative biopsies from the right atrial appendage and free walls from patients who have AF reveal severe alterations in collagen 1 and 3 synthesis/degradation associated with disturbed MMP/TIMP systems. TGF-beta-1 contributes to the development of atrial fibrosis. These processes culminate in accumulations of fibrillar and nonfibrillar collagens, leading to excessive atrial fibrosis and maintenance of AF.[51]

Serum markers of collagen type 1 turnover differ significantly between patients who have AF and those who have sinus rhythm. PICP and CITP are reported to be significantly higher in patients who have AF than in control subjects. Patients who have persistent AF have higher levels of PICP but not CITP, compared with those who have paroxysmal AF. Patients with persistent AF have lower levels of MMP-1 but increased levels of TIMP-1 compared with patients who have paroxysmal AF. TIMP-1 levels are significantly lower in control subjects compared with those patients in both paroxysmal and persistent AF.[52] These results suggest that the intensity of extracellular synthesis and degradation of collagen type 1 may be related to the burden or type of AF. A similar study, however, found inconsistent results with raised CITP levels and no changes in PIIINP and the N-terminal fragment of collagen type 3.[53] Another report found raised CITP levels and no change in PINP, the N-terminal fragment of collagen type 1.[54] Circulating levels of CITP vary with the type and duration of AF. Interestingly, the same authors of this report assessed the impact of the angiotensin-converting enzyme (ACE) insertion (I)/deletion (D) polymorphisms on circulating levels of CITP in hypertensive patients who had AF and in patients who had arterial hypertension in sinus rhythm. They found that the presence of the D allele in hypertensive patients who have AF is associated with attenuation of type 1 collagen degradation and that therapy with an ACE inhibitor increases degradation of collagen type 1.[55]

The relationship between ECCM serum markers, BNP, high-sensitivity C-reactive protein (hsCRP), and ventricular arrhythmias has been investigated in patients implanted with cardioverter defibrillators for spontaneous sustained ventricular tachycardia and a history of MI.[56] In multivariate analysis, a LV ejection fraction less than 0.35, an increased serum BNP, hsCRP and PINP, and a decreased PIIINP were associated with an increased incidence of ventricular tachycardia.

INFLUENCE OF THERAPY ON EXTRACELLULAR CARDIAC MATRIX BIOMARKERS

The ability of antihypertensive and HF treatment to reduce myocardial fibrosis may be monitored by the measurement of various serum peptides arising from the metabolism of collagen.[7]

Angiotensin Converting Enzyme Inhibitors and Angiotensin Receptor Blockers

Blockade of the angiotensin 2 type 1 receptor has been shown to be associated with inhibition of collagen type 1 synthesis and regression of myocardial fibrosis in hypertensive patients. In a study comparing losartan with amlodipine, biopsy-proven myocardial fibrosis decreased concomitantly with a reduction in serum procollagen type I peptides in losartan-treated patients, while neither collagen volume fraction nor serum procollagen type I peptides changed significantly in amlodipine-treated patients. These results suggest that the ability of antihypertensive treatment to regress fibrosis in patients who have essential hypertension is independent of its antihypertensive efficacy.[7]

A substudy of the Losartan Intervention for Endpoint Reduction in Hypertension Study trial compared the effects of an angiotensin 2 receptor antagonist with a beta-blocker on myocardial collagen volume (assessed by echo reflectivity and serum collagen markers) in 219 hypertensive patients who had echocardiographically documented LVH. Echo reflectivity, previously shown to correlate directly with collagen volume fraction on endomyocardial biopsy, was measured concomitantly with serum markers of collagen synthesis (PICP, PIIINP) or degradation (ICTP) as secondary outcome variables. Losartan but not atenolol was associated with an increase in echo reflectivity. Collagen markers also changed in the direction of decreased collagen in patients receiving losartan, but the differences between groups were not statistically significant.[57] In another small trial, Swedish Irbesartan in Left Ventricular Hypertrophy Investigation Versus

Atenolol in patients who had hypertensive LVH, irbesartan and atenolol reduced PICP similarly. Only in the irbesartan group, however, did changes in PICP relate to changes in isovolumic relaxation time and LVM. These findings with irbesartan suggest a role for angiotensin 2 in the control of myocardial fibrosis and diastolic function in patients who have hypertension and LVH.[24] In patients who have HF, however, there is as yet no clinical report concerning the effects of either ACE inhibitors or angiotensin receptor blockers on ECCM biomarkers.

Beta-blocker Therapy

Despite evidence of the involvement of the sympathetic system in LVH, cardiac remodeling, and fibrosis, there is relatively little information on the effects of beta- blocker therapy on preventing cardiac fibrosis in experimental models or clinical studies of hypertension, HF, or MI.

Aldosterone Antagonists

Aldosterone has been shown to promote cardiac fibrosis in experimental models and in people,[58,59] and aldosterone antagonists have beneficial effects on LVH in patients who have hypertension.[60] In a small number of patients who had essential hypertension treated with spironolactone and an ACE inhibitor for 24 weeks, both blood pressure and serum PIIINP levels were decreased significantly, and there was a statistical significant correlation between the changes in LVMI and PIIINP. These results suggest that spironolactone limits cardiac collagen turnover in patients who have high baseline PIIINP levels. Larger studies may provide more definitive evidence for the involvement of aldosterone in LVH in patients who have abnormally high PIIINP levels.[61]

A sample of 261 patients from the Randomized Aldactone Evaluation Study (RALES) was randomized to placebo or spironolactone (12.5 to 50 mg daily). At 6 months, serum PICP and PIIINP markers decreased in the spironolactone group but remained unchanged in the placebo group. The effect of spironolactone on mortality was significant only in patients who had baseline levels of collagen markers above the median. These results suggest that limitation of excessive extracellular matrix turnover may be one of the important extrarenal mechanisms contributing to the beneficial effects of spironolactone in patients who have congestive heart failure (CHF).[45]

More recently, Izawa and colleagues[14] investigated the effects of spironolactone in patients who had dilated cardiomyopathy. The patients were divided into two groups on the basis of the serum PIP/CITP ratio less than or equal to 35, group A, n = 12; greater than 35, group B, n = 13, an index of myocardial collagen accumulation. LV diastolic chamber stiffness, collagen volume fraction, and abundance of collagen type 1 and 3 mRNAs in biopsy tissue were greater, and the LV early diastolic strain rate (tissue Doppler echocardiography) was smaller in group B than in group A at baseline. These differences and the difference in PIP/CITP were reduced after treatment with spironolactone in patients in group B, whereas treatment had no effect on these parameters in patients in group A. The collagen volume fraction was correlated significantly with PIP/CITP, LV early diastolic strain rate, and LV diastolic chamber stiffness for all patients before and after treatment with spironolactone. Therefore, spironolactone ameliorated LV diastolic dysfunction and reduced chamber stiffness in association with regression of myocardial fibrosis in mildly symptomatic patients who had DCM. Interestingly, these effects appeared limited to patients who had increased myocardial collagen accumulation.

In summary, a particularly important determinant for the therapeutic benefit of mineralocorticoid receptor antagonists seems to be their ability to prevent and reverse cardiac fibrosis. Mineralocorticoid receptor antagonists improve clinical outcome only in HF patients with high cardiac collagen deposition, and patient prognosis correlates with the extent by which cardiac collagen levels are reduced. This raises the interesting hypothesis that patients most likely to benefit from mineralocorticoid receptor antagonists may be screened by the measurement of ECCM biomarkers.[2,62]

In patients who had acute myocardial Infarction (AMI), Hayashi and colleagues[13] found that aldosterone was extracted through the heart and that extracting aldosterone stimulated postinfarct LV remodeling. They randomized 134 patients who had a first anterior acute MI to receive potassium canreonate (the active metabolite of spironolactone) on top of an ACE inhibitor or control treatment. LV ejection fraction was improved significantly, and LV end diastolic volume dilatation was suppressed significantly in the aldosterone antagonist group compared with the control group. Transcardiac extraction of aldosterone through the heart was suppressed significantly, and plasma PIIINP levels were significantly lower in the aldosterone antagonist group. The authors suggest that aldosterone antagonist therapy combined with an ACE inhibitor can prevent postinfarct LV remodeling better than an ACE inhibitor alone in association with the suppression of a marker of collagen synthesis.

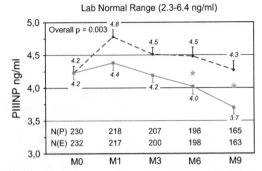

Fig. 5. Kinetics of procollagen type III N-terminal peptide PIIINP serum levels during 9-month follow-up, in a substudy of EPHESUS. Acute changes in PIIINP were blunted with the use of eplerenone, and PIIINP was lowered by eplerenone during long-term follow-up. (*From* Iraqi W, Rossignol P, Angioi M, et al. Extracellular cardiac matrix biomarkers in patients with acute myocardial infarction complicated by left ventricular dysfunction and heart failure: insights from the Eplerenone Post-Acute Myocardial Infarction Heart Failure Efficacy and Survival Study (EPHESUS) study. Circulation 2009;119:2471–9; with permission.)

In a substudy of EPHESUS, important changes in biomarkers levels occurred within the first month after AMI, were blunted with the use of eplerenone, and remained lower in the eplerenone than the placebo group throughout long-term follow-up, implying that treatment with eplerenone suppresses collagen turnover (**Fig. 5**).[39] Therefore, the results of this substudy with eplerenone are consistent with and extend the results of previous experimental and clinical observations with aldosterone antagonists in HF and after AMI and suggest that the effect of aldosterone receptor blockade on ECCM remodeling may contribute to the clinical benefits of this therapy.

Statins

In one recent study, atorvastatin decreased serum N-terminal telopeptide of type 1 collagen in patients who had hypercholesterolemia, which was interpreted to be the result of a beneficial effects on bone metabolism,[63] but could have been related to an effect on cardiovascular ECCM. This study points out the nonspecificity of serum ECCM biomarkers. In another study,[64] valsartan/simvastatin combination did not alter fibrosis markers as compared with valsartan in patients who had hyperlipidemia and hypertension. Thus, the role of statins on ECCM biomarkers remains to be determined.

Limitations of the Use of Extracellular Cardiac Matrix Biomarkers in Cardiovascular Disease

MMPs and TIMPs are synthesized within various tissue types; therefore changes in circulating levels may not reflect changes occurring within the myocardium. This is of a particular concern in patients who have multiple disease processes such as pregnancy, cancer, infectious diseases, inflammatory connective disease, kidney disease, and bone disorders.[65] Similarly, increased circulating levels of collagen peptides have been reported in patients presenting with cancer, bone diseases, liver diseases, and inflammatory connective diseases.[66] Thus, it is important to evaluate these potentially confounding conditions before attempting to use these biomarkers in a patient who has HF at an individual or epidemiologic level. Many of the clinical studies performed to date have attempted to control for these potential confounding factors through the use of exclusion criteria; however, this is a concern in large-scale long-term studies. There are several preanalytical potential pitfalls that should be taken into account. For example, serum and plasma MMP-9 levels differ significantly, the former being higher because of the release of MMP-9 by polymorphonuclear cells during blood clotting.[67] Another potential problem is the as yet unknown influence of long-term freezing and storage. Additionally, the anticoagulant used to sample blood may alter MMP/TIMP plasma levels.[68] At the analytical level, as pointed out by Zucker, among the difficulties in comparing results using different commercial ELISA kits is the absence of individual purified MMP standards for use in producing calibration curves.[69] Likewise, quantifying MMP/TIMP and collagen fragment measurements can give different absolute results depending on the specific antibody combinations employed in the assay kit.[69,70] Thus, it is crucial to define standardized procedures before using these experimental biomarkers in clinical practice.

SUMMARY

Given the importance of myocardial fibrosis in myocardial dysfunction, the noninvasive assessment of fibrosis could prove to be clinically useful in patients who have HF. Biomarkers reflecting collagen formation and or degradation may be used for:

Early detection of otherwise subclinical disease
Diagnostic assessment of acute or chronic clinical syndromes

Risk stratification of patients who have confirmed disease

Selection of appropriate therapeutic interventions

Monitoring the response to these interventions

ECCM biomarkers in patients who have HF may detect early changes in heart and large vessel structure and function, the transition to HF, and prognosis. The ability of treatment to reduce myocardial fibrosis in patients who have HF may be monitored by the measurement of various serum peptides arising from the metabolism of collagen types. Characterization of patients according to the severity of cardiac fibrosis, as assessed by ECCM biomarkers, may prove useful for selecting appropriate drug regimens. The available data set the stage for large-scale long-term randomized trials to validate this approach. Before widespread application of this approach, however, it will be necessary to standardize the various measurements of ECCM biomarkers and to recognize their limitations. In part, these limitations may be overcome by the concomitant use of new imaging techniques to localize myocardial fibrosis such as radionuclide angiography with labeled integrins and MRI.

REFERENCES

1. Bishop JE, Laurent GJ. Collagen turnover and its regulation in the normal and hypertrophying heart. Eur Heart J 1995;16:38–44.

2. Zannad F, Dousset B, Alla F. Treatment of congestive heart failure: interfering the aldosterone–cardiac extracellular matrix relationship. Hypertension 2001;38:1227–32.

3. D'Armiento J. Matrix metalloproteinase disruption of the extracellular matrix and cardiac dysfunction. Trends Cardiovasc Med 2002;12:97–101.

4. Visse R, Nagase H. Matrix metalloproteinases and tissue inhibitors of metalloproteinases: structure, function, and biochemistry. Circ Res 2003;92:827–39.

5. Laviades C, Varo N, Fernandez J, et al. Abnormalities of the extracellular degradation of collagen type I in essential hypertension. Circulation 1998;98:535–40.

6. Weber KT. Monitoring tissue repair and fibrosis from a distance. Circulation 1997;96:2488–92.

7. Lopez B, Gonzalez A, Querejeta R, et al. The use of collagen-derived serum peptides for the clinical assessment of hypertensive heart disease. J Hypertens 2005;23:1445–51.

8. Risteli J, Risteli L. Analysing connective tissue metabolites in human serum. Biochemical, physiological, and methodological aspects. J Hepatol 1995;22:77–81.

9. Jensen LT, Horslev-Petersen K, Toft P, et al. Serum aminoterminal type III procollagen peptide reflects repair after acute myocardial infarction. Circulation 1990;81:52–7.

10. Querejeta R, Varo N, Lopez B, et al. Serum carboxy-terminal propeptide of procollagen type I is a marker of myocardial fibrosis in hypertensive heart disease. Circulation 2000;101:1729–35.

11. Querejeta R, Lopez B, Gonzalez A, et al. Increased collagen type I synthesis in patients with heart failure of hypertensive origin: relation to myocardial fibrosis. Circulation 2004;110:1263–8.

12. Diez J, Querejeta R, Lopez B, et al. Losartan-dependent regression of myocardial fibrosis is associated with reduction of left ventricular chamber stiffness in hypertensive patients. Circulation 2002;105:2512–7.

13. Hayashi M, Tsutamoto T, Wada A, et al. Immediate administration of mineralocorticoid receptor antagonist spironolactone prevents postinfarct left ventricular remodeling associated with suppression of a marker of myocardial collagen synthesis in patients with first anterior acute myocardial infarction. Circulation 2003;107:2559–65.

14. Izawa H, Murohara T, Nagata K, et al. Mineralocorticoid receptor antagonism ameliorates left ventricular diastolic dysfunction and myocardial fibrosis in mildly symptomatic patients with idiopathic dilated cardiomyopathy: a pilot study. Circulation 2005;112:2940–5.

15. Lopez B, Gonzalez A, Querejeta R, et al. Alterations in the pattern of collagen deposition may contribute to the deterioration of systolic function in hypertensive patients with heart failure. J Am Coll Cardiol 2006;48:89–96.

16. Lalu MM, Pasini E, Schulze CJ, et al. Ischaemia–reperfusion injury activates matrix metalloproteinases in the human heart. Eur Heart J 2005;26:27–35.

17. Inokubo Y, Hanada H, Ishizaka H, et al. Plasma levels of matrix metalloproteinase-9 and tissue inhibitor of metalloproteinase-1 are increased in the coronary circulation in patients with acute coronary syndrome. Am Heart J 2001;141:211–7.

18. Carver W, Nagpal ML, Nachtigal M, et al. Collagen expression in mechanically stimulated cardiac fibroblasts. Circ Res 1991;69:116–22.

19. Mukherjee D, Sen S. Collagen phenotypes during development and regression of myocardial hypertrophy in spontaneously hypertensive rats. Circ Res 1990;67:1474–80.

20. Nakahara T, Takata Y, Hirayama Y, et al. Left ventricular hypertrophy and geometry in untreated essential hypertension is associated with blood levels of aldosterone and procollagen type III amino-terminal peptide. Circ J 2007;71:716–21.

21. Ahmed SH, Clark LL, Pennington WR, et al. Matrix metalloproteinases/tissue inhibitors of met-alloproteinases: relationship between changes in proteolytic determinants of matrix composition and structural, functional, and clinical manifestations of hypertensive heart disease. Circulation 2006;113:2089–96.

22. Martos R, Baugh J, Ledwidge M, et al. Diastolic heart failure: evidence of increased myocardial collagen turnover linked to diastolic dysfunction. Circulation 2007;115:888–95.

23. Lindsay MM, Maxwell P, Dunn FG. TIMP-1: a marker of left ventricular diastolic dysfunction and fibrosis in hypertension. Hypertension 2002;40:136–41.

24. Muller-Brunotte R, Kahan T, Lopez B, et al. Myocardial fibrosis and diastolic dysfunction in patients with hypertension: results from the Swedish Irbesartan Left Ventricular Hypertrophy Investigation versus Atenolol (SILVHIA). J Hypertens 2007;25:1958–66.

25. Poulsen SH, Andersen NH, Heickendorff L, et al. Relation between plasma amino-terminal propeptide of procollagen type III and left ventricular longitudinal strain in essential hypertension. Heart 2005;91:624–9.

26. Gonzalez-Vilchez F, Ayuela J, Ares M, et al. Oxidative stress and fibrosis in incipient myocardial dysfunction in type 2 diabetic patients. Int J Cardiol 2005;101:53–8.

27. Alla F, Kearney-Schwartz A, Radauceanu A, et al. Early changes in serum markers of cardiac extracellular matrix turnover in patients with uncomplicated hypertension and type II diabetes. Eur J Heart Fail 2006;8:147–53.

28. Berg TJ, Snorgaard O, Faber J, et al. Serum levels of advanced glycation end products are associated with left ventricular diastolic function in patients with type 1 diabetes. Diabetes Care 1999;22:1186–90.

29. Quilliot D, Alla F, Bohme P, et al. Myocardial collagen turnover in normotensive obese patients: relation to insulin resistance. Int J Obes (Lond) 2005;29:1321–8.

30. Diez J. Arterial stiffness and extracellular matrix. Adv Cardiol 2007;44:76–95.

31. Ishikawa J, Kario K, Matsui Y, et al. Collagen metabolism in extracellular matrix may be involved in arterial stiffness in older hypertensive patients with left ventricular hypertrophy. Hypertens Res 2005;28:995–1001.

32. Kitahara T, Takeishi Y, Arimoto T, et al. Serum carboxy-terminal telopeptide of type I collagen (ICTP) predicts cardiac events in chronic heart failure patients with preserved left ventricular systolic function. Circ J 2007;71:929–35.

33. Jugdutt BI. Ventricular remodeling after infarction and the extracellular collagen matrix: when is enough enough? Circulation 2003;108:1395–403.

34. Jugdutt BI. Remodeling of the myocardium and potential targets in the collagen degradation and synthesis pathways. Curr Drug Targets Cardiovasc Haematol Disord 2003;3:1–30.

35. Radauceanu A, Moulin F, Djaballah W, et al. Residual stress ischaemia is associated with blood markers of myocardial structural remodeling. Eur J Heart Fail 2007;9:370–6.

36. Uusimaa P, Risteli J, Niemela M, et al. Collagen scar formation after acute myocardial infarction: relationships to infarct size, left ventricular function, and coronary artery patency. Circulation 1997;96:2565–72.

37. Poulsen SH, Host NB, Jensen SE, et al. Relationship between serum amino-terminal propeptide of type III procollagen and changes of left ventricular function after acute myocardial infarction. Circulation 2000;101:1527–32.

38. Papadopoulos DP, Moyssakis I, Makris TK, et al. Clinical significance of matrix metalloproteinases activity in acute myocardial infarction. Eur Cytokine Netw 2005;16:152–60.

39. Iraqi W, Rossignol P, Fay R, et al. Extracellular cardiac matrix biomarkers in patients with acute myocardial infarction complicated by left ventricular dysfunction and heart failure: insights from the EPHESUS study. Circ J 2009;119:2471–9.

40. Murakami T, Kusachi S, Murakami M, et al. Time-dependent changes of serum carboxy-terminal peptide of type I procollagen and carboxy-terminal telopeptide of type I collagen concentrations in patients with acute myocardial infarction after successful reperfusion: correlation with left ventricular volume indices. Clin Chem 1998;44:2453–61.

41. Cerisano G, Pucci PD, Sulla A, et al. Relation between plasma brain natriuretic peptide, serum indexes of collagen type I turnover, and left ventricular remodeling after reperfused acute myocardial infarction. Am J Cardiol 2007;99:651–6.

42. Webb CS, Bonnema DD, Ahmed SH, et al. Specific temporal profile of matrix metalloproteinase release occurs in patients after myocardial infarction: relation to left ventricular remodeling. Circulation 2006;114:1020–7.

43. Mukherjee D, Sen S. Alteration of collagen phenotypes in ischemic cardiomyopathy. J Clin Invest 1991;88:1141–6.

44. Klappacher G, Franzen P, Haab D, et al. Measuring extracellular matrix turnover in the serum of patients with idiopathic or ischemic dilated cardiomyopathy and impact on diagnosis and prognosis. Am J Cardiol 1995;75:913–8.

45. Zannad F, Alla F, Dousset B, et al. Limitation of excessive extracellular matrix turnover may contribute to survival benefit of spironolactone therapy in patients with congestive heart failure: insights from the Randomized Aldactone Evaluation

Study (RALES). RALES Investigators. Circulation 2000;102:2700–6.

46. Radauceanu A, Ducki C, Virion JM, et al. Extracellular matrix turnover and inflammatory markers independently predict functional status and outcome in chronic heart failure. J Card Fail 2008;14:467–74.

47. Nishio Y, Sato Y, Taniguchi R, et al. Cardiac troponin T vs other biochemical markers in patients with congestive heart failure. Circ J 2007;71:631–5.

48. Rossi A, Cicoira M, Bonapace S, et al. Left atrial volume provides independent and incremental information compared with exercise tolerance parameters in patients with heart failure and left ventricular systolic dysfunction. Heart 2007;93: 1420–5.

49. Bonapace S, Rossi A, Cicoira M, et al. Aortic stiffness correlates with an increased extracellular matrix turnover in patients with dilated cardiomyopathy. Am Heart J 2006;152(93):e1–6.

50. Everett TH 4th, Olgin JE. Atrial fibrosis and the mechanisms of atrial fibrillation. Heart Rhythm 2007;4:S24–7.

51. Polyakova V, Miyagawa S, Szalay Z, et al. Atrial extracellular matrix remodeling in patients with atrial fibrillation. J Cell Mol Med 2008;12:189–208.

52. Kallergis EM, Manios EG, Kanoupakis EM, et al. Extracellular matrix alterations in patients with paroxysmal and persistent atrial fibrillation: biochemical assessment of collagen type-I turnover. J Am Coll Cardiol 2008;52:211–5.

53. Shimano M, Shibata R, Tsuji Y, et al. Circulating adiponectin levels in patients with atrial fibrillation. Circ J 2008;72:1120–4.

54. Tziakas DN, Chalikias GK, Papanas N, et al. Circulating levels of collagen type I degradation marker depend on the type of atrial fibrillation. Europace 2007;9:589–96.

55. Tziakas DN, Chalikias GK, Stakos DA, et al. Effect of angiotensin-converting enzyme insertion/deletion genotype on collagen type I synthesis and degradation in patients with atrial fibrillation and arterial hypertension. Expert Opin Pharmacother 2007;8: 2225–34.

56. Blangy H, Sadoul N, Dousset B, et al. Serum BNP, hs-C-reactive protein, procollagen to assess the risk of ventricular tachycardia in ICD recipients after myocardial infarction. Europace 2007;9: 724–9.

57. Ciulla MM, Paliotti R, Esposito A, et al. Different effects of antihypertensive therapies based on losartan or atenolol on ultrasound and biochemical markers of myocardial fibrosis: results of a randomized trial. Circulation 2004;110:552–7.

58. Funder JW. Minireview: aldosterone and the cardiovascular system: genomic and nongenomic effects. Endocrinology 2006;147:5564–7.

59. Young MJ. Mechanisms of mineralocorticoid receptor-mediated cardiac fibrosis and vascular inflammation. Curr Opin Nephrol Hypertens 2008;17:174–80.

60. Pitt B, Reichek N, Willenbrock R, et al. Effects of eplerenone, enalapril, and eplerenone/enalapril in patients with essential hypertension and left ventricular hypertrophy: the 4E-left ventricular hypertrophy study. Circulation 2003;108:1831–8.

61. Sato A, Takane H, Saruta T. High serum level of procollagen type III amino-terminal peptide contributes to the efficacy of spironolactone and angiotensin-converting enzyme inhibitor therapy on left ventricular hypertrophy in essential hypertensive patients. Hypertens Res 2001;24:99–104.

62. Zannad F, Radauceanu A. Effect of MR blockade on collagen formation and cardiovascular disease with a specific emphasis on heart failure. Heart Fail Rev 2005;10:71–8.

63. Majima T, Komatsu Y, Fukao A, et al. Short-term effects of atorvastatin on bone turnover in male patients with hypercholesterolemia. Endocrinol Jpn 2007;54:145–51.

64. Rajagopalan S, Zannad F, Radauceanu A, et al. Effects of valsartan alone versus valsartan/simvastatin combination on ambulatory blood pressure, C-reactive protein, lipoproteins, and monocyte chemoattractant protein-1 in patients with hyperlipidemia and hypertension. Am J Cardiol 2007;100: 222–6.

65. Zucker S, Hymowitz M, Conner C, et al. Measurement of matrix metalloproteinases and tissue inhibitors of metalloproteinases in blood and tissues. Clinical and experimental applications. Ann N Y Acad Sci 1999;878:212–27.

66. Garnero P, Bianchi F, Carlier MC, et al. [Biochemical markers of bone remodeling: pre-analytical variations and guidelines for their use. SFBC (Societe Francaise de Biologie Clinique) Work Group. Biochemical markers of bone remodeling]. Ann Biol Clin (Paris) 2000;58:683–704.

67. Fontaine V, Jacob MP, Houard X, et al. Involvement of the mural thrombus as a site of protease release and activation in human aortic aneurysms. Am J Pathol 2002;161:1701–10.

68. Jung K, Nowak L, Lein M, et al. Role of specimen collection in preanalytical variation of metalloproteinases and their inhibitors in blood. Clin Chem 1996;42:2043–5.

69. Zucker S, Doshi K, Cao J. Measurement of matrix metalloproteinases (MMPs) and tissue inhibitors of metalloproteinases (TIMP) in blood and urine: potential clinical applications. Adv Clin Chem 2004;38: 37–85.

70. Cremers S, Garnero P. Biochemical markers of bone turnover in the clinical development of drugs for osteoporosis and metastatic bone disease: potential uses and pitfalls. Drugs 2006;66:2031–58.

Index

Note: Page numbers of article titles are in **boldface** type.

Heart Failure Clin 5 (2009) 601–604
doi:10.1016/S1551-7136(09)00064-6

United States Postal Service

Statement of Ownership, Management, and Circulation
(All Periodicals Publications Except Requestor Publications)

1. Publication Title	2. Publication Number								3. Filing Date
Heart Failure Clinics of North America	0	2	5	-	0	5	5		9/15/09

4. Issue Frequency	5. Number of Issues Published Annually	6. Annual Subscription Price
Jan, Apr, July, Oct	4	$193.00

7. Complete Mailing Address of Known Office of Publication (Not printer) (Street, city, county, state, and ZIP+4®)

Elsevier Inc.
360 Park Avenue South
New York, NY 10010-1710

Contact Person
Stephen Bushing

Telephone (Include area code)
215-239-3688

8. Complete Mailing Address of Headquarters or General Business Office of Publisher (Not printer)

Elsevier Inc., 360 Park Avenue South, New York, NY 10010-1710

9. Full Names and Complete Mailing Addresses of Publisher, Editor, and Managing Editor (Do not leave blank)

Publisher (Name and complete mailing address)

John Schrefer, Elsevier, Inc., 1600 John F. Kennedy Blvd. Suite 1800, Philadelphia, PA 19103-2899

Editor (Name and complete mailing address)

Barbara Cohen-Kligerman, Elsevier, Inc., 1600 John F. Kennedy Blvd. Suite 1800, Philadelphia, PA 19103-2899

Managing Editor (Name and complete mailing address)

Catherine Bewick, Elsevier, Inc., 1600 John F. Kennedy Blvd. Suite 1800, Philadelphia, PA 19103-2899

10. Owner (Do not leave blank. If the publication is owned by a corporation, give the name and address of the corporation immediately followed by the names and addresses of all stockholders owning or holding 1 percent or more of the total amount of stock. If not owned by a corporation, give the names and addresses of the individual owners. If owned by a partnership or other unincorporated firm, give its name and address as well as those of each individual owner. If the publication is published by a nonprofit organization, give its name and address.)

Full Name	Complete Mailing Address
Wholly owned subsidiary of	4520 East-West Highway
Reed/Elsevier, US holdings	Bethesda, MD 20814

11. Known Bondholders, Mortgagees, and Other Security Holders Owning or Holding 1 Percent or More of Total Amount of Bonds, Mortgages, or Other Securities. If none, check box ▶ None

Full Name	Complete Mailing Address
N/A	

12. Tax Status (For completion by nonprofit organizations authorized to mail at nonprofit rates) (Check one)
The purpose, function, and nonprofit status of this organization and the exempt status for federal income tax purposes:
☐ Has Not Changed During Preceding 12 Months
☐ Has Changed During Preceding 12 Months (Publisher must submit explanation of change with this statement)

PS Form 3526, September 2007 (Page 1 of 3 (Instructions Page 3)) PSN 7530-01-000-9931 PRIVACY NOTICE: See our Privacy policy in www.usps.com

---

13. Publication Title	14. Issue Date for Circulation Data Below
Heart Failure Clinics of North America	April 2009

15. Extent and Nature of Circulation		Average No. Copies Each Issue During Preceding 12 Months	No. Copies of Single Issue Published Nearest to Filing Date
a. Total Number of Copies (Net press run)		599	497
b. Paid Circulation (By Mail and Outside the Mail)	(1) Mailed Outside-County Paid Subscriptions Stated on PS Form 3541. (Include paid distribution above nominal rate, advertiser's proof copies, and exchange copies)	99	96
	(2) Mailed In-County Paid Subscriptions Stated on PS Form 3541 (Include paid distribution above nominal rate, advertiser's proof copies, and exchange copies)		
	(3) Paid Distribution Outside the Mails Including Sales Through Dealers and Carriers, Street Vendors, Counter Sales, and Other Paid Distribution Outside USPS®	35	32
	(4) Paid Distribution by Other Classes Mailed Through the USPS (e.g. First-Class Mail®)		
c. Total Paid Distribution (Sum of 15b (1), (2), (3), and (4))	▶	134	128
d. Free or Nominal Rate Distribution (By Mail and Outside the Mail)	(1) Free or Nominal Rate Outside-County Copies Included on PS Form 3541	64	71
	(2) Free or Nominal Rate In-County Copies Included on PS Form 3541		
	(3) Free or Nominal Rate Copies Mailed at Other Classes Through the USPS (e.g. First-Class Mail)		
	(4) Free or Nominal Rate Distribution Outside the Mail (Carriers or other means)		
e. Total Free or Nominal Rate Distribution (Sum of 15d (1), (2), (3) and (4))	▶	64	71
f. Total Distribution (Sum of 15c and 15e)	▶	198	199
g. Copies not Distributed (See instructions to publishers #4 (page #3))	▶	401	298
h. Total (Sum of 15f and g)	▶	599	497
i. Percent Paid (15c divided by 15f times 100)		67.68%	64.32%

16. Publication of Statement of Ownership

☐ If the publication is a general publication, publication of this statement is required. Will be printed in the October 2009 issue of this publication.   Publication not required

17. Signature and Title of Editor, Publisher, Business Manager, or Owner

[signature]
Stephen Bushing – Executive Director of Subscription Services

Date
September 15, 2009

I certify that all information furnished on this form is true and complete. I understand that anyone who furnishes false or misleading information on this form or who omits material or information requested on the form may be subject to criminal sanctions (including fines and imprisonment) and/or civil sanctions (including civil penalties).

PS Form 3526, September 2007 (Page 2 of 3)

Moving?

Make sure your subscription moves with you!

To notify us of your new address, find your **Clinics Account Number** (located on your mailing label above your name), and contact customer service at:

E-mail: elspcs@elsevier.com

800-654-2452 (subscribers in the U.S. & Canada)
314-453-7041 (subscribers outside of the U.S. & Canada)

Fax number: 314-523-5170

Elsevier Periodicals Customer Service
11830 Westline Industrial Drive
St. Louis, MO 63146

*To ensure uninterrupted delivery of your subscription, please notify us at least 4 weeks in advance of move.

ELSEVIER